Abdominal Trauma:
Surgical and Radiologic Diagnosis

Abdominal Trauma:
Surgical and Radiologic Diagnosis

Harry M. Delany
Professor of Surgery
Albert Einstein College of Medicine

Director of Surgery
North Central Bronx Hospital

Robert S. Jason
Assistant Professor of Radiology
Albert Einstein College of Medicine

Associate Attending Radiologist
North Central Bronx Hospital

With Contributions by
Nino Carnevale, Walter Delph, Charles M. Moss, and Amiel Rudavsky

Foreword by
Drs. Harold G. Jacobson and Marvin L. Gliedman

With 259 Illustrations

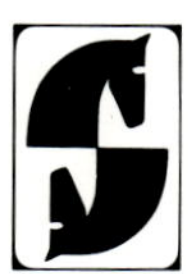

Springer-Verlag
New York Heidelberg Berlin

Harry M. Delany, M.D., F.A.C.S.
Department of Surgery
and
Robert S. Jason, M.D.
Department of Radiology
North Central Bronx Hospital
Kossuth Avenue
Bronx, New York 10467, U.S.A.

Sponsoring Editor: Larry W. Carter
Production: Abe Krieger
Design: Russell Till

The color illustration on the front cover was rendered by Robert Demerest.

Prints of the radiographs and nuclear scans were made by Michael Carlin.

Library of Congress Cataloging in Publication Data
Delaney, Harry M.
Abdominal trauma.
Bibliography: p.
Includes index.
1. Abdomen—Wounds and injuries. 2. Abdomen—Surgery.
3. Abdomen—Radiography. 4. Diagnosis, Radioscopic.
I. Jason, Robert. II. Title. [DNLM: 1. Abdominal injuries—Radiography. 2. Abdominal injuries—Surgery.
WI 900 D337a]
RD540.D34 617'.55044 81-5707
AACR2

Printed in the United States of America

9 8 7 6 5 4 3 2 1

ISBN 0-387-90502-2 Springer-Verlag New York Heidelberg Berlin
ISBN 3-540-90502-2 Springer-Verlag Berlin Heidelberg New York

The authors wish to dedicate this book to our wives, Ms. Barbara Delany and Dr. Susan Jason, for their love, indulgence, and understanding during the preparation of this work.

Contents

3

Specific Diagnostic Techniques 35

Foreword

Trauma to the abdomen, both accidental and willful, has become increasingly common in this era of increasing violence. Large numbers of patients all over the country are admitted to emergency rooms because of abdominal trauma of varying degrees of severity. All too often the correct diagnosis is suspected belatedly or not at all, so that proper treatment is not initiated in sufficient time to be lifesaving. Not infrequently, the injured patient is examined by an intern or an insufficiently experienced resident physician. Even in instances where more senior internists and surgeons are available, detailed knowledge about the necessary methodology to establish the correct diagnosis and institute the appropriate treatment is lacking.

This monograph, representing the felicitous collaboration of a surgeon and a radiologist together with several other contributors, is timely and important. The authors (and their contributors) have approached their subject with a wealth of clinical experience obtained in several very active acute-care municipal hospitals in the largest city in this country. They have observed and treated a very large number of patients with a multitude of traumatic causes, including firearm injuries, stab wounds, vehicular accidents, falls, and assaults.

The authors have divided this work into four main sections: General Perspectives on Abdominal Injury, Types of Abdominal Injuries, Specific Diagnostic Techniques, and Specific Organ or Supporting-Structure Injury.

Physical examination and history-taking are by no means ignored, but considerable stress is placed on the appropriate radiological techniques employed and evaluation of the findings on these radiological studies. The radiological features in the various types of abdominal trauma affecting the abdominal organs (and structures) are described in detail and well-illustrated. Comparison of the operative findings with the changes observed radiologically are skillfully documented.

The emphasis on appropriate radiological studies and the need for accurate interpretation are matched by a truly first-rate dissertation of the surgical principles involved in caring for patients with abdominal trauma.

The section on Specific Diagnostic Techniques is particularly noteworthy, dealing with a large variety of special techniques other than the radiological examination.

The section on Specific Organ or Supporting-Structure Injury again details diagnostic methods as well as principles of treatment relating to injuries to such organs as the liver and spleen and the various segments of the gastrointestinal tract.

This volume is noteworthy for the very considerable amount of information it imparts about an important subject, much of which is seldom appreciated by the average physician observing a patient for the first time after trauma to the abdomen. On reading this book it is evident that the principles of diagnosis and treatment which are stressed, if followed by the examining physician, will enhance his (her) ability to deal with many difficult situations arising from trauma to the abdomen, undoubtedly resulting in a significantly lowered mortality and morbidity.

A large number of case histories is incorporated, illustrating in each section the definitive points which the authors stress. An excellent, relevant list of References is included at the end of each section.

This pragmatic work constitutes an important effort and should prove highly rewarding to every physician, including house staff, and medical students interested in the subject. It will be particularly valuable to those physicians who must deal with a significant number of individuals who have experienced trauma to the abdomen.

The authors are to be congratulated for documenting their considerable experiences at a time when patients with abdominal trauma are encountered in great numbers throughout the country in emergency settings. Thus, a timely book has been written on a very timely subject at an appropriate time. Since trauma to the abdomen is so exceedingly common, a comprehensive knowledge of the various diagnostic techniques which may be utilized (particularly radiological) in such patients, plus an intimate knowledge of the surgical principles involved in their treatment, will clearly spell the difference in many instances between the life and death of a given individual.

Harold G. Jacobson
Marvin L. Gliedman

Preface

This book is designed to state the currently accepted principles in the surgical and radiologic diagnosis of abdominal trauma. Some of the material is fundamental and will be of special value to students and residents. Some more advanced principles are introduced for the physician who has limited exposure to the type and volume of injuries described here.

Despite its prevalence, trauma has not gained the attention it deserves in the training programs of our medical schools and hospitals. As a result of inadequate experience and training, many physicians are not familiar with the variability in clinical manifestations produced by hemoperitoneum, retroperitoneal, and visceral injury. There is a high incidence of error in the early diagnosis of both blunt and penetrating abdominal injury, and a significant morbidity and mortality for many abdominal injuries can be directly attributed to inaccurate or delayed diagnosis.

A physician examining a patient should be aware of the currently available techniques for the diagnosis of abdominal trauma. A laparotomy is the ultimate and final diagnostic measure and is only justified if careful assessment and the appropriate, modern, sophisticated diagnostic tools have been carefully applied to the evaluation of the patient. Avoiding unnecessary surgery is as important in managing trauma as it is in the management of other medical disorders.

With the increasing incidence of urban injury, civilian emergency centers are replacing the battlefields of war as the source of surgical experience in trauma. The Morrisania City Hospital in New York City was a typical urban public medical facility that changed from a voluntary hospital serving a middle-class population to a municipal facility serving a poor community. Over several years and up until its closing, the Morrisania City Hospital rendered care to increasing numbers of urban trauma victims. The authors of this book were members of the hospital staff and used their accumulated experience in the management of trauma as material for the preparation of this text.

An extrapolation from the military to the urban experience is appropriate, especially in terms of the diagnostic assessment of penetrating injury, the transportation of trauma victims, and the organization of medical care and resources in hospital emergency receiving areas. The techniques for expeditious transport of combat victims developed in World War II, Korea, and Vietnam made a unique contribution to the organization of civilian emergency services. When it was appreciated that rapid transportation of injured patients significantly affected survival rates, it became evident that civilian receiving facilities required reorganization. The early, postinjury arrival of civilian trauma victims necessitated the use of organized, team-structured resuscitative measures with rapid fluid-volume infusion and aggressive respiratory care. Today, emergency room personnel throughout the United States are finally being trained to respond quickly to the trauma emergency.

In spite of the parallel between urban trauma care and the military model, the military principles do not universally apply to the civilian situation. The wartime necessity for a pragmatic approach to the management of abdominal trauma derives from limitations imposed on military surgeons by equipment and personnel shortages and the need for speed. Thus, maximum attention was given to "emergency treatment" and little attention to diagnosis. Since comparable material limitations do not exist in modern civilian hospitals, the original concept of triage, with some patients discarded as beyond salvage, does not have a place in civilian emergency care.

The current surge of interest in civilian abdominal trauma has resulted from newer concepts and diagnostic techniques, coupled with modern technology. The selective observation of penetrating abdominal injury, the use of preoperative antibiotics, the exteriorization and suture repair of colonic injury, laparoscopy, peritoneal lavage, radionuclide scanning, ultrasound, arteriography, and endovascular occlusive procedures are advances that took origin from the resources and experience of physicians in modern civilian emergency facilities.

We would like to take this opportunity to thank Mr. Lawrence Klosk of the Michael Foundation, Dr. Harold G. Jacobson for his editorial assistance, the staff of the department of radiology of Montefiore Hospital and Medical Center, Dr. Marvin L. Gliedman, and members of the department of surgery of Montefiore Hospital and Medical Center. We would like to give special acknowledgment to Audrey Tobar, Marjory Mitchell, Nettie Morrison, and Carole Badalati for their assistance in the preparation of the manuscript.

Harry M. Delany
Robert S. Jason

Introduction

The change in the social and economic character of the Morrisania community in the mid- and late 1960s is demonstrated by the emergence of the colloquial name "Fort Apache" to designate the police precinct responsible for the protection of the community. Dramatic shifts in population, the flight of the stable middle class, coupled with and followed by the rapid influx of the poor were associated with a dramatic increase in violence and victims of violent acts. There are enumerable economic and cultural factors involved in the change in the Morrisania Hospital district and similar changes seen in most of the large cities in this country. The written teachings of one of the schools of martial arts located in this same community aptly summarize the local philosophy toward violence.

> Approximately (4) million years ago, if one is to accept the prevailing thought in behavior sciences, Man emerged on the plains of the African Savanna, as a creature like none other in nature. . . . Quite uninspiring in physical appearance, almost comical, he possessed not a single visible attribute requisite to survival in a world forbidding and hostile beyond our comprehension. . . . Irrespective of his unimposing size, Man developed techniques of violence unparalleled in nature; schooled offspring in the violent ways to ensure future replication; and refined each method as a direct function of a superior and inventive intellect. Understood in context, violence is but one trait, a single strand among numerous which define and characterize the behavior of the species. However, Man . . . the child of wonder in evolution . . . when viewed in isolation from his art, science, technology; and, most importantly, his romantic self-evaluation, often steeped in conceit and illusion has for (4) million years ruled by a single consistent principle . . . might! For the moment, assuming the foregoing analysis of Man's nature is accurate, consider the potential for destruction such a creature could possess after several million years of practicing, refining, and manipulating violence as a function of survival, territorial expansion, mastery, and diversion from boredom. Additionally, arm him with a modern hunting knife, chain, tire tool, or handgun and relocate him in a city street in 20th century America. Under these conditions it is difficult, if not imaginary, to exaggerate the actual threat this creature represents individ-

ually or in concert if motivated to act in opposition to your person, family, or property.

Viewed in this light, it is not the poor, a particular race, or members of a particular political or religious persuasion who are the enemy. It is each and every one of us. For each and every one of us, given the appropriate circumstances, may lash out in violence and victimize another. The art and science of medicine began as an effort to counteract the violence inherent in nature. Until some means are found to restrain and control both the violent acts of nature and man, the physician will be called on to treat and promote the survival of the victims of these acts. It is hoped that the information contained in this text will be of some benefit in achieving this goal.

1

General Perspectives on Abdominal Injury

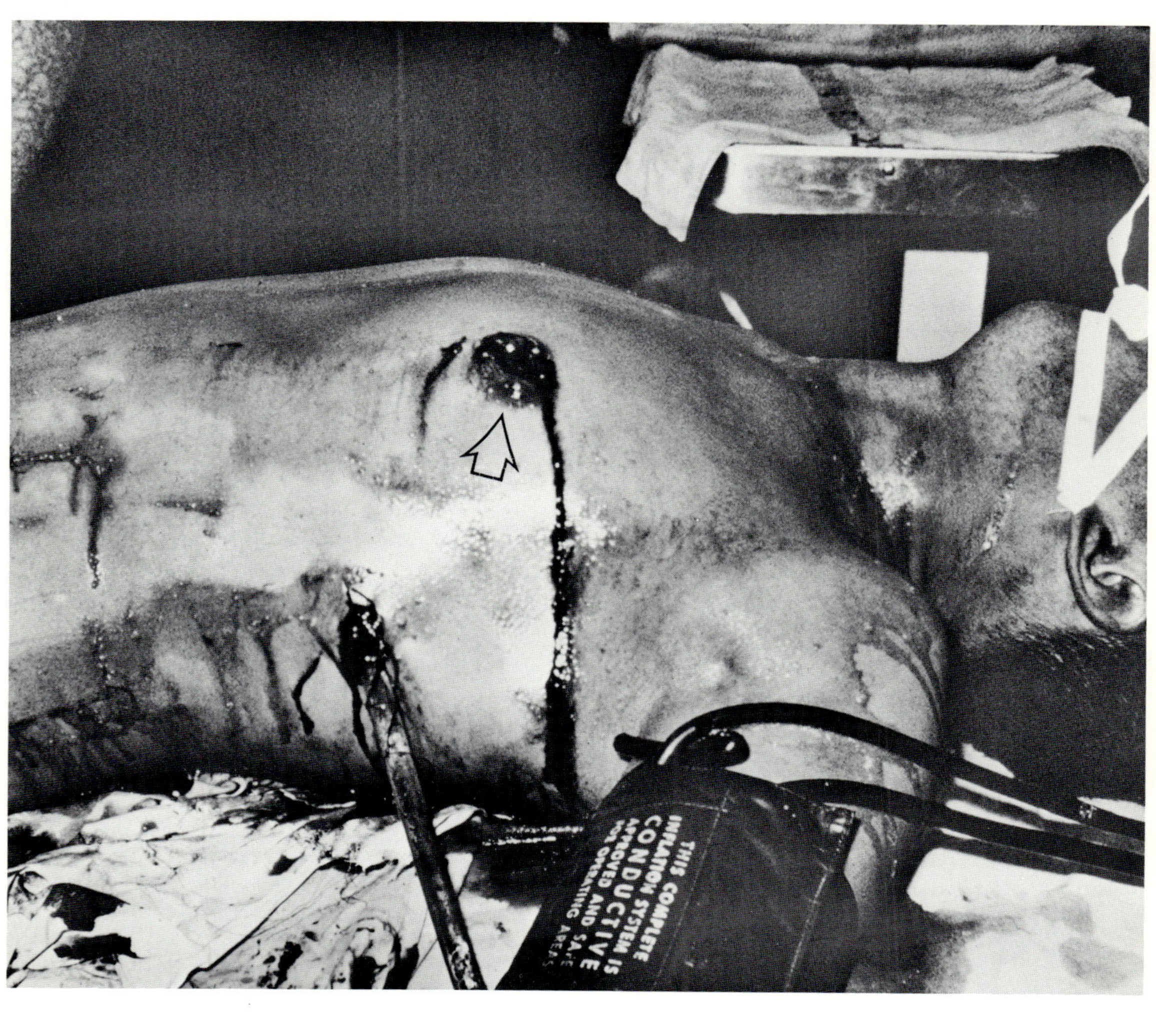

INCIDENCE OF ABDOMINAL INJURIES

Diagnosis and admission data for patients entering any civilian hospital will depend on the community served by the institution and its geographic location. Allen and Curry, reporting from the Hurley Hospital in Michigan in 1956, stated that patients with abdominal trauma of all types represented 0.2% of all patients hospitalized and 2.2% of all patients entering the hospital with injury [1]. In 1973, 19.8% of patients admitted for injuries at the Morrisania Hospital in New York City suffered from abdominal trauma as the primary diagnosis (see Table 1.1).

Nonpenetrating abdominal trauma, at least in the American experience, is one of the clearest examples of man as a victim of his own technology. Whereas abdominal trauma constitutes only 7% [13] of all auto injuries, 50% [15] to 70% [1] of blunt trauma is due to the automobile. In children, the auto is the offending agent in 75% of cases, whereas 10% are due to playground accidents and 15% are attributed to either the battered-child syndrome or birth trauma [21].

TABLE 1.1. Civilian trauma, all types[a]

Site	% patients
Head and neck	28.4
Thorax	11.2
Abdomen	19.8
Upper extremities	8.4
Lower extremities	20.0
Spine	1.6

[a] Data from Morrisania City Hospital, trauma-related admissions (primary diagnosis), 499 patients, 1973.

Between 1960 and 1966, nonpenetrating abdominal trauma occurred in 19.8% of reported automobile driver injuries (Table 1.2). This incidence fell to 16.5% between 1967 and 1969 [17] as a result of improved auto design and safety. In a 1970 study of traffic fatalities reported from Philadelphia [23], 20.2% of patients had abdominal injuries, and 4.8% of deaths were related to these injuries (Table 1.3).

The incidence of abdominal injury resulting from falls from heights, urban riots, and combat activity is lower than for vehicle-related trauma. Reporting on persons falling from heights or "sky divers," Reynolds et al. found a 5.3% incidence of abdominal injury [20]. Lewis et al., in a similar study, but including persons dead on arrival (DOAs), found a 12.2% incidence of significant abdominal-organ injury [12]

TABLE 1.2. Vehicular passenger injuries

	Injuries per 100 patients	
	1960–1966	1967–1969
Head and neck	91.0	105.5
Thorax	35.6	33.8
Abdomen	19.8	16.5
Upper extremities	28.8	35.7
Lower extremities	51.4	50.0
Mortality	10.4	4.0

Source: Nahum AM, Siegel AW (1971) The changing panorama of collision injury. Surg Gynecol Obstet 133: 783

TABLE 1.3. Philadelphia traffic fatalities, 311 cases

	Fatal accidents			Primary cause of death, victim dying within 24 h	
Site[a]	No. of fatalities	% of group	Incidence of involvement	No. of fatalities	% of fatalities
Head or neck	157	50.5	1 of 2	87	28.0
Heart or great vessels	56	18.0	1 of 5	18	5.8
Chest	72	23.2	1 of 4	14	4.5
Abdomen	63	20.2	1 of 5	15	4.8
Major fractures[b]	80	25.8	1 of 4	31	10.0
External hemorrhage[c]	6	1.9	1 of 50	2	0.6
Miscellaneous				13	4.2
"Multiple" injuries				131	42.1
				311	100.0

[a] Table 1.3 includes two or more sites of injury in many patients.
[b] Excluding skull, chest, and minor fractures.
[c] Of life-threatening extent.
Source: Spelman JW, Bordner KK, Howard JM (1970) Traffic fatalities in Philadelphia. J Trauma 10: 885

TABLE 1.4. Falls (jumpers): 200 patients, 360 injuries

	% injuries	% patients
Head and neck	15.8	28.5
Chest	5.3	9.5
Abdomen	5.3	9.5
Upper extremities	23.3	42.0
Lower extremities	29.4	53.0
Spine	11.1	20.0
Pelvis	9.7	17.5
Mortality	17	

Source: Reynolds BM, Balsam NA, Reynolds FX (1971) Falls from heights. A surgical experience of 200 consecutive cases. Ann Surg 174: 304

(Table 1.4). Robb and Mathews have reported a 5.7% incidence of abdominal injury from the urban riot activity in Belfast [22]. The Vietnam combat experience was described separately by Feltis [5] and Heaton [9]. They found abdominal trauma in 14.4% and 7.1% of injuries in their respective reports (Table 1.5).

VARIABLES AFFECTING MORBIDITY AND MORTALITY

General

The introduction of improved communication techniques and the rapid transportation of the trauma vic-

TABLE 1.5. Military trauma, all types

Site	**A.** Regional distribution of wounds in Vietnam, % injuries[a]	**B.** Evacuation hospital in Vietnam, % injuries[b]
Head and neck	12.0	11.3
Thorax	7.2	10.1
Abdomen	7.1	14.0
Upper extremities	22.4	29.9
Lower extremities	40.6	34.7
Other[c]	10.7	

[a] Of 7869 hospital admissions, October 1965 to June 1966.
[b] Of 6927 patients, 1971.
[c] Flanks, back, buttocks, genitalia, and unidentified as to location.
Source: **(A)** Heaton LD (1966) Military surgical practices of the United States Army in Vietnam. Curr Probl Surg, Year Book Publishers (November 1966) Chicago, Ill.; **(B)** Feltis JM (1979) Surgical experience in a combat zone. Am J Surg 119: 275

tim, the use of antibiotics, aggressive resuscitative techniques using blood and colloid administration, the monitoring of functioning circulatory blood volume by venous pressure measurements, teams of skilled abdominal surgeons, and better coordination of operating room and paramedical emergency personnel have all contributed to a significant reduction in the morbidity and mortality of patients who sustain trauma to the abdomen.

The mortality for abdominal injuries sustained in military combat has declined from a reported 53.5% during World War I to 25% for World War II, 12% for Korea, and finally 8.5% for the Vietnam conflict. There has been a similar reduction in mortality of civilian abdominal injury from 50% in 1943 [1] to 14% in 1960 [27]. Although the mortality rate for nonpenetrating abdominal injury still ranges from 10.4% to 45.7% [18,19], the mortality for penetrating abdominal injury, particularly from stab wounds, has shown a gradual reduction. Billings and Walkling, in 1931, reported a mortality for civilian abdominal stab wounds of 22% [3]. Forty-seven years later, McAlvanah and Shaftan found the mortality to be approximately 1% [14]. Aside from the form of injury, penetrating vs nonpenetrating, there are other variables that play a role in the morbidity and mortality of the patient.

Age and Sex

Although the problem of abdominal injury affects all age groups, approximately 67% of patients are between 10 and 39 years of age [1,28]. Of patients who require surgical treatment or who die from their injury, 75.9% are in the first to fourth decade, with the highest incidence (25.9%) in the third decade [25] (Table 1.6).

Nonpenetrating trauma is the etiology in 77.5% to 79% of patients with injury to the abdomen [24,28]. The male to female ratio ranges from 3 : 1 to 22 : 1 for blunt trauma [8]; however, in children, the male/female ratio is more nearly equal at 6 : 4 [21]. Of the patients, 60% are under the age of 30 [27], and 70% are between 20 and 50 years old [8].

With penetrating injuries, 91% of patients are between the ages of 11 and 40, with a peak incidence in the second decade. Seventy-eight to eighty-one percent of all patients are male [19,29]. Thus, trauma is a disease of the younger population, and males are more commonly affected than females.

Condition of the Patient prior to the Trauma

Vulnerability to abdominal trauma may vary with the condition of the abdominal organs. Minimal trauma in children can result in serious injury owing to the high incidence of preexisting visceral lesions. Richardson [21] found that one-half of pediatric injury-related renal lesions occurred in abnormal organs. In addition, Baker and Berdon [2] have found that a specific organ injury may frequently be superimposed on or lead to the diagnosis of a previously silent, serious abnormality.

Patient mental awareness is always significant to the outcome of a violent or potentially violent situation. Innumerable studies have shown that many accidents could have been avoided except for some correctable aspect of mental awareness. Such a circumstance may also increase the delay between in-

TABLE 1.6. Age distribution of abdominal trauma in Connecticut in 1971

Decade	No. of patients[a]	% of patients[a]	No. of deaths[b]	% of deaths[b]
0–9	42	(12.2)	0	(0)
10–19	67	(19.5)	9	(19.1)
20–29	89	(25.9)	9	(19.1)
30–39	63	(18.3)	6	(12.8)
40–49	31	(9.0)	4	(8.5)
50–59	28	(8.1)	6	(12.8)
60–69	15	(4.4)	7	(14.9)
70–79	8	(2.3)	4	(8.5)
80–89	1	(0.3)	1	(2.1)
Total	344	(100.0)	46	(97.8)

[a] One patient (0.8%) of unknown age is not listed.

[b] One death (2.1%) in patient of unknown age is not listed.

Source: Strauch GO (1973) Major abdominal trauma in 1971. A study of Connecticut by the Connecticut Society of American Board Surgeons and the Yale Trauma Program. Am J Surg 125: 413–418

jury and treatment with significant increase in morbidity and mortality.

Multiple-System and Multiple Abdominal Organ Injury

Extraabdominal injuries will frequently mask or complicate the diagnosis and treatment of visceral trauma. Williams and Zollinger [28] found that 40% of patients with abdominal trauma had complications from extraabdominal-system trauma. In a series of 200 nonpenetrating abdominal trauma patients reported by Fitzgerald et al. in 1960, a comparison was made between patients dead on arrival (DOA) at the hospital and patients who arrived alive (Table 1.7). Abdominal injuries alone occurred in only 15.5% of patients in the series. Of the 167 patients with multiple-system injuries, 97 were dead before hospital admission and 17 were dead before therapy could be initiated. Extraabdominal injuries were present in 97% of patients admitted DOA and in 70% of patients admitted alive [6].

Allen and Curry found that there was multiple visceral involvement associated with 14% of nonpenetrating and 62% of penetrating injuries [1]. The factor of multiplicity of organ injury as a predictive index for prognosis has been established by a number of clinical reports. The significance of multiple visceral involvement with blunt trauma was described in 1961 by Kleinert and Romero [11]. They found that the mortality rate with one organ involved was 8%, with two organs 38%, and with three or more organs 70%. Wilson and Sherman described a similar but less dramatic progression of mortality rate for civilian penetrating injuries. Feltis confirmed the same pattern in military penetrating injuries [5,29] (Tables 1.8 and 1.9).

TABLE 1.8. Civilian penetrating wounds of abdomen: Multiple organs and mortality, 275 cases

No. of organs	Stab	Gunshot	Total deaths	Total deaths, %
1	0	0	0	0
2	4	1	5	23.8
3	1	5	6	28.6
4	1	3	4	19.0
Over 4	0	6	6	28.6
Total	6	15	21	100

Source: Wilson H, Sherman R (1961) Civilian penetrating wounds of the abdomen. Factors in mortality and differences from military wounds in 494 cases. Ann Surg 153: 639

TABLE 1.9. Relation of number of organs injured to mortality in combat

No. of organs injured	No. of patients	% of patients	No. of deaths	% mortality
1	419	64.3	27	6.5
2	166	25.4	23	13.6
3	45	6.9	11	24.4
4 or more	22	3.4	18	81.8
Total	652		79	12.1

Source: Feltis JM (1979) Surgical experience in a combat zone. Am J Surg 119: 275

The collected mortality figures of Williams and Zollinger [28] reveal that as many as two-thirds of patients dying with intraabdominal injury had serious extraabdominal trauma, and of this group at least 14.4% may have had an altered course if an early diagnosis of abdominal injury had been made. Van Wagoner's 1961 analysis of 606 healthy adult males who were injured

TABLE 1.7. Associated injury in 200 patients with nonpenetrating abdominal injury

Injury	Entire series		Dead on arrival		Living on arrival		Survival (group admitted alive)	
	No.	%	No.	%	No.	%	No.	%
Rib fractures	108	54	71	71	37	37	21	57
Long-bone fractures	74	37	45	45	29	29	17	59
Craniocerebral	62	31	44	44	18	18	5	28
Pulmonary	62	31	50	50	12	12	4	33
Pelvic fracture	40	20	21	21	19	19	13	68
Spinal fracture	29	14.5	25	25	4	4	2	50
Heart and great vessels	19	9.5	19	19	0	0	0	0
Urethra	4	2	0	0	4	4	4	100
None	33	16.5	3	3	30	30	28	93

Source: Fitzgerald JB, Crawford ES, DeBakey ME (1960) Surgical consideration of nonpenetrating abdominal injuries. An analysis of 200 cases. Am J Surg 100: 22

TABLE 1.10. Where death occurred in 159 patients dying as a result of auto accidents

	Total no. patients	Salvageable	Nonsalvageable	Possible salvage
Death at scene	75	7	64	4
Death in transit	24	9	14	1
Death in hospital	60	12	44	4

Source: Frey CF, Huelke DF, Gikas PW (1969) Resuscitation and survival in motor vehicle accidents. J Trauma a(4): 292–301

and died within 2 weeks after their admission to the hospital adds a more worrisome fact. He found that one of three patients in whom the main cause of death was abdominal trauma had the diagnosis made at postmortem examination [26].

Condition of the Patient following Trauma

Rapid transport of trauma victims makes the condition of the patient at the time of hospital arrival a better index of survival than in earlier times. The experience, in both military and civilian settings, indicates that trauma mortality is high in the early hours of hospitalization of the critically injured patient. A series of auto accident fatalities was reported by Frey et al. [7] (Table 1.10).

Strauch [25] reviewed the cumulative experience with abdominal trauma in Connecticut and noted that in a group of 345 patients, the mortality was 13.6%. The deaths of eleven patients, or 23.4%, occurred prior to operation. Eight patients died during surgery and twenty-eight patients died subsequent to surgery. Twenty-three of the forty-two patients died of hemorrhage and shock.

In Fitzgerald et al.'s series of patients with blunt trauma, 93% of patients with a blood pressure recording initially of greater than 90 mmHg (systolic) survived, whereas the survival was only 47% in patients with a systolic blood pressure of less than 90 mmHg [6]. Faris and Dudley, in reporting a series of patients with closed liver injury, noted a mortality of 83.3% if the initial blood pressure was less than 50 mmHg (systolic); 34.2% if the blood pressure was between 50 and 100 mmHg; and 4.7% if the blood pressure was greater than 100 mmHg [4].

REFERENCES

1. Allen RB, Curry GJ (1957) Abdominal trauma. A study of 297 consecutive cases. Am J Surg 93: 398–404
2. Baker DH, Berdon WE (1966) Special trauma problems in children. Radiol Clin North Am 4(2): 289–305
3. Billings AE, Walkling A (1931) Penetrating wounds to the abdomen. Ann Surg 94: 1018–1043
4. Faris IB, Dudley HAF (1973) Closed liver injury. An assessment of prognostic factors. Br J Surg 60: 227
5. Feltis JM (1979) Surgical experience in a combat zone. Am J Surg 119: 275
6. Fitzgerald JB, Crawford ES, DeBakey ME (1960) Surgical consideration of nonpenetrating abdominal injuries. An analysis of 200 cases. Am J Surg 100: 22
7. Frey CF, Huelke DF, Gikas PW (1969) Resuscitation and survival in motor accidents. J Trauma 4: 292–301
8. Griswold RA, Collier HS (1961) Collective review: Blunt abdominal trauma. Surg Gynecol Obstet (Int Abstr Surg 112: 309–329)
9. Heaton LD (1966) Military surgical practices of the United States Army in Vietnam. Curr Probl Surg, Year Book Publishers
10. Jett HH, VanHoy JM, Hamit HF (1972) Clinical and socioeconomic aspects of 254 admissions for stab and gunshot wounds. J Trauma 12: 577–580
11. Kleinert AE, Romero J (1961) Blunt abdominal trauma. Review of cases admitted to a general hospital over a 10 year period. J Trauma 1: 226–247
12. Lewis WS, Lee AB, Grantham AS (1965) Jumpers syndrome. J Trauma 5: 812
13. Lim RC, Glickman MG, Hunt TK (1972) Angiography in patients with blunt trauma to the chest and abdomen. Surg Clin North Am 52(3): 551–565
14. McAlvanah MJ, Shaftan GW (1978) Selective conservatism in penetrating abdominal wounds: A continuing reappraisal. J Trauma 18: 206–212
15. Martin JD (1969) Trauma to the Thorax and Abdomen. Charles C Thomas, Springfield, Ill.
16. Mullen JT (1974) The magnitude of the problem and trauma. J Trauma 14(12): 1070–1072
17. Nahum AM, Siegel AW (1971) The changing panorama of collision injury. Surg Gynecol Obstet 133: 783
18. Nelson JF (1966) The roentgenologic evaluation of abdominal trauma. Radiol Clin North Am 4(2): 415–431
19. Perry JF (1965) A five year survey of 152 acute abdominal injuries. J Trauma 5: 53
20. Reynolds BM, Balsam NA, Reynolds FX (1971) Falls from heights: A surgical experience of 200 consecutive cases. Ann Surg 174: 304
21. Richardson JD (1972) Blunt abdominal trauma in children. Ann Surg 176: 213–216
22. Robb JDA, Mathews JGW (1971) The injuries and man-

agement of riot casualties admitted to the Belfast Hospital wards, August to October 1969. Br J Surg 58: 413
23. Spelman JW, Bordner KK, Howard JM (1970) Traffic fatalities in Philadelphia. J Trauma 10: 885
24. Stivelman RL, Glaubitz JP, Crampton RS (1963) Laceration of the spleen due to nonpenetrating trauma. One hundred cases. Am J Surg 106: 888–891
25. Strauch GO (1973) Major abdominal trauma in 1971: A study of Connecticut by the Connecticut Society of American Board Surgeons and the Yale Trauma Program. Am J Surg 125: 413–418
26. Van Wagoner FA (1961) Died in hospital: A three year study of deaths following trauma. J Trauma 1: 401–408
27. Watkins GL (1960) Blunt trauma to abdomen. Arch Surg 80: 187–191
28. Williams RD, Zollinger RM (1959) Diagnostic and prognostic factors in abdominal trauma. Am J Trauma 97: 575–581
29. Wilson H, Sherman R (1961) Civilian penetrating wounds of the abdomen: Factors in mortality and differences from military wounds in 494 cases. Ann Surg 153: 639

2

Types of Abdominal Injury

Violence (is) a "Face-Dancer": Inherently possessing the capacity to modify expressions, as the chameleon is able to change its colors. [31]

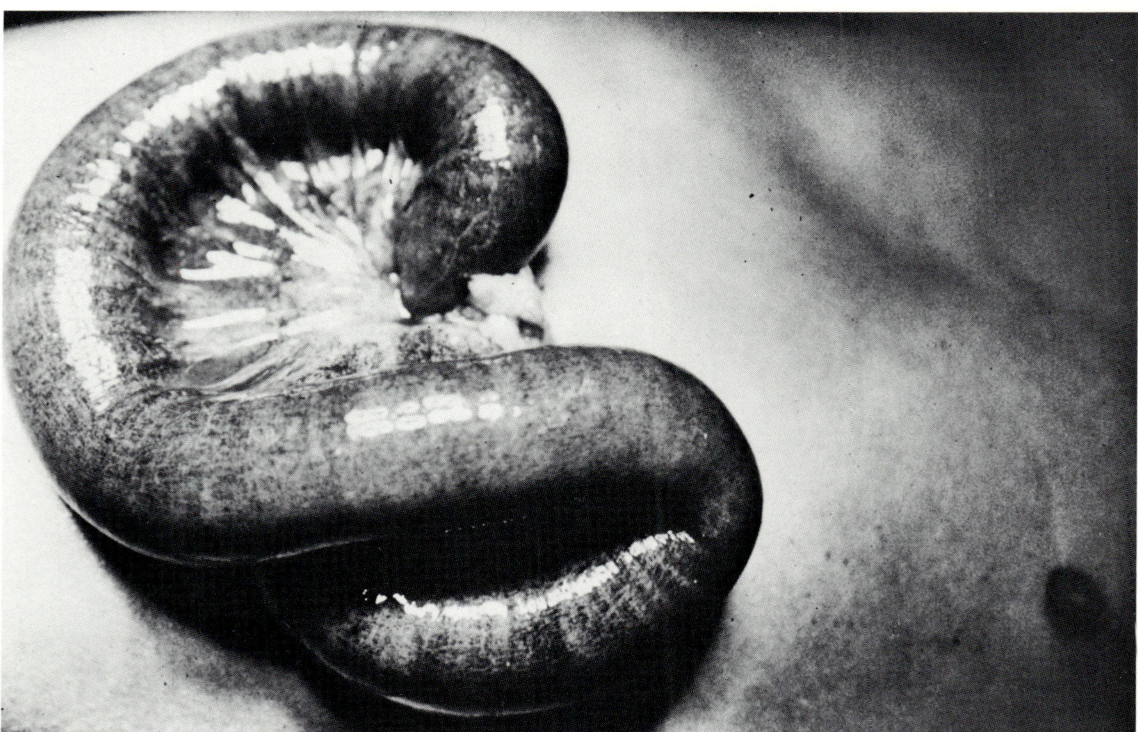

PENETRATING INJURY

Historic View and Changing Mortality Rate

The severity of penetrating abdominal injury varies with the injuring agent and the organs affected. The variety of injuries that can be produced is a challenge to the diagnostic and therapeutic skills of the physicians involved in the patient's care. Accidents, animal attacks, environmental upheavals, and wars (using relatively low-velocity missiles such as rocks, knives, spears, and arrows) accounted for most visceral trauma prior to the introduction of gunpowder. However, since the introduction of gunpowder in the fourteenth century, there has been a progressively increasing incidence of injury from relatively high-velocity missiles, causing extensive soft-tissue and osseous injury.

Eviscerating abdominal wounds are frightening and dramatic. Prior to modern surgery, the victims of such injury were doomed to suffer a slow, painful death. Because of the horror of such deaths, this form of injury was incorporated into the procedure of formal punishment and execution for very serious crimes. In thirteenth-century England, drawing and quartering included opening the abdomen and evisceration. The entrails were then burned in front of the victim's eyes!

The traditional approach to the therapy for penetrating abdominal trauma was to make decisions based solely on the initial clinical assessment of the patient. Emergency diagnostic procedures were not considered in the evaluation of such injuries until the last few years.

Nonoperative management of penetrating injuries was accepted until the late nineteenth century. During that pre-Listerian, preanesthesia era, the mortality for penetrating injuries to the abdomen was over 90%. The death of President Garfield in 1881 from a penetrating wound to the abdomen stirred interest in the problem of surgical treatment for penetrating abdominal injury. The newly accepted surgical excision of pelvic tumors and the possibility of laparotomy for gunshot wounds was discussed by J. Marion Sims in 1882 [40]. A number of other surgeons wrote on the subject of penetrating injury. Coley, in 1891, reported a mortality of 67% for 165 abdominal injuries [3]. Stimson reported a mortality of 81% for 4958 cases managed nonoperatively [43]. The mortality for penetrating abdominal injury during World War I was high and the civilian experience was not better. Loria reported a 62.3% mortality from the Charity Hospital in New Orleans for the period between 1901 and 1930 [21].

The subsequent improvement in the results of surgery for penetrating injury paralleled the progress in medical and surgical science. World War II marked the beginning of the current era in the management of penetrating abdominal injuries—a period characterized by favorable surgical results, with the aid of antibiotics, blood transfusions, preoperative preparation, and appropriate diagnostic techniques. Poer has summarized this progress and stated that improvement in surgical results during World War II was initiated

TABLE 2.1. Mortality for penetrating abdominal wounds, civilian

Series	Date	No. of patients	% mortality
Sherman	1956	212	7.8
McComb	1958	307	6.4
Moore	1959	109	6.4
Shaftan	1960	180	6.4
Wilson	1960	430	5.8
Perry	1970	129	3.5
McAlvanah	1978	829	2.5

Source: Adapted from Wilson H, Sherman R (1961) Civilian penetrating wounds of the abdomen. Factors in mortality and differences from military wounds in 494 cases. Ann Surg 153: 639–649

by the introduction of prompt surgical intervention using field hospitals, avoidance of long-distance transport of patients, and the concept of triage [32].

The declining mortality rate for civilian penetrating injuries to the abdomen has been encouraging. The sequentially reported overall mortality figures show a decline from 7.8% in 1956 to 2.5% in 1978 (Table 2.1).

The pattern of penetrating injuries in civilian life has changed in recent years. Pridgen et al. reported a 70% incidence of stab wounds and a 30% incidence of gunshot wounds in a series of 776 cases, but noted an increase in gunshot wounds in the later years of the study [34] (Table 2.2). The reports of civilian penetrating injuries by Wilson and Sherman [50], Netterville and Hardy [30], Ryzoff et al. [37], and Steichen et al. [42] present a significant and increasing incidence of gunshot wounds of the abdomen.

Etiology

In 1971, Strauch reported a large series of abdominal injuries from the state of Connecticut; 16.6% of the injuries were knife wounds and 13.7% were gunshot wounds [44] (Table 2.3). DeFore et al. reported 1590 liver injuries in 1976 and showed a progressive increase

TABLE 2.2. Penetrating wounds of the abdomen: Type and location

	No. of cases			
	1950–1956	1957–1966	Total	%
Stab wound	247	297	544	70
Gunshot wound	64	168	232	30

Source: Pridgen JE, Aust JB, Fisher GW (1970) Penetrating Wounds of the Abdomen. Charles C Thomas, Publisher, Springfield, Ill.

TABLE 2.3. Abdominal trauma, 1971

Type of injury	No. of cases	%
Blunt	229	66.6
Knife	57	16.6
Gunshot	47	13.7
Other perforating	11	3.2
	344	

Source: Strauch GO (1973) Major abdominal trauma in 1971. A study of Connecticut by the Connecticut Society of American Board Surgeons and the Yale Trauma Program. Am J Surg 125: 413–418

in the incidence of gunshot wounds to the liver over a 35-year period [5]. Between 1971 and 1974, there were 322 gunshot wounds to the liver as compared with 100 stab wounds. McAlvanah and Shaftan reporting from New York described 221 gunshot wounds and 590 stab wounds in a total series of 829 penetrating injuries up to 1978 [26] (Table 2.4). The weapons used to inflict penetrating injuries in the civilian population are documented in several of the foregoing series (Tables 2.5, 2.6).

The penetrating abdominal injury of military combat has been largely the result of fragments projected from exploding grenades, bombs, and shells. Bullets

TABLE 2.4. Abdominal trauma: Type of injury

Penetrating		Blunt	
Type	No.	Type	No.
Stab wounds	590	Pedestrian auto	63
Gunshot wounds	221	Occupant auto	65
Other penetrating	18	Major falls	30
		Other	49
Total	829	Total	207

Source: McAlvanah MJ, Shaftan GW (1978) Selective conservatism in penetrating abdominal wounds. A continuing appraisal. J Trauma 18: 206

TABLE 2.5. Agent producing penetrating injury

Agent	No. of cases
Bullet	83
Knife	59
Shotgun	9
Broken glass	2
Broken chain link	1
Ice pick	1
Total	155

Source: Netterville RE, Hardy JD (1967) Analysis of 155 cases with problems in management. Ann Surg 166: 232–237

TABLE 2.6. Agent producing penetrating injury

Agent	No. of cases
Shotgun	49
Pistol	101
Ice pick	14
Butcher knife	15
Rifle	26
Switchblade knife	17
Pocket knife	44
Total	206

Source: Wilson H, Sherman R (1961) Civilian penetrating wounds of the abdomen. Factors in mortality and differences from military wounds in 494 cases. Ann Surg 153: 639

were responsible for approximately one-third of abdominal injuries prior to the Vietnam conflict. In addition to the magnitude of the intraabdominal injury produced by the high-velocity force of the military missiles, multiplicity adds to the overall complexity, morbidity, and mortality of the military penetrating injury.

Age, Sex, and Race

The traditional involvement of ethnic minorities in the "urban trauma" phenomenon is a reflection of the population distribution. The ultimate effect of urban violence, alcoholism, and drug abuse on the productivity of minority youth is nonmeasurable but unmistakably significant. The ready availability of drugs will ultimately foster the spread of violence and has profound and untold effects on the potential of minority youth to participate in the "normal" pattern of educational and psychological development. The series presented by Wilson and Sherman [50] in 1961 gives the age, sex, and race distribution in 452 penetrating injury cases (Table 2.7). Lowe et al. from Chicago reported that 88.1% of the 362 patients with gunshot wounds were black, with an average age of 27.8 years [22]. The Brooklyn, New York series published in 1978 by McAlvanah and Shaftan included 829 patients suffering penetrating injuries. Of the patients, 65% were black, 19% were Puerto Rican, and 16% were white [26]. Fifty-two percent of the patients were between 18 and 29 years of age. A specific study of penetrating abdominal injuries in children and adolescents was reported by Tunell et al. [48]. They described a series of 132 patients up to 16 years of age. There were 5 deaths and 35 complications.

Stab Wounds

Mortality

The abdominal stab wound has been extensively studied. Many clinical reports list organ injuries, mortality, and principles of management. The civilian experience, documented between 1931 and 1978, has had an overall decline in mortality [28] (Table 2.8).

Penetrating stab injuries produce a somewhat predictable course. When injured by a sharp penetrating object, the abdominal organs are split or lacerated, not perforated and blown apart as in gunshot wounds. Surgical repair of stab wounds is easier than is surgical repair of organs injured by explosion-released projectiles.

TABLE 2.8. Abdominal stab wounds

Series	Date	No. of patients	% mortality
Billings	1931	77	22.0
McGowen	1935	100	21.0
Wright	1939	184	13.5
Rippy	1942	156	10.9
McComb	1958	243	2.5
Moss	1960	550	1.1
Kazarian	1971	500	1.1
McAlvanah	1978	590	1.1

Source: Adapted from Moss LK, Schmidt FE, Creech O Jr (1962) Analysis of 550 stab wounds of abdomen. Am Surg 28: 483

TABLE 2.7. Penetrating abdominal wounds: Age, sex, and race distribution, 1948–1959, 452 cases

Type	Male	Female	Negro	White	Peak age (extremes)	Total
Stab	215	17	248	14	20–30 (4–64)	262
Gunshot	152	38	172	18	20–30 (3–67)	190
Totals	367	85	420	32	20–30 (1–67)	452

Source: Wilson H, Sherman R (1961) Civilian penetrating wounds of the abdomen. Factors in mortality and differences from military wounds in 494 cases. Ann Surg 153: 639

Site of Injury

The site of a stab injury may vary in appearance from a small ice-pick wound to a large defect with evisceration (see section on physical examination, p. 44). The appearance of the external wound is considered of limited clinical value in determining the extent and severity of abdominal injury.

Abdominal stab wounds have a predictable pattern based on the fact that the injuries are most often inflicted from the front and by right-handed assailants [17,26]. Such stab wounds more commonly occur on the left side of the body and are two to three times more likely to involve the upper as opposed to the lower abdominal quadrants. This pattern of injury for civilian stab wounds is described by Hopson et al. [17] and, more recently, by McAlvanah and Shaftan. The location and incidence of penetration given by Hopson et al. (Table 2.9) show that penetration of the full thickness of the abdominal wall occurs in 65% to 80% of cases [17]. However, penetration and visceral injury are obviously not synonymous and patients may sustain penetration of the abdomen without significant organ injury.

The percentage distribution of organ injury from stab wounds differs from that of gunshot wounds. Stab wounds are accompanied by a lower incidence of small-bowel and colonic injury. This difference can be explained by the tendency of intestinal loops to move away from a penetrating object forced through the abdominal wall at a relatively slow speed. There is also a lower incidence of multiple-organ injury with stab wounds (Table 2.10).

Although evisceration of omentum or bowel and

TABLE 2.9. Stab wounds: 297 cases

					Mid		Back		
	RUQ[a]	RLQ	LUQ	LLQ	Upper	Lower	R	L	Total
No penetration	18	5	35	13	21	3	2	2	99
Penetration but no injury	17	4	30	12	18	1	2	2	86
Penetration and visceral injury	26	11	46	14	12	6	0	6	121
Total	61	20	111	39	51	10	4	10	306

Key: RUQ, right upper quadrant; RLQ, right lower quadrant; LUQ, left upper quadrant; LLQ, left lower quadrant.
Source: Hopson WB, Sherman RJ, Sanders JW (1966) Stab wounds of the abdomen. 5 year review of 297 cases. Am J Surg 32: 213

TABLE 2.10. Civilian penetrating wounds of the abdomen: Organ-injury distribution and mortality, 279 cases

	Type					
Injury	Stab	GSW[a]	Cases	Wounds	Deaths	% Mortality
Aorta	0	2	2	2	2	100
Vena cava	1	2	3	3	1	33.3
Biliary	2	4	6	6	2	33.3
Duodenum	2	17	19	22	5	26.3
Pancreas	7	3	10	10	2	20
Urinary bladder	0	12	12	14	2	16.7
Kidney	6	14	20	20	3	15
Vascular	12	9	17	17	2	11.8
Colon	18	68	86	98	10	11.6
Small bowel	34	58	92	521	10	10.9
Spleen	9	10	19	19	2	10.5
Stomach	35	19	54	67	5	9.3
Liver	63	44	107	112	7	6.5
Uterus	1	2	3	3	0	0

[a] Gunshot wound.
Source: Wilson H, Sherman R (1961) Civilian penetrating wounds of the abdomen. Factors in mortality and differences from military wounds in 494 cases. Ann Surg 153: 639

leaking of small-bowel contents through an abdominal-wall wound clearly imply full-thickness wall injury and visceral trauma, the clinical differentiation of non-penetrating, penetrating, and penetrating wounds with visceral trauma is difficult without an exploratory laparotomy. In the past, radiology has played its least significant role in this population of patients, since early surgical exploration was frequent. In addition, Wilson and Sherman [50] suggest that, in terms of the diagnosis of perforation, radiologic studies were helpful in only 8.3% of patients, produced false-positive diagnoses in 2.4%, and were of no diagnostic value in 89.6%. However, the identification of entry and exit stab wounds with lead markers prior to the radiologic evaluation of the abdomen may be helpful, not only in suggesting peritoneal penetration, but also in suggesting possible visceral injury. Entry and exit stab wounds in close proximity to one another or flank wounds may suggest a benign injury, but associated hemoperitoneum or trauma to an organ must be ruled out.

The Selective Approach to Surgery

The decision to explore all patients with stab wounds is controversial. A clinically selective approach to the management of these wounds has been proposed and vigorously espoused by a number of authors. The current emphasis on clinical judgment in deciding the course of management of civilian stab wounds of the abdomen is a noteworthy advance in therapy. It has focused attention on the need to view the abdominal trauma patient as a diagnostic challenge.

In 1960 Shaftan reported on 180 abdominal trauma patients from the Kings County Hospital. Only 53 of these patients were explored, and there was only 1 death as a result of this selective approach [38]. Printen et al. reported on 267 patients with stab wounds from Cook County Hospital. In this series, 52.9% of patients were observed without surgical exploration with no mortalities [33]. Nance and Cohn published a retrospective comparative series of 600 patients [29]. Between 1964 and 1967, 92% of 480 patients had exploratory laparotomy. Only one-third of patients explored required repair of an intraabdominal injury. In a later, second series of 120 patients treated with a selective approach, 72 patients escaped surgery. Thus, the surgical exploration rate for stab wounds decreased from 92% to 40%. There were no complications in the conservatively managed group, and the average hospital stay was 2.1 days [29] (Table 2.11).

Certain authors favor continuing a policy of mandatory exploration of all abdominal stab wounds. Mathewson [25] and Forde and Ganepola [12] are representative of this group. They have emphasized the low morbidity and mortality in laparotomies with no significant findings, and stress the dangers of observing patients with initially negative abdominal examinations.

However, there is a mortality and morbidity associated with negative laparotomy. Lowe et al. reported on the problem and presented a morbidity figure of 19% for patients with no visceral injury and 23% for patients with minor visceral injury [23]. The figure for morbidity in a no-injury group explored at the Charity Hospital between 1964 and 1967 is given in Table 2.12 [29].

In supporting the selective approach, Nance and Cohn documented the low mortality from peritonitis in a large collected review of series of stab wounds (Table 2.13). The emphasis on adjunctive diagnostic procedures in managing penetrating injury is stressed by Lowe et al. [22] and McAlvanah and Shaftan [26]. The use of such techniques should reduce the incidence of negative exploration and thereby decrease the mor-

TABLE 2.11. Management of stab wounds

	1964–1967 480 cases			1967–1969 120 cases		
Disposition	No. patients	%		No. patients	%	
No exploration	38	8		72	60	
Exploration, no injury	250	52	92%	12	10	40%
Injury, no repair necessary	46	9		3	3	
Injury, repair required	146	31		33	27	
Total	480	100		120	100	

Source: Nance CF, Cohn I Jr (1969) Surgical judgment in the management of stab wounds of the abdomen. A retrospective and prospective analysis based on a study of 600 stabbed patients. Ann Surg 170(4): 569–580

TABLE 2.12. Complications following exploration for stab wounds, 1964–1967

Complication	Laparotomy no injury	Injury, no repair required	Injury, repair required
Wound infection	25	4	10
Temp, 101°	21	4	20
Evisceration	5	0	5
Spleen injury	4	0	0
Intra. abd. abscess	3	0	3
Torn small bowel	3	0	0
Obstruction	2	1	4
Prolonged ileus	1	0	2
Pneumonia	2	1	4
Atelectasis	1	4	4
Fecal fistula	0	1	0
Death	1	0	1

Source: Nance CF, Cohn I Jr (1969) Surgical judgment in the management of stab wounds of the abdomen. A retrospective and prospective analysis based on a study of 600 stabbed patients. Ann Surg 170(4): 569–580

bidity and mortality associated with it. Recent figures for the operative indications, morbidity and mortality of the selective management of penetrating injury are presented by McAlvanah and Shaftan [26] (Tables 2.14–2.16).

Guernsey and Ganchrow have reported an experience with exploratory laparotomy in patients with multiple-system injury during the Vietnam conflict. Of 700 patients with multiple injury, 561 had intraabdominal injury [15]. The morbidity in the 139 patients with negative findings was 2%.

The "selective" approach to abdominal stab wounds starts with a complete initial examination of the patient including radiologic and laboratory studies. If the patient does not have findings indicating the need for laparotomy at that time, the patient is admitted to the hospital for close observation including the frequent determination of vital signs and repeated physical examination by a competent physician. If there is any change in the patient's condition or the development of any of the criteria for intervention, exploratory laparotomy is carried out. The clinical criteria for mandatory exploration reported and listed by Richter and Zachy [36] differ little from the criteria used by Nance and Cohn [29] or by Shaftan [39] (see Table 2.17).

Although the presence of free intraperitoneal air is strong evidence for peritoneal penetration and possible visceral injury, Ryzoff et al. describe a single case of penetrating injury with free air and no abdominal signs that did not have visceral injury at the time of exploration [37].

The presence of evisceration of bowel or omentum suggests that there should be mandatory exploration. However, 6 of 19 stab-wound patients with evisceration reported by Steichen et al. did not have a visceral injury [42]. Of 25 cases with evisceration of the omen-

TABLE 2.13. Peritonitis, a rare cause of death: Deaths from abdominal sepsis following stab wounds of abdomen (collected series)

Institution	Policy	No. cases	No. died	Died of peritonitis
Charity Hospital	Explore	1783	14	0
John Gaston	Explore	297	4	1
John Gaston	Explore	256	8	2
Robert B. Green	Explore	243	6	1
Lincoln Hosp., N.Y.	Explore	158	7	1
Univ. Mississippi	Explore	60	0	0
Manchester, England	Explore	43	3	1
Univ. Illinois	Selective	127	0	0
Kings County	Selective	477	10	0
Cook County	Selective	267	2	0
L. A. County	Selective	369	6	2
Joint Diseases	Selective	159	3	0
Kansas City Gen.	Selective	326	3	0
Baragwanath Hospital	Selective	340[a]	13	4
Baragwanath Hospital	Selective	100	1	0
		5005	72 (1.44%)	12 (0.24%)

[a] Includes gunshot wounds.

Source: Nance CF, Cohn I Jr (1969) Surgical judgment in the management of stab wounds of the abdomen. A retrospective and prospective analysis based on a study of 600 stabbed patients. Ann Surg 170(4): 569–580

TABLE 2.14. Operative indications—Penetrating trauma

	Stab	Gunshot	Other
Initial peritoneal signs	26 (14.7)[a]	27 (22.5)	1 (16.7)
Development of signs	41 (23.2)	17 (14.1)	
Positive tap/lavage	82 (46.5)	49 (40.8)	1 (16.7)
Shock/bleeding	6 (3.3)	14 (11.7)	2 (33.3)
Bowel evisceration	13 (7.3)	1 (0.8)	1 (16.7)
Ancillary	6 (3.4)	6 (4.9)	1 (16.7)
Routine	2 (1.1)	6 (5.0)	—
	176	120	6

[a] Figures in parentheses are percentages.
Source: McAlvanah MJ, Shaftan GW (1978) Selective conservatism in penetrating abdominal wounds. A continuing appraisal. J Trauma 18: 206

TABLE 2.15. Mortality—Penetrating trauma

	Total number		Total deaths		%	
Stab wounds	590		7		1.1	
Stab nonoperated		414		3[a]		0.7[a]
Stab operated		176		4		2.2
Gunshot wounds	221		12		5.4	
GSW nonoperated		101		4[a]		4.0[a]
GSW operated		120		8		6.6
Other penetrating	18		2		11.1	
Nonoperated		12		0		0
Operated		6		2		33.3

[a] Includes moribund patients dying before treatment.
Source: McAlvanah MJ, Shaftan GW (1978) Selective conservatism in penetrating abdominal wounds. A continuing appraisal. J Trauma 18: 206

TABLE 2.16. Morbidity—Penetrating trauma

	Total number		With complications		%	
Stab wounds	590		69		11.7	
Stab nonoperated		414		12		2.9
Stab operated		176		57		32.4
Gunshot wounds	221		64		29	
GSW nonoperated		101		3		3.0
GSW operated		120		61		50.8
Other penetrating	18		5		27.8	
Nonoperated		12		1		8.3
Operated		6		4		66.7

Source: McAlvanah MJ, Shaftan GW (1978) Selective conservatism in penetrating abdominal wounds. A continuing appraisal. J Trauma 18: 206

tum reported by Ryzoff et al., 11 had surgery and no visceral injury was present [37]. In 8 of these cases, only ligation and reduction of the omentum was performed. In the presence of omental protrusion, clinical signs were an accurate indication of the need for laparotomy.

A large series of patients with evisceration of omentum and bowel was presented by Thavendran et al. (Table 2.18).

A relatively small number of their patients had a negative laparotomy when omental protrusion was present [46]. Evisceration of bowel or omentum indi-

TABLE 2.17. Indications for laparotomy: Stab wounds of the abdomen

A	B
Mandatory laparotomy: One or more of the following: 1. Peritoneal signs a. Absent bowel sounds b. Rebound tenderness c. Abdominal rigidity 2. Shock or systolic BP below 90 mmHg 3. Gastrointestinal bleeding 4. Urinary-tract bleeding 5. Free intraperitoneal air 6. Evisceration of bowel 7. Uncontrolled bleeding from the wound	1. If patient has evisceration, shock, or obvious peritonitis, do not delay appropriate treatment. 2. Exploratory laparotomy will be carried out on the following indications: a. Evisceration of an intraperitoneal structure such as omentum of bowel b. Signs of intraperitoneal injury—particularly diffuse guarding or tenderness, rebound, or decreased or absent bowel sounds c. Blood in the nasogastric tube or on rectal examination d. Definitely positive peritoneal aspiration e. Air under the diaphragm on X-ray 3. All other patients will be observed for a period of 48 h.

Source: **(A)** Richter RM, Zachy MH (1967) Selective conservative management of penetrating abdominal wounds. Ann Surg 166: 238–244; **(B)** Nance CF, Cohn I Jr (1969) Surgical judgment in the management of stab wounds of the abdomen. A retrospective and prospective analysis based on a study of 600 stabbed patients. Ann Surg 170(4): 569–580

TABLE 2.18. 226 abdominal stab wounds: Significance of evisceration of bowel and omental protrusion

	Omental protrusion	Evisceration of bowel
No. of patients	48	10
No. died	1	0
Operation	47	10
Operative deaths	0	0
Negative laparotomy	5	2

Source: Thavendran A, Vijaygragavan A, Rasaretnam R (1975) Selective surgery for abdominal stab wounds. Br J Surg 62: 750–752

cates penetration of the abdominal wall and peritoneal cavity, and wounds of this size require operative repair in almost all instances to avoid abdominal-wall hernias. The question that remains is whether abdominal-wall repair should be accompanied by complete exploratory laparotomy. If general anesthesia is required for the repair, then laparotomy adds little further insult to the patient.

Roentgenographic Evaluation by Stab-Wound Contrast Injection

The use of direct contrast injection under radiologic control to study penetrating abdominal wounds was introduced by Cornell et al. in 1965 [4]. To perform this examination, a catheter is snugly fitted into the penetrating abdominal wound and secured to the wound edges by surgical suture material; 50–60 cc of urographic water-soluble contrast material is then injected under pressure through the catheter and into the wound. Penetrating injury to the abdominal cavity can be demonstrated by the intraperitoneal spread of contrast to outline loops of bowel and other abdominal viscera. In experienced hands the examination has an accuracy rate of 90%. However, certain limitations do exist. First, the procedure is quite painful. Second, serial abdominal examinations may be precluded by the presence of residual contrast and/or air secondary to the infusion. Third, the examination only indicates entrance of the peritoneal cavity which does not necessarily indicate visceral injury or penetration. Fourth, there is a significant false-positive rate of 6.7% as well as a significant false-negative rate. False negatives are attributed to (a) the use of peritoneal lavage prior to this examination, (b) the presence of multiple penetrating wounds, (c) insufficient volume of contrast and injection pressure, and (d) the unreliability of the technique when the pleura has been entered.

Steichen et al., at Lincoln Hospital in New York City, compared clinical selective management of patients with penetrating injury to those observed with radiologic diagnosis and management in a randomly selected prospective group of 267 patients. In the stab-wound group, the radiologic diagnosis resulted in a

15.9% incidence of unnecessary laparotomies. Clinically selective management resulted in a 7.3% incidence [42]. For gunshot wounds, Steichen et al. found that clinical signs were manifested early, and radiologic diagnosis was relied on in only 6 patients. Five patients did not have evidence of penetration of the peritoneal cavity and were treated without laparotomy. The other gunshot-wound patients were treated by selective management. Of these, 5 were treated conservatively because of a lack of clinical findings, and did not require exploratory laparotomy (Tables 2.19, 2.20).

Although the concept of using physical findings

TABLE 2.19. Stab wounds: Radiographic examination vs selective management (7/1/66–8/31/68)

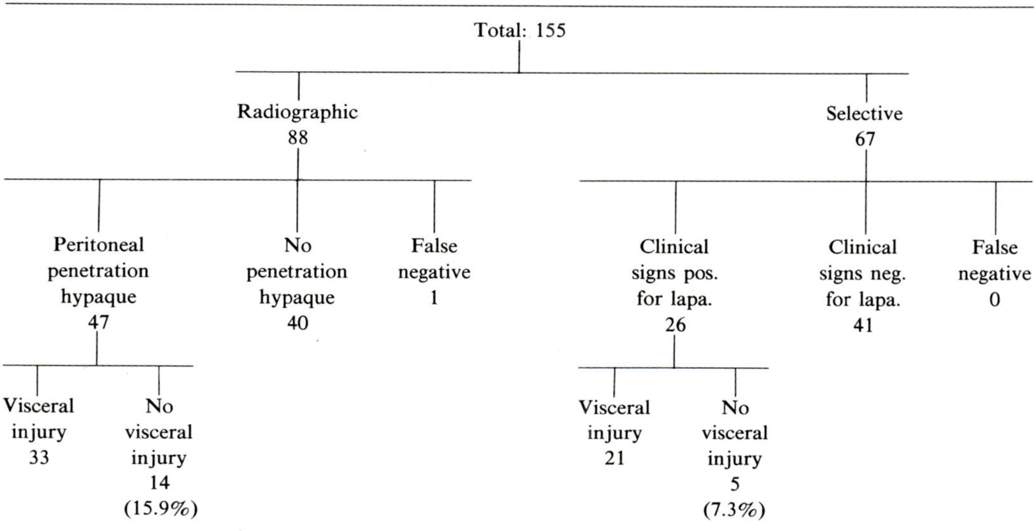

Source: Steichen FM, Efron G, Pearlman DM, Weil PH (1969) Radiographic diagnosis vs selective management in penetrating wounds of the abdomen. Ann Surg 170(6): 978–983

TABLE 2.20. Gunshot wounds: Radiographic examination vs selective management (7/1/66–8/31/68)

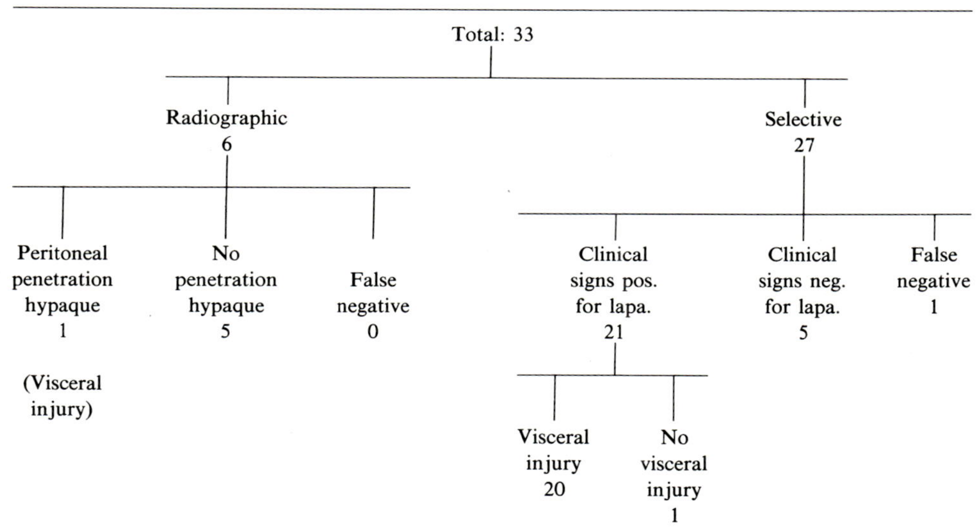

Source: Steichen FM, Efron G, Pearlman DM, Weil PH (1969) Radiographic diagnosis vs selective management in penetrating wounds of the abdomen. Ann Surg 170(6): 978–983

as the basis for operative intervention appears to be current, debate over the proper approach to penetrating abdominal injuries has existed for many years. The present debate over selectivity and the conservative management of stab wounds has been accompanied by rapid progress in the development of adjunctive diagnostic techniques applicable to patients suffering abdominal trauma. The proponents of selectivity find favor in the fact that a great deal of information about the condition of the abdominal injury can now be obtained without a surgical procedure.

Gunshot Wounds

The Weapon

Two and one-half million handguns are sold in the United States each year. Firearms are five times more deadly than knives, and of the 20,000 homicides in the United States in 1974, 54% were the result of handgun injuries [2]. Recently there has been a significant change in the pattern of homicides. In the past, the percentage of murders by strangers was relatively low. At the present, reports from New York and Washington, D.C. describe a significant increase in such murders, nearly reaching the 50% mark. The handgun homicide rate in the United States is 3.5 to 10 times that of similar homicide rates of at least 10 other major countries.

Wounding Potential

The wounding potential of a bullet is dependent on its caliber (diameter expressed in millimeters), weight, construction, and velocity. Information about the weapon used in producing a gunshot wound may help in appreciating the extent of injury to organs and adjacent tissues produced by the passage of the bullet through the patient. The variability of wounding potential of a number of different bullets with similar weight is shown in Table 2.21 [6].

The two most important features of the bullet, with respect to wounding potential, are its velocity and construction. The kinetic energy of the bullet, produced by its forward motion and rotation, is expended in the tissues along the wound tract. These tissues become secondary missiles which move outward at enormous speeds, creating a cavity. The size of the cavity is directly proportional to the energy absorbed by the expanding medium. This energy absorption increases with increases in specific gravity of the tissues involved. Thus, the lung will suffer less bullet-wound damage than will the liver, spleen, or kidney. Bullet construction is also important in the degree of tissue damage. An expanding bullet, which can enlarge several times

TABLE 2.21. Variability between energy (wounding potential) in bullets of similar caliber

Projectile	Weight (g)	Muzzle velocity (approx. ft/s)	Energy (muzzle) (ft-lb)
.22 Caliber runfire	40	1145	116
.220 Swift	55	4100	2000
30–30	170	2100	1660
30–'06	180	2800	3130
.32 Pistol (new colt)	98	785	134
.32 Special (rifle)	170	2100	1660
.38 Colt (pistol)	150	680	154
.38 Special (pistol)	158	855	256
.375 H&H Magnum	270	2740	4500

Source: DeMuth WmE (1968) High velocity bullet wounds of the thorax. Am J Surg 115: 616–625

its normal caliber, will allow greater energy transfer and thus result in a far larger cavity. The wound produced will have a cone configuration from entrance to exit. This cone of tissue injury is much greater in volume than the injury produced by jacketed, nonexpanding bullets which allow less energy transfer. Jacketed bullets, however, have greater penetrating power than expanding ones. Fortunately, most of the handguns available in the urban communities are poorly made, have low caliber and muzzle velocity, use bullets which do not readily expand, and are of poor accuracy. Considerable imagination has been used in the construction of weapons that are easily concealed. The gun in the form of a fountain pen is an example (Fig. 2.1).

The general clinical effect of low-velocity versus high-velocity wounds is evident in the difference in mortality between military and civilian bullet-wound injuries. A high-velocity missile will cause extensive damage to tissue adjacent to the missile tract. The passage of a high-velocity bullet into or through the abdomen will cause widespread bursting injury to any organ near the bullet. Low-velocity missiles will often change trajectory at interfaces between tissues of different density. For this reason, the path of the bullet through the abdomen in urban injury can be unpredictable, and a thorough and complete abdominal exploration is necessary in surgically assessing bullet wounds of the abdomen. A bullet-produced abdominal injury may be characterized by a small, innocuous entry wound, and radiologic evaluation will be required to judge the course of the bullet and to locate the position of the missile in the abdominal cavity or adjacent areas.

The increasing incidence of gunshot wounds has been documented many times. The only compensation

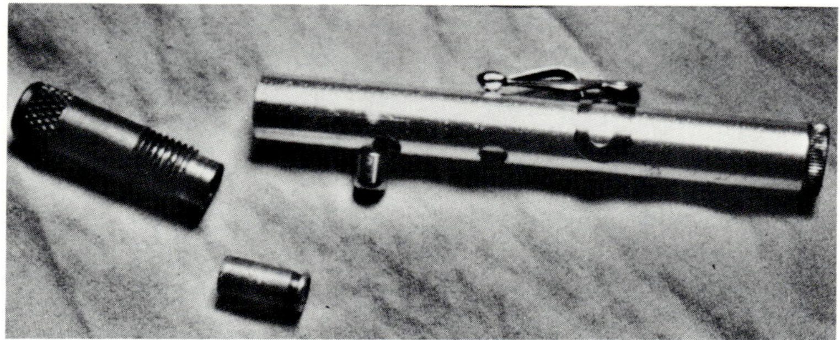

FIG. 2.1. Disguised weapons may be in unusual forms. A gun disguised as a fountain pen is shown in the figure. The device holds a single 22-caliber bullet.

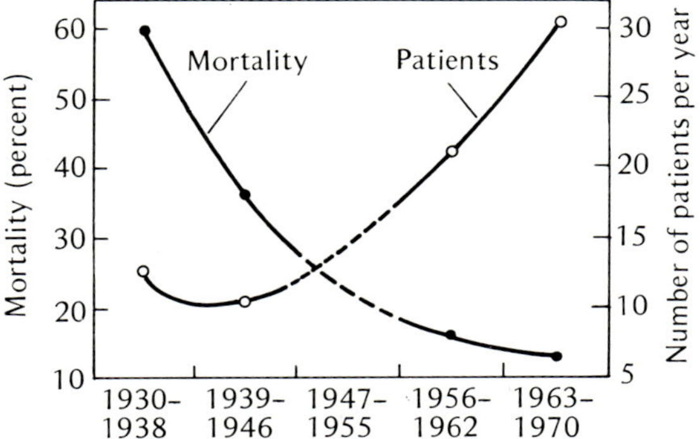

FIG. 2.2. Graphic representation of mortality and incidence of gunshot wounds of the abdomen. From Taylor FW (1973) Ann Surg 177: 174–177

for the increasing problem of missile injury is the declining mortality and morbidity from such trauma. Surgical-trauma experience and education in the diagnostic aspects and medical management of the problem have contributed to the favorable current outlook—especially in civilian life. It is of note that the current mortality for gunshot wounds relates more to vascular than to bowel injury. Taylor has published a retrospective review of gunshot-wound mortality going back to 1930. The changing pattern of organ injury and its contribution to mortality is also well documented by Taylor [45] (Fig. 2.2, Table 2.22).

Shotgun Injury

Shotgun wounds can be classified into three categories on the basis of the amount of tissue injury produced. Aside from the multiple small missiles of the shotgun blast, the potential for tissue injury is more determined by the distance between the weapon and the victim than for regular gunshot injury. Type 1 injury is produced from the shotgun 7 or more yards away from the victim. The injury is usually one of penetration of the subcutaneous tissues and deep fascia. Type 2 injuries result when the patient is shot within a range of 3–7 yards and the wound shows perforation beneath the deep fascia. Type 3 injury is sustained when the shotgun is less than 3 yards away, resulting in massive injury and disorganization and devitalization of tissue. In civilian shotgun injuries, there is often close proximity between the victim and the assailant, and severely damaging wounds are inflicted. Most accidental or

TABLE 2.22. Mortality percent resulting from various injured organs

	1930–1938	1938–1946	1946–1955	1955–1962	1962–1970
Stomach-small	45	0	—	15	2.38
Colon-rectum	33	33.0	—	0	11.80
Gut + solid viscus	84	70.0	—	36	11.90
Solid viscus	70	5.3	—	13	11.10
Great vessel					
Aorta, renal a. portal v.	—	—	—	75	62.00
Iliacs, vena cava	—	—	—	45	20.00

Source: Taylor FW (1973) Gunshot wounds of the abdomen. Ann Surg 177: 174–177

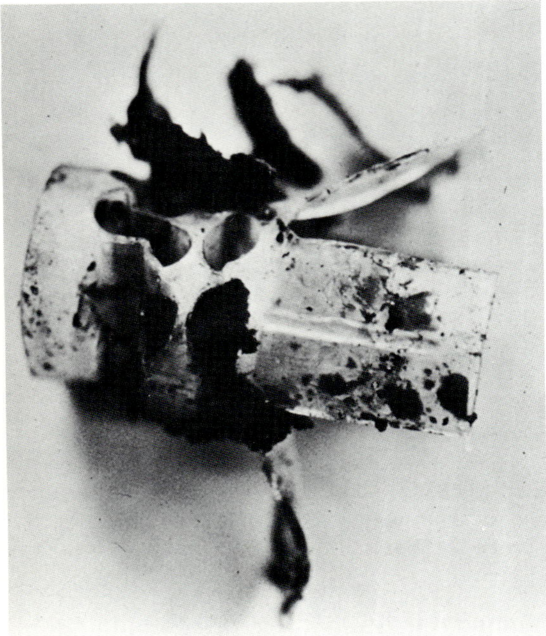

FIG. 2.3. Close proximity shotgun wounds produce extensive soft-tissue injury. In addition to the shredding effect of multiple missiles, injury is often inflicted by the plastic wadding from the shotgun shell. This figure is a photo of plastic wadding removed from the right lobe of the liver in a patient who sustained a close-range shotgun injury to the right upper quadrant with laceration of the liver, colon, diaphragm, and lung. A right hepatic lobectomy was required.

assault shotgun injuries are sustained at 20 yards or less, and the injured patient is struck by the full load of the shot. Shotgun wounds produce a shredding effect on the tissues and introduce clothing debris as well as shell wadding or plastic caps into the substance of the wound (see Fig. 2.3).

Fitzgerald et al. studied 1487 civilian gunshot wounds of which 154 of the injuries were from shotguns. One hundred and three patients had truncal injuries. Multiple-organ and multiple-system injury was common, as were cases with thoracoabdominal or body-wall defects. A high percentage of patients died from complications subsequent to the initial treatment. Reconstructive surgery was frequently necessary and was associated with prolonged hospitalization [11] (Tables 2.23, 2.24).

Mandatory Surgical Intervention and Selectivity

Abdominal gunshot wounds require surgical exploration immediately after the patient's condition is fully evaluated and stabilized. This approach is modified if it is proven that abdominal-wall penetration has not occurred. The gunshot-wound victim may present with a tangential wound or a flank or back wound without definite penetration of the peritoneal cavity. The innocuous nature of such missile injuries must be proven by the examining physician.

An important difference between abdominal stab wounds and gunshot wounds is a low incidence of significant injury in the former and a high incidence

TABLE 2.23. Classification of 103 truncal shotgun wounds

	Total no. of patients	No. of survivors	No. of deaths	Survival rate (%)
Group I				
Observation	12	12	0	100
Group II				
Observation and tube thoracostomy	11	11	0	100
Group III				
General anesthesia	19	16	3	84
Major procedure				
Extrapleural or extraperitoneal				
Group IV				
General anesthesia	61	42	19	69
Major procedure				
Thoracotomy or laparotomy				
Total	103	81	22	79

Source: Fitzgerald JB, Quast DC, Beahl AC, DeBakey ME (1965) Surgical experience with 103 truncal shotgun wounds. J Trauma 5: 72

TABLE 2.24. Major organs injured (group IV)

Organ	Number
Colon	32
Small intestine	32
Lung	23
Liver	19
Stomach	15
Kidney	14
Diaphragm	13
Major artery	12
Spleen	10
Major vein	8
Pancreas	7
Mesentery	7
Rectum	3
Bladder	3
Heart	2
Esophagus	2
Appendix	2
Gallbladder	1
Omentum	1
Uterus	1
Ureter	1
Total	208

Source: Fitzgerald JB, Quast DC, Beahl AC, DeBakey ME (1965) Surgical experience with 103 truncal shotgun wounds. J Trauma 5: 72

in the latter. Lowe et al. reviewed the problem of selectivity in the management of gunshot-wound patients [22]. Aside from a lower mortality, stab wounds had a one-third incidence of significant abdominal injury in their series. Abdominal gunshot wounds had an incidence of significant organ injury in 69.9% of 362 patients, with a mortality rate of 11.8%. These figures and a similar high incidence of severe injury from abdominal gunshot wounds in other series justify a more aggressive surgical approach in patients with gunshot wounds (Table 2.25).

TABLE 2.25. Disposition of 747 patients with abdominal gunshot and stab wounds

Disposition	Gunshot wounds	Stab wounds
Not explored	55 (15.2%)	207 (53.8%)
Explored-negative	54 (14.9%)	59 (15.3%)
Explored-positive	253 (69.9%)	119 (30.9%)
Total	362	385

Source: Lowe RJ, Salletta JD, Read DR, Radhakrishnan J, Moss GS (1977) Sould laparotomy be mandatory or selective in gunshot wounds of the abdomen. J Trauma 17: 903–907

TABLE 2.26. Results of explorations done in the absence of clinical indications for surgery

Group		Patients
No injury found		24 (58.5%)
Injury found		17 (41.5%)
Organs injured		
Diaphragm	7	
Liver	5	
Spleen	3	
Colon	3	
Stomach	2	
Major veins	2	
Pancreas	2	

Source: Lowe RJ, Salletta JD, Read DR, Radhakrishnan J, Moss GS (1977) Should laparotomy be mandatory or selective in gunshot wounds of the abdomen. J Trauma 17: 903–907

Lowe et al. performed exploratory surgery on 41 patients with gunshot wounds who did not have preoperative clinical findings of visceral injury. They found that 17 patients had significant organ injuries found at the time of surgery, and 24 patients did not [22] (Table 2.26). Peritoneal signs were present in 30 of a total of 54 patients with negative exploratory surgery. Lowe et al. emphasized the value of assessment of the bullet wound to determine whether there has been penetration of the peritoneal cavity by the missile. In the presence of such penetration, only 2.4% of patients fail to show a visceral injury (Tables 2.27–2.29). Thus, careful diagnostic study of the wound to determine the extent of abdominal-wall and peritoneal injury is important. Tangential abdominal-wall gunshot wounds can produce enough local effect to cause the typical tenderness, rigidity, and rebound of peritonitis. The morbidity rate in trauma for simple abdominal laparotomy, when no significant visceral injury is found, is reported as significant [23]. These morbidity and mortality rates are strong arguments for selectivity and careful preoperative assessment of all penetrating injury cases. In addition to the prevention of unwarranted surgical intervention and its associated compli-

TABLE 2.27. Reliability of abdominal-cavity penetration as a predictor of injury

Missile course	No. cases	% with injuries
Intraabdominal	259	97.6
Extraabdominal	48	0

Source: Lowe RJ, Salletta JD, Read DR, Radhakrishnan J, Moss GS (1977) Should laparotomy be mandatory or selective in gunshot wounds of the abdomen. J Trauma 17: 903–907

TABLE 2.28. Abdominal gunshot wounds: Major indications for surgery

Indication	Injury found	No injury found
Peritoneal signs	197	30
Absent bowel sounds	80	4
Shock	59	0
Positive IVP or cystogram	35	3
Blood in the GI tract	23	0
Pneumoperitoneum	15	0
Evisceration	3	0
None	17	24

Source: Lowe RJ, Salletta JD, Read DR, Radhakrishnan J, Moss GS (1977) Should laparotomy be mandatory or selective in gunshot wounds of the abdomen. J Trauma 17: 903–907

TABLE 2.29. Essential characteristics of patients undergoing negative laparotomies for abdominal gunshot wounds

Missile path	
Extraperitoneal	48 (88.9%)
Intraperitoneal	6 (11.1%)
Preoperative findings	
Shock	0
Peritoneal signs	30
Absent bowel sounds	4
Positive IVP	3
None	24
Average hospital stay	7.8 days

Source: Lowe RJ, Salletta JD, Read DR, Radhakrishnan J, Moss GS (1977) Should laparotomy be mandatory or selective in gunshot wounds of the abdomen. J Trauma 17: 903–907

cations, a selective approach to abdominal injuries often results in a shortened hospital stay and financial savings.

The Military Experience

The most recent military experience with injuries to the abdomen has been almost exclusively with penetrating wounds. Heaton states that penetration or perforation occurred in 98.2% of wounds in Vietnam. This was the same pattern observed in World War II and the Korean War. However, the nature of the penetrating agent in Vietnam differed from previous wars in that 71.8% of the injuries were the result of bullets and 26.4% resulted from fragments [16]. The incidence of fragment injury was higher in the previous conflicts (Fig. 2.4). Heaton also states that in World War II there were a total of 4893 organ injuries in 3154 patients or 1.55 injuries per patient. For Vietnam, the organ-injury/patient ratio was 1.67. In other words, the Vietnam conflict resulted in more multiple-

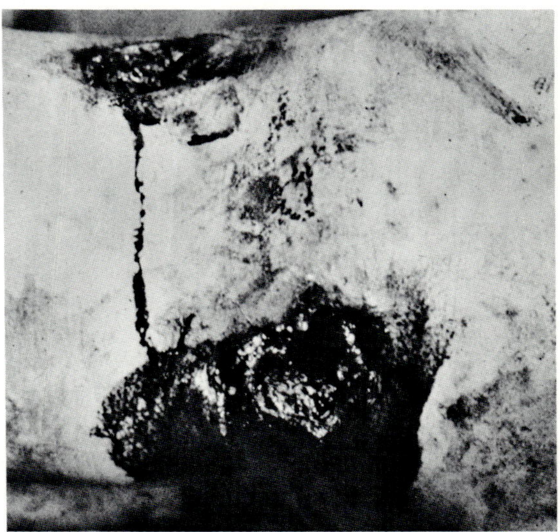

FIG. 2.4. The soldier depicted in this figure received a shrapnel injury to the right lower quadrant during the Vietnam War. There was damage to the cecum and terminal ileum. The large size of the exit wound is typical for this type of injury. Abdominal shrapnel wounds were more common during World War II than during the Vietnam War.

organ injuries (Table 2.30). The extensive use of lightweight, low-caliber, high-velocity bullets probably accounts for this increase in organ injury.

Feltis, in his report from Vietnam, emphasized the high mortality during the first 24 h after military injury [9]; 56.2% of deaths occurred in that period and 33.8% occurred in the operating room (Table 2.31). Feltis reviewed 769 laparotomies and found that there were positive findings in 652 or 84.8% of patients. The incidence of organ injury was 1.5 organ injuries per positive laparotomy. There were 79 deaths in the positive laparotomy group for an overall mortality of 12.1%. The mortality correlated directly with the number of organs injured, and the highest mortality was in patients with major intraabdominal vascular injuries. In the mortality group, the most common organ injury was the colon, with the small intestine second (Tables 2.32–2.34).

BLUNT, NONPENETRATING INJURIES

Incidence and Mortality

The victim of a gunshot wound or an eviscerating stab wound of the abdomen will attract the prompt attention of hospital staff. The blunt-trauma victim may be handled with less concern because the abdominal wall is intact, the symptoms and findings are vague, the initial vital signs may be satisfactory, and the sever-

TABLE 2.30. Distribution of injured organs in operated casualties

	World War II (3154 patients)		Vietnam (1966) (201 patients)	
	No.	%	No.	%
Total organs injured	4893	155.0	336	167.0
Stomach	416	13.2	34	16.9
Small intestine	1286	40.8	111	55.2
Colon and rectum	1222	36.5	64	32.3
Liver	829	26.3	51	25.4
Spleen	341	10.8	29	14.4
Kidney	427	13.5	15	7.5
Bladder	155	4.9	16	7.9
Pancreas	62	2.0	9	4.5
Great vessels	75	2.4	4	2.0
Gallbladder	53	1.7	1	0.5
Ureter	27	0.9	2	0.5
Exploration, no injury	333	10.6	27	13.4
Organ injuries/patient		1.55		1.67

Source: Heaton LD (1966) Military surgical practices of the United States Army in Vietnam. Curr Probl Surg, Year Book Publishers, Chicago, Ill.

TABLE 2.31. Time of death

Time	No.	%
Operating room	41	33.8
First postoperative day	27	22.3
Second to fifth postoperative day	21	17.5
Beyond fifth postoperative day	32	26.4

Source: Feltis JM (1970) Surgical experience in a combat zone. Am J Surg 119: 275

TABLE 2.32. Mortality related to organ injured

Organ	No. injured	No. of deaths	% mortality
Major vessels	16	11	68.7
Liver	125	38	30.4
Kidney	70	15	21.5
Colon	254	43	16.9
Stomach	85	15	17.6
Bladder	50	6	12.0
Small bowel	242	38	15.7
Spleen	101	8	7.9

Source: Feltis JM (1970) Surgical experience in a combat zone. Am J Surg 119: 275

TABLE 2.33. Mortality associated with single organ

Organ	No.	%
Liver	13	48.2
Colon	6	22.2
Major vessels	5	18.5
Spleen	2	7.0
Stomach	1	3.7

Source: Feltis JM (1970) Surgical experience in a combat zone. Am J Surg 119: 275

TABLE 2.34. Causes of death after first 24 h

Cause	No.	%
Sepsis	20	37.8
Pulmonary embolus	14	26.4
Hemorrhage	6	11.3
Upper gastrointestinal bleeding	4	7.5
Respiratory failure	4	7.5
Fat embolism	4	7.5
Renal failure	1	1.8
Total	53	43.8

Source: Feltis JM (1970) Surgical experience in a combat zone. Am J Surg 119: 275

TABLE 2.35. Types of trauma producing nonpenetrating abdominal injury

Cause	No. of cases
Auto accident	259
Pedestrian accident	125
Blows to the abdomen	72
Falls	48
Other or unknown	14

Source: D'Vincenti FC, Rives JD, LaBorde EJ, Fleming ID, Cohn I Jr (1968) Blunt abdominal trauma. J Trauma 8(a): 1004–1010

ity of the injury is uncertain. A delay in the institution of vigorous diagnostic and therapeutic measures for the blunt-trauma patient can result from this deceptive initial appearance.

The incidence of error in the diagnosis of blunt abdominal injury is high. The reported mortality rate varies from 6% to 45%. The wide range in mortality is due to the fact that some authors report on patients who die prior to arrival at a hospital. A high percentage (40% to 50%) of these injuries are related to the automobile, and the balance of cases are the result of accidents, falls, athletic injuries, etc. (Table 2.35). The etiology, mortality, and associated injuries in a series of 518 blunt-abdominal-trauma patients has been presented by d'Vincenti et al. [8] (Table 2.36).

The proportion of patients admitted to a modern urban trauma service with blunt injury is given in the figures of the Kings County Hospital in New York City. Between July 1, 1963 and December 1971, 207 adult patients were admitted with blunt abdominal trauma and 829 with penetrating injuries [26]. Most suburban and rural hospitals have a much higher percentage of patients with blunt trauma. The male/female ratio was 3:1 or greater, and approximately 70% of patients were between 20 and 50 years of age [14].

TABLE 2.36. Nonpenetrating abdominal injuries, admissions 1951–1966

	No. of cases	% mortality
Total	518	23
Died before treatment	53	
Salvageable patients	465	
Nonoperative management	106	18
Treated surgically	359	
Died during or after surgery	49	14
Treated surgically and survived	310	

Source: D'Vincenti FC, Rives JD, LaBorde EJ, Fleming ID, Cohn I Jr (1968) Blunt abdominal trauma. J Trauma 8(a): 1004–1010

The extent of injury from blunt trauma is related to the speed of the blow, the organs injured, and the condition of the abdominal wall. Lewis and Pirruccello [20] and Trimble and Eason [47] have made the observation that circumscribed forces are more likely to produce injuries to the intestinal viscera and kidney, whereas diffuse forces are more apt to cause hepatic, splenic, pancreatic, and vascular lesions. A solid organ is more vulnerable to contusion than is a hollow viscus, and the elastic, mobile organs of children are more resistant to blunt trauma than are the organs of the adult. A tight, rigid abdominal wall is protective against blows, whereas if it is in a relaxed state, the abdominal organs are more readily injured [14].

Large, fixed organs with an abundant blood supply, such as the liver and spleen, are frequently injured in serious blunt trauma. It is this fact that accounts for the subtle and sometimes catastrophic nature of this injury. Blunt trauma with liver injury is more frequently associated with mortality than is similar trauma with splenic injury. Liver injury was present in 70% of deaths in the Fitzgerald et al. series of patients with nonpenetrating abdominal injuries [10] (Table 2.37).

Multiple Injury

The presence of associated head, chest, and limb trauma significantly increases the mortality of blunt abdominal injury. In the Bolton et al. series of 59 blunt-abdominal-trauma cases, multiple injuries occurred in 47 patients. The mortality increased with the number of systems injured. With four involved systems, the mortality was 45% [1] (Table 2.38). In the Fitzgerald et al.'s series of 100 patients with blunt trauma who died before hospital admission, 97% had extraabdominal injuries. Death occurred in only 3 patients with injuries limited to the abdomen. In addition to the correlation between systems injured and mortality in blunt trauma, there is also some correlation between the number of organs injured and mortality. Of patients who died before admission, 40% had multiple abdominal-organ injuries; of patients alive at the time of admission only 20% had the same findings [10].

The failure to properly diagnose abdominal-organ injury and delayed organ rupture are especially characteristic of the blunt-injury situation. A vigilant diagnostic approach is a prerequisite to the proper management of the blunt-abdominal-trauma patient. Gertner et al., reporting from Baltimore, reviewed 33 patient fatalities involving drivers, pedestrians, and passengers

TABLE 2.37. Abdominal organs injured in 200 patients with blunt abdominal trauma

Organ	Entire series		Dead on arrival		Living on arrival		Survival (group admitted alive)	
	No.	%	No.	%	No.	%	No.	%
Liver	105	52.5	74	74	31	31	13	42
Spleen	93	46.5	42	42	51	51	35	69
Small bowel	18	9	5	5	13	13	10	77
Mesentery	16	8	2	2	14	14	10	71
Diaphragm	16	8	8	8	8	8	5	62
Colon	10	5	5	5	5	5	3	60
Kidney	9	4.5	5	5	4	4	3	75
Bladder	8	4	4	4	4	4	3	75
Abdominal wall	4	2	0	0	4	4	4	100
Stomach	2	1	1	1	1	1	0	0
Pancreas	2	1	0	0	2	2	1	50
Omentum	2	1	0	0	2	2	2	100
Renal artery	2	1	1	1	1	1	0	0
Inferior vena cava	2	1	1	1	1	1	0	0
Gallbladder	1	0.5	0	0	1	1	1	100
Torn adhesion	1	0.5	0	0	1	1	1	100

Source: Fitzgerald JB, Crawford ES, DeBakey ME (1960) Surgical consideration of nonpenetrating abdominal injuries. An analysis of 200 cases. Am J Surg 100: 22

[13] (Table 2.39). The patients had sustained only abdominal-organ injury, and none of the patients died in less than 1 h from the time of injury. Almost three-fourths of the deaths occurred 6 h or longer after the injury. Forty percent of the patients were not operated upon, and there were errors in diagnosis or delay in treatment of 21 of the 33 patients. There was a delay in diagnosis in 7 cases and failure to render adequate volume-replacement or to perform the appropriate surgery in the remaining patients.

TABLE 2.38. Associated injuries and mortality

Sites of injury	No. of patients	No. of deaths	% mortality
Abdominal alone	12	0	0
Abdominal—orthopedic[a]	12	0	0
Abdominal—craniocerebral[b]	8	1	13
Abdominal—thoracic	3	0	0
Abdominal—orthopedic —craniocerebral	6	1	17
Abdominal orthopedic —thoracic	3	0	0
Abdominal—craniocerebral —thoracic	4	1	25
Abdominal—craniocerebral —thoracic—orthopedic	11	5	45
Total	59	8	14

[a] Orthopedic injury: Fracture of one or more long bones or the pelvis.

[b] Craniocerebral injury: Includes facial fracture and scalp and facial lacerations. One had cerebral injury.

Source: Bolton PW, Wood CB, Quartey-Papafio JB, Blumgart LH (1973) Blunt abdominal injury: A review of 59 consecutive cases undergoing surgery. Br J Surg 60(8): 657–663

TABLE 2.39. Area of injury and apparent errors in management

Organs injured	Delay in diagnosis and surgery	Inadequate resuscitation	Inadequate resuscitation plus delay	Operative error	No major error	Total
Spleen	2	1	3[a]		1	7
Kidney		1				1
Liver			1			1
Liver + other solid viscera	1[a]	1			3	5
Spleen + pancreas				1		1
Bladder		1	1			2
Intestine	1		1		2	4
Solid + hollow viscera	2		1		3	6
Major vessel		1[a]			1	2
Major vessel + viscera	1			1[a]	2	4
Total	7	5	7	2	12	33

[a] One person in each of these categories would have had a poor chance of survival even with optimum care.

Source: Gertner HR, Baker SP, Rutherford RB, Spitz WV (1972) Evaluation of the management of vehicular fatalities secondary to abdominal injury. J Trauma 12: 425

Gertner et al.'s study is important because it emphasizes the subtle nature of isolated blunt abdominal injury and clearly demonstrates that the failure to evaluate such patients aggressively has unfortunate and ominous consequences.

A combination of diagnostic procedures can be quite useful in blunt-trauma patients if there is the slightest evidence of intraabdominal injury or hemodynamic instability. Injuries to the lower rib cage, on either side, justify a very cautious clinical observation. When rib or pelvic fractures are present, investigative measures may be necessary to detect the presence of occult or nonobvious abdominal injury.

Falls from Heights

The jumper or "sky diver" is nearly always found in the urban setting. Patients who suffer severe trauma from a fall from a height present very serious and difficult clinical problems since they usually experience complicated and dramatic multiple blunt injuries. A significant percentage of these patients are children because children commonly play near open, unprotected windows. Abdominal injuries are reported to occur in 10% to 40% of patients of this type. Reynolds et al. [35] and Lewis et al. [19], in two separate reports, have found a high instance of multiple-organ and -system injuries associated with a high mortality (Fig. 2.5). Despite the large number of patients who suffer death or major injury from falls from heights, relatively little attention has been directed to the problem. In 1963, 748 persons died of falls in New York City; 290 were suicides and 458 were accidental falls [19]. Lewis et al. reported 53 patients from the Harlem Hospital Center in New York City [19]. All patients either jumped or fell from a height of three or more stories. More than one-third of the patients survived. Of the 26 patients admitted alive, 22 lived and 4 died. All patients who died expired 15 min to 3 h following admission. Ten patients were in shock. In the Lewis series, accident was more frequently the cause of the fall than crime, suicide, or undetermined etiologies, and the incidence was greatest during the summer. Reynolds et al. in a series of 200 cases from the Misericordia and Fordham Hospitals in the Bronx, found that the age of incidence for such falls was highest in the first through the third decades of life [35]. There was a direct correlation between the height of the fall and the incidence of mortality (Fig. 2.6). The major variables for survival in such patients are the age of the patient (Table 2.40), the orientation of the patient's body, and the surface encountered. The presence of associated pelvic and skull fractures increase the mortality. Because the series consisted of patients admitted alive between January 1965 and November 1967, the overall mortality rate for the Reynolds et al. report was 17% as compared to an almost 50% mortality in the Lewis et al. series. Survival after very high falls has been reported in rare instances. Kazarian et al. reported the survival of a 17-year-old boy after a 17-story fall [18]. The patient landed on a steel fence, bushes, and mud.

Seat-Belt Injuries

The use of seat belts has reduced the mortality from automobile accidents by approximately 35% [27]. Properly adjusted seat belts seldom cause injury except

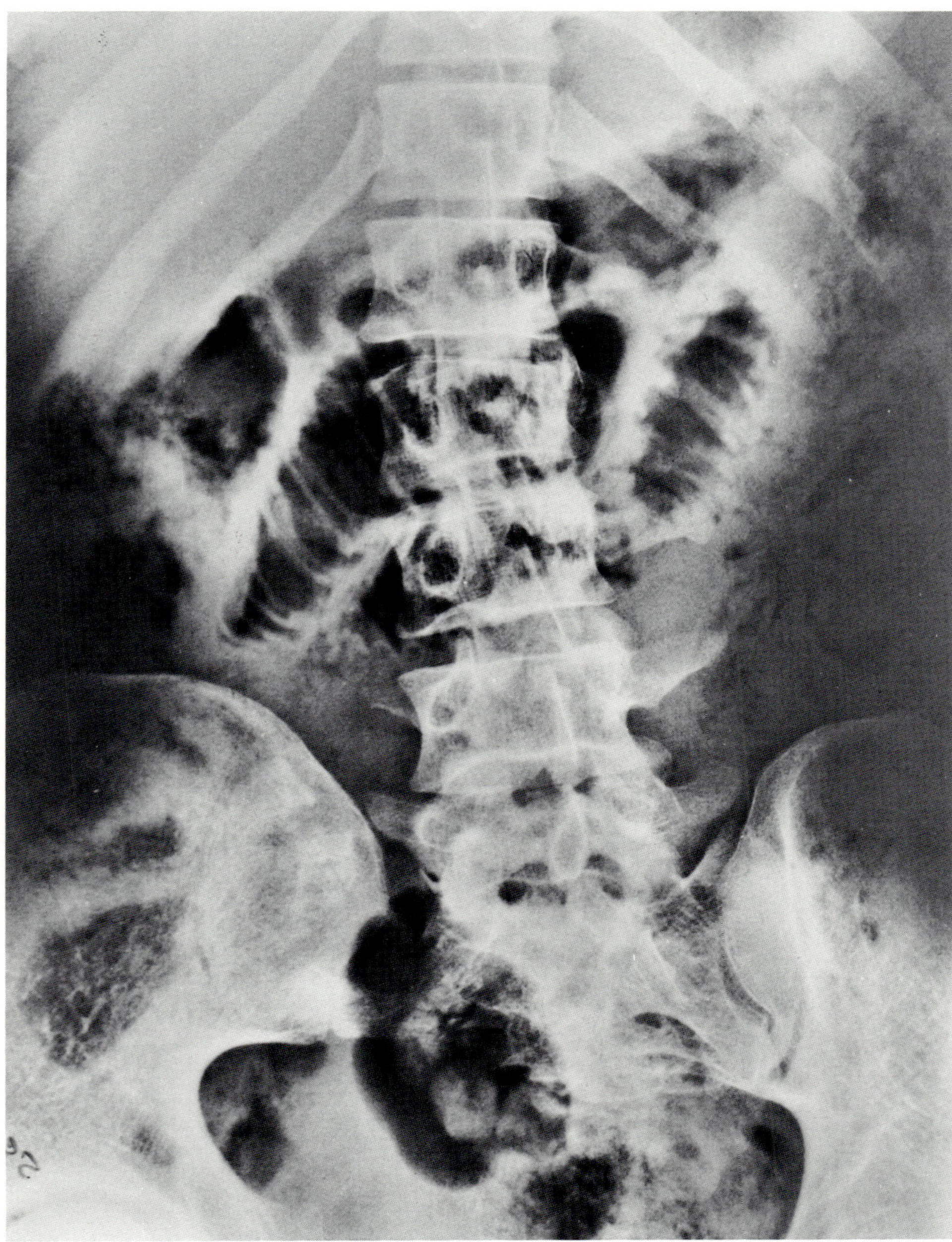

A

FIG. 2.5. This young male patient was admitted after falling from a fourth-floor apartment window. The anteroposterior, supine view of the abdomen **(A)** reveals dextrorotary scoliosis of the lumbar spine secondary to a compression fracture of the left side of L2. The pelvic film from his IVP **(B)** shows extensive fractures of the anterior right pelvis and left sacrum. There is contrast extravasation into the retroperitoneal soft tissues of the right pelvis. The retrograde cystogram **(C)** confirms the presence of contrast extravasation. At exploration, a tear of the right anterolateral wall of the urinary bladder was found and repaired. *(Continued on p. 30.)*

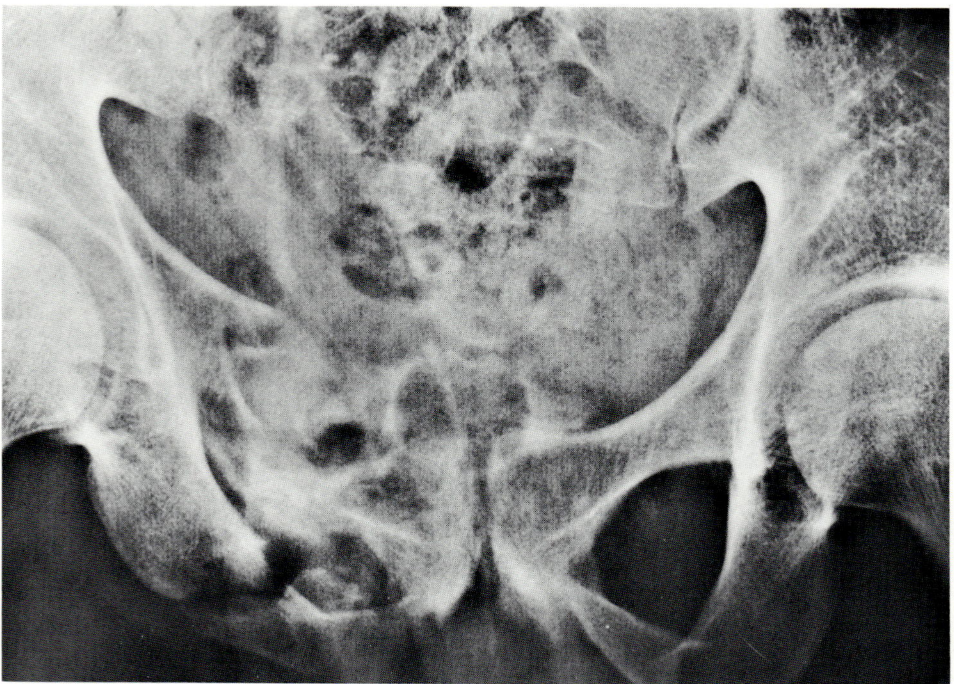

B

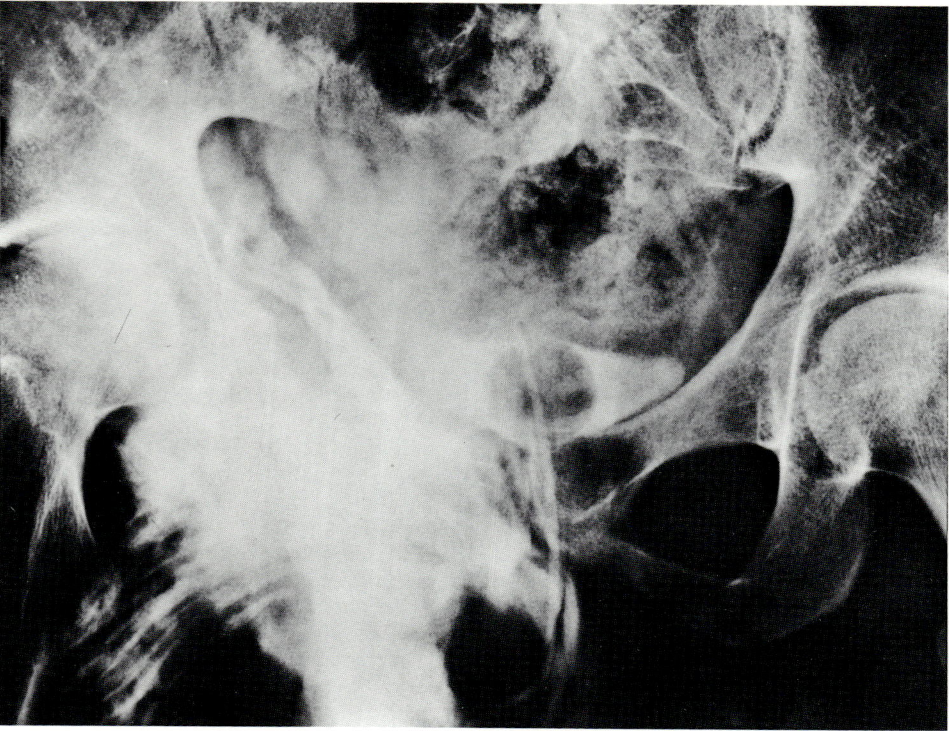

C

FIG. 2.5. *(Continued from p. 29.)*

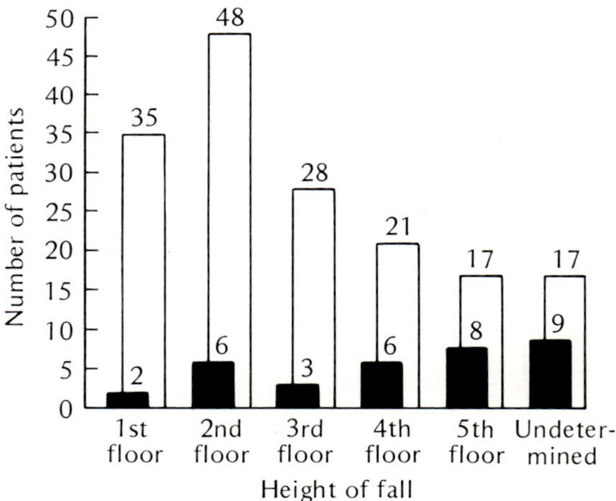

FIG. 2.6. Relation of height of fall to survival. *Clear bars,* survivors; *solid bars,* nonsurvivors. From Reynolds BM, Balsam NA, Reynolds FX (1971) Falls from heights: A surgical experience of 200 consecutive cases. Ann Surg 174: 304

when the applied forces exceed the stress resistance of the musculoskeletal system [24]. Improper placement, including the use of only the lap strap, is a source of injury not only to the anterior abdominal wall but also to intraabdominal structures. The use of only the lap strap can result in Chance fractures of the lumbar spine as well as tears of the posterior spinal ligaments and separation of the zygoapophyseal joints of the spine [27]. Small-bowel perforation and mesentery tears frequently accompany these lumbar-spine injuries. In general, the mechanism for injury by seat belts is through direct violence, shearing or torsion, entrapment, or a combination of these forces [24].

The special problem of seat-belt injury was reviewed by Williams and Kirkpatrick [49] and by Snyder [41]. They emphasized the association of other injuries and the dangers of delay in making the diagnosis. Abdominal paracentesis was thought to be unreliable. The presence of a contused band around the lower abdomen as a diagnostic physical finding was described by Snyder. Apparently, the best vehicular passenger safety is provided by the three-point-fixation lap belts and shoulder harness. However, bowel injuries have been reported with this equipment as well [41,49] (Tables 2.41–2.45).

TABLE 2.40. Relation of age to mortality

	No. of cases		
Age	Survivors	Non-survivors	% mortality
0–5	38	9	19
6–10	33	5	13
11–20	29	0	
21–30	33	4	11
31–40	17	2	11
41–50	8	0	
51 & over	8	14	64
Total overall mortality	166	34	17

Source: Reynolds BM, Balsam NA, Reynolds FX (1971) Falls from heights: A surgical experience of 200 consecutive cases. Ann Surg 174: 304

TABLE 2.41. Lap belt: Intestinal and mesenteric injuries

Injury	Small intestine	Large intestine	
Contusion	3	4	
Seromuscular tear	11	4	
Perforation	26	4	
Mesenteric tear	23	7	
Subtotal	63	19	
Total			82

Source: Williams JS, Kirkpatrick JR (1971) The nature of seat belt injuries. J Trauma 11(3): 207–218

TABLE 2.42. Lap belt: Lumbar-spine injuries

Compression fracture	9
Subluxation	7
Fracture articular process	7
Fracture lamina and pedicles	2
Complete anterior subluxation	2
Horizontal (Chance Fx L_2 or L_3) (10)	10
Transverse process fracture	2
Rotational fracture	2
Disk rupture	2
Posterior ligamentous tear	2
Unknown	6
Total	51

Source: Williams JS, Kirkpatrick JR (1971) The nature of seat belt injuries. J Trauma 11(3): 207–218

TABLE 2.43. Lap-belt accidents: Additional injuries

Soft tissue	
Abdominal wall	8
Spleen	4
Omentum	2
Pancreas	2
Uterus	2
Urethra	1
Iliac artery	1
Rupture diaphragm	1
Liver	1
Fractures	
Extremities	6
Pelvis	4
Facial	3
Total	35

Source: Williams JS, Kirkpatrick JR (1971) The nature of seat belt injuries. J Trauma 11(3): 207–218

TABLE 2.44. Shoulder-restraint injuries

Fractures	
Ribs	9
Cervical spine	4
Thoracic spine	3
Lumbar spine	1
Sternum	3
Skin and soft tissue	
Contusion, hematoma, and abrasion	5
Ligamentous injury, cervical spine	2
Fat necrosis	1
Diaphragmatic tear	1
Organs	
Larynx	2
Liver	2
Liver and spleen	1
Kidney	1
Major vessel	2
Spleen	1

Source: Williams JS, Kirkpatrick JR (1971) The nature of seat belt injuries. J Trauma 11(3): 207–218

TABLE 2.45. Three-point-belt injuries

Fractures	
Rib, single	20
Rib, multiple	8
Sternum	4
Clavicle	5
Abdomen	
Organs unknown	3
Jejunum, perforation	1
Duodenum, perforation	3
Contusions and abrasions	
Chest	11
Lap area	5
Shoulder	4
Neck	4
Back	2
Other	1

Source: Williams JS, Kirkpatrick JR (1971) The nature of seat belt injuries. J Trauma 11(3): 207–218

REFERENCES

1. Bolton PM, Wood CB, Quartey-Papafio JB, Blumgart LH (1973) Blunt abdominal injury: A review of 59 consecutive cases undergoing surgery. Br J Surg 60(8): 657–663
2. Browning C (1978) Handguns and homicide—A public health problem. JAMA 236(19): 2198
3. Coley WB (1891) The treatment of penetrating wounds of the abdomen. Am J Med Sci 101: 243
4. Cornell WP, Ebert PA, Zuidema GD (1965) X-ray diagnosis of penetrating wounds of the abdomen. J Surg Res 5: 142–146
5. DeFore WW, Mattox KL, Jordon GL Jr, Beall AC (1976) Management of 1,590 consecutive cases of liver trauma. Arch Surg 111: 493–497
6. DeMuth WE (1968) High velocity bullet wounds of the thorax. Am J Surg 115: 616–625
7. DeMuth WE (1966) Bullet velocity and design as determinants of wounding capability; an experimental study. J Trauma 6(2): 222–232
8. D'Vincenti FC, Rives JD, LaBorde EJ, Fleming ID, Cohn I Jr (1968) Blunt abdominal trauma. J Trauma 8(a): 1004–1010
9. Feltis JM (1970) Surgical experience in a combat zone. Am J Surg 119: 275
10. Fitzgerald JB, Crawford ES, DeBakey ME (1960) Surgical consideration of non-penetrating abdominal injuries: An analysis of 200 cases. Am J Surg 100: 22
11. Fitzgerald JB, Quast DC, Beahl AC, DeBakey ME (1965) Surgical experience with 103 truncal shotgun wounds. J Trauma 5: 72

12. Forde KA, Ganepola AP (1974) Is mandatory exploration for penetrating abdominal trauma extinct? The morbidity and mortality of negative exploration in a large municipal hospital. J Trauma 14(9): 764
13. Gertner HR, Baker SP, Rutherford RB, Spitz WV (1972) Evaluation of the management of vehicular fatalities secondary to abdominal injury. J Trauma 12: 425
14. Griswold RA, Collier HS (1961) Collective review: Blunt abdominal trauma. Surg Gynecol Obstet (Int Abstr Surg) 112: 309–329
15. Guernsey JM, Ganchrow MI (1975) Diagnostic laparotomy in the patient with multiple injuries. J Trauma 15(12): 1053–1055
16. Heaton LD (1966) Military surgical practices of the United States Army in Viet Nam. Curr Probl Surg Year Book Publishers, Chicago, Ill.
17. Hopson WB, Sherman RJ, Sanders JW (1966) Stab wounds of the abdomen: 5 year review of 297 cases. Am J Surg 32: 213
18. Kazarian K, Bole P, Smith KA, Mersheimer WL (1976) High flyer syndrome: Survival after 17 story fall. NY State J Med 76(6): 982–985
19. Lewis WS, Lee AB, Grantham AS (1965) Jumpers syndrome. J Trauma 5: 812
20. Lewis LI, Pirruccello R (1973) Use of angiography to diagnose subcapsular hematoma of the spleen before rupture. Am Surg 39: 587
21. Loria FL (1932) The influence of hemorrhage in abdominal gunshot injuries. Ann Surg 96: 169
22. Lowe RJ, Saletta JD, Read DR, Radhakrishnan J, Moss GS (1977) Should laparotomy be mandatory or selective in gunshot wounds of the abdomen. J Trauma 17: 903–907
23. Lowe RJ, Boyd DR, Folk FA, Baker RJ (1972) The negative laparotomy for abdominal trauma. J Trauma 12: 853–860
24. Martin JD (1969) Trauma to the Thorax and Abdomen. Charles C Thomas, Springfield, Ill.
25. Mathewson C Jr (1969) Routine exploration of stab wounds of the abdomen. J Trauma 9: 1028–1030
26. McAlvanah MJ, Shaftan GW (1978) Selective conservatism in penetrating abdominal wounds: A continuing appraisal. J Trauma 18: 206
27. McCort JJ (1973) Abdominal trauma. In: Margulis AR, Burhenne HJ (eds) Alimentary Tract Roentgenology, Vol. I. C.V. Mosby Co, St. Louis, pp 228–270
28. Moss LK, Schmidt FE, Creech O Jr (1962) Analysis of 550 stab wounds of the abdomen. Am Surg 28: 483
29. Nance CF, Cohn I Jr (1969) Surgical judgment in the management of stabwounds of the abdomen: A retrospective and prospective analysis based on a study of 600 stabbed patients. Ann Surg 170(4): 569–580
30. Netterville RE, Hardy JD (1967) Analysis of 155 cases with problems in management. Ann Surg 166: 232–237
31. Pereira AP, Lewis JJ (1973) Introduction to Miyama Ryu Jujutsu. Tremont School of Judo, Karate and Jujutsu Inc., New York
32. Poer DH (1948) The management of penetrating abdominal injuries—Comparative military and civilian experiences. Ann Surg 127: 1092
33. Printen KJ, Freeark RJ, Shoemaker WC (1968) Conservative management of penetrating abdominal wounds. Arch Surg 96: 899
34. Pridgen JE, Aust JB, Fisher GW (1970) Penetrating Wounds of the Abdomen. Charles C Thomas, Springfield, Ill.
35. Reynolds BM, Balsam NA, Reynolds FX (1971) Falls from heights: A surgical experience of 200 consecutive cases. Ann Surg 174: 304
36. Richter RM, Zachy MH (1967) Selective conservative management of penetrating abdominal wounds. Ann Surg 166: 238–244
37. Ryzoff RI, Shaftan GW, Herbsman H (1966) Selective conservatism in penetrating abdominal trauma. Surgery 59: 650–653
38. Shaftan GW (1960) Indications for operation in abdominal trauma. Am J Surg 99: 657–664
39. Shaftan GW (1969) Editorial: Selective conservatism in penetrating abdominal trauma. J Trauma 9(12): 1026–1028
40. Sims JM (1882) The treatment of gunshot wounds of the abdomen in relation to modern peritoneal surgery. Br Med J 302
41. Snyder CJ (1972) Bowel injuries from automobile seat belts. Am J Surg 123: 312–316
42. Steichen FM, Efron G, Pearlman DM, Weil PH (1969) Radiographic diagnosis versus selective management in penetrating wounds of the abdomen. Ann Surg 170(6): 978–983
43. Stimson LA (1889) NY Med J Quoted by Coley [3]
44. Strauch GO (1973) Major abdominal trauma in 1971. A study of Connecticut by the Connecticut Society of American Board Surgeons and the Yale Trauma Program. Am J Surg 125: 413–418
45. Taylor FW (1973) Gunshot wounds of the abdomen. Ann Surg 177: 174–177
46. Thavendran A, Vijaygragavan A, Rasaretnam R (1975) Selective surgery for abdominal stab wounds. Br J Surg 62: 750–752
47. Trimble C, Eason FJ (1972) A complication of splenosis. J Trauma 12: 358–361
48. Tunell WP, Knast J, Nance FC (1975) Penetrating abdominal injuries in children and adolescents. J Trauma 15(8): 720–725
49. Williams JS, Kirkpatrick JR (1971) The nature of seat belt injuries. J Trauma 11(3): 207–218
50. Wilson H, Sherman R (1961) Civilian penetrating wounds of the abdomen: Factors in mortality and differences from military wounds in 494 cases. Ann Surg 153: 639
51. Worth MH Jr (1976) Abdominal trauma. JAMA 235(8): 853–854

3

Specific Diagnostic Techniques

There are few concerted efforts that succeed in making the public aware of the magnitude of the problem of trauma. As a result, the federal budget for study of these diseases during the past several years has averaged $220 for each cancer patient, $74 for each cardiovascular patient, and 24¢ for each trauma victim. [77]

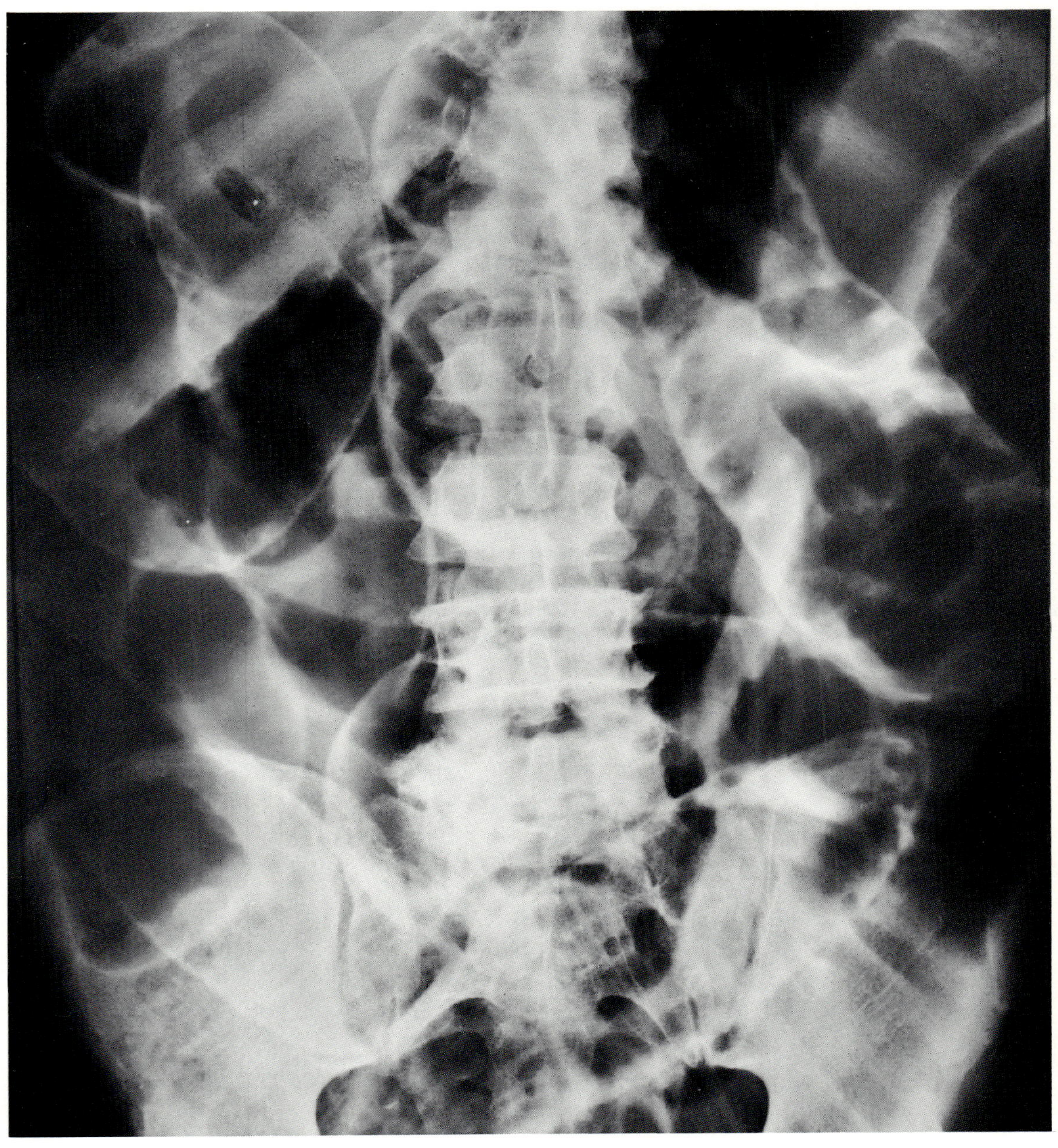

HISTORY TAKING

General Considerations

History taking is considered by many to be of limited value in patients with abdominal trauma; and yet, very often, relevant information can be obtained by careful questioning. Usually the circumstances surrounding an abdominal injury are such that the patient cannot recall exactly what happened. In the case of an assault, the victim will frequently be frightened and intimidated and unable to describe where the assailant stood or the nature of the weapon used. Automobile accidents occur so suddenly that the injured occupants or pedestrian will recall little of the sequence of events.

In patients with small, penetrating wounds, the history may be vital to a diagnosis. Deep penetration can occur with almost no identifiable skin defect. The "pig-stick" needle and ice-pick wounds are examples of this type of injury and are notoriously difficult to identify. Because such penetrating trauma are common among prisoners and criminals, the patient may purposely deny the occurrence of the assault for fear of retribution from others.

Information describing the direction from which a gunshot wound was inflicted, as well as the proximity of the patient to the assailant, is of value to the surgeon. A statement about the number of injuries is also important in such a situation. There is a tendency to focus attention on obvious areas of injury and to ignore the less dramatic secondary sites of trauma. However, careful questioning can call attention to significant associated injuries.

Medicolegal

The medicolegal aspect of most trauma cases has bearing not only on the economics of this situation but also on the apprehension and conviction of assailants. Members of medical emergency teams often neglect the details of the trauma incident that are of importance to the police and the legal profession. Godley and Smith have emphasized the value of retrieving the relevant information at first assessment of trauma patients. Proper description of clothing, weapons, and missiles is essential. Obtaining the proper information and documenting the location of penetrating or blunt injury may play an important role in subsequent legal action [39] (Table 3.1).

TABLE 3.1. Missile-wound checklist

1. Circumstances (accident, unknown, etc.)
2. Range
3. Time of injury
4. Weapon (type, caliber, model, brand name, country or origin)
5. Ammunition (type, caliber)
6. Missile (description, weight in grams, photograph, specimen in coin envelope)
7. Clothing of victim (dried and packaged; description of holes, burns, blood, etc.)
8. External wounds (type, i.e., contact, close-up, distant, high-velocity, low-velocity; also, location, dimensions in millimeters, photographs)
9. Additional documentation
   a. X-rays
   b. Photographs of wounds, weapon, missile
   c. Formalin-fixed tissue of "entrance" and "exit" wounds for spectrographic and/or microscopic study

Source: Godley DR, Smith TK (1977) Some medicolegal aspects of gunshot wounds. J Trauma 17: 866–871

Subtle Injuries

The wound from a bullet or knife can be overlooked at the time of physical examination if a very careful search is not made. A penetrating injury can be sustained through the mouth, buttock, genitalia, rectum, or umbilicus without obvious external signs; and a history of pain or description of the assault may be the only clue to the nature of the injury. Spitting or coughing of blood can be contributory in the diagnosis of oral, gastroesophageal, or pulmonary injury. Similarly, blood passed by rectum after either penetrating or blunt trauma indicates the need for proctoscopy and sigmoidoscopy. Rectal injuries can obviously occur with penetrating trauma. However, their occurrence after blunt trauma is not generally appreciated. Rectal bleeding after blunt injuries may indicate direct rectal laceration or mesenteric vascular trauma [48].

Abdominal injury does not always produce abdominal pain corresponding to the anatomic location of the organ or combination of organs injured. Injury to the liver or spleen may produce pain in the epigastrium or flank, but there may also be pain in the shoulders from diaphragmatic irritation. If the hepatic or splenic injury is localized to the posterior surfaces, it may irritate the undersurfaces of the diaphragm with very little associated peritoneal reaction; thus, a history of shoulder pain, difficulty in breathing, or shortness of breath in the abdominal injury case has special significance. The referral of pain to the tip of the shoulder was described by Kehr as an important diagnostic sign in patients with splenic injury [58]. Blood from a lacerated liver or spleen can track down the lateral paracolic gutter on either or both sides and cause lower abdominal pain. Patients have suffered splenic or hepatic injury and subsequently presented with lower abdominal pain suggesting primary lower-abdominal inflammatory disorders. Patients have also presented with signs suggesting acute appendicitis and have subsequently been found to have had a ruptured spleen.

Delayed Manifestations of an Old Injury

The loss of large volumes of blood from a ruptured or lacerated spleen or the rupture of a subcapsular splenic hematoma can be catastrophic and will produce the classic findings of acute hemoperitoneum and hypovolemic shock. However, delayed splenic rupture can occur at a time remote from the initial trauma [86]. It is stated that in 50% of delayed splenic rupture cases the symptoms manifest themselves in less than 1 week, 75% in 2 weeks or less, and 90% within 4 weeks. The balance of patients may have a rupture up to 150 days following injury. The criterion for a diagnosis of delayed splenic rupture consists of a period of at least 36 to 48 h before the appearance of signs of intraperitoneal hemorrhage. Recently, doubt has been expressed whether time "delay" in rupture of the spleen does occur or whether the problem is really a delay in diagnosis [8,84].

A history of trauma is therefore quite important in the evaluation of the patient's condition. Despite the fact the trauma may seem quite incidental in the history of a patient's previous medical problems, there are a number of conditions that relate to previous blunt or penetrating injuries. Splenic bleeding or marked enlargement of the spleen can, on rare occasions, result from trauma sustained many years before the presentation to a hospital. Clark et al. reported a case of spontaneous delayed splenic rupture occurring 5 years after the initial trauma [18]. A case of giant splenic enlargement with secondary esophageal obstruction was reported by Garvey and Delany [34] (Fig. 3.1). The patient was found to have an acquired cyst of the spleen secondary to trauma 11 years prior to the development of significant symptoms.

Intraabdominal traumatic injury can occur following vigorous coughing and changes in body position in patients especially vulnerable to splenic tear. This form of splenic rupture is usually associated with preexisting splenomegaly. Eighteen well-documented cases of splenic rupture associated with mononucleosis without trauma are described in the literature [100]. A history of mononucleosis, sickle cell disease, malaria, or severe recent infectious disease may be relevant to the patient's presenting problem. The presence of enlarged or cystic abdominal organs will increase the vulnerability of the patient to blunt trauma. Pathologically enlarged kidneys in children are prone to injury when subject to trauma (see pp. 176–193 on genitourinary system).

Thoracoabdominal penetrating injuries, especially stab wounds, can produce minimal initial findings and clinical manifestations without requiring surgical intervention. The later occurrence of diaphragmatic hernia though the stab-wound defect is a well-known clinical phenomenon. A history of a thoracoabdominal penetrating injury may be the key to the diagnosis of intestinal obstruction and acute respiratory distress secondary to incarcerated intraabdominal contents. Trauma to the relaxed abdomen is more likely to produce significant intraabdominal injury than trauma to the tense, rigid abdomen. Thus the immediate condition under which blunt injury is sustained, especially the patient's awareness and anticipation, may influence the degree of injury.

A history of medication and drug ingestion will also bear on the patient's response to trauma, especially long-term medication with steroids or anticoagulants. A tendency to excessive bleeding may change a minor episode of trauma into a major hemorrhage.

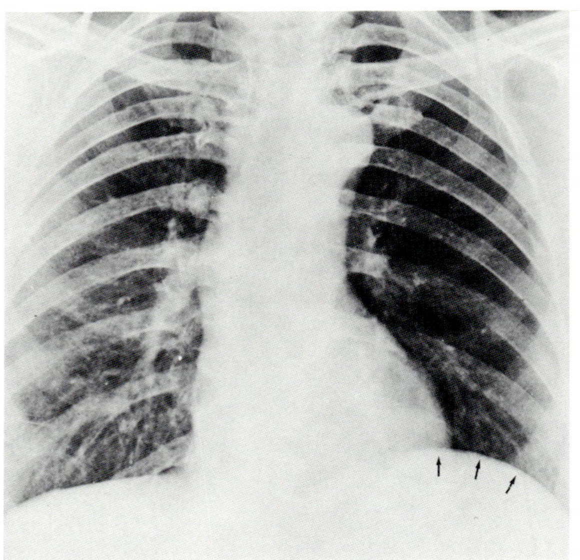

A

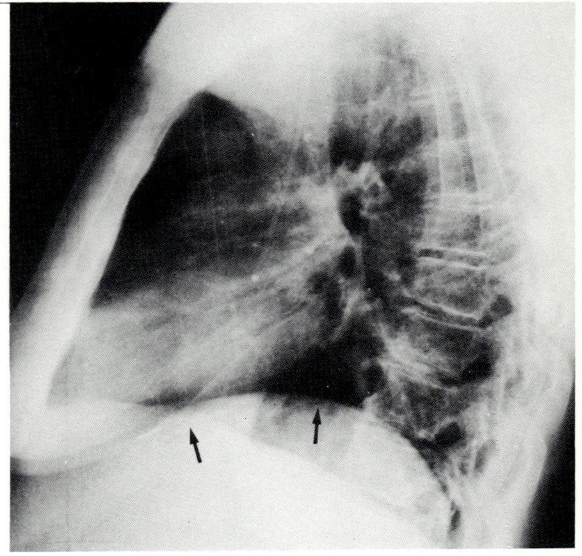

B

C

FIG. 3.1. This 56-year-old female was admitted to the Morrisania Hospital in October 1971 with the chief complaint of a 4-month history of dysphagia and vomiting. Her past history revealed a fall from a porch, 11 years prior to her present admission, from which she sustained lower left rib contusions. The **(A)** frontal and **(B)** lateral projections of the chest reveal left diaphragmatic elevation with a crescentic linear calcification beneath the diaphragm *(solid arrows)*. A large calcified LUQ mass is seen on the **(C)** AP supine view of the abdomen.

(Continued on p. 40)

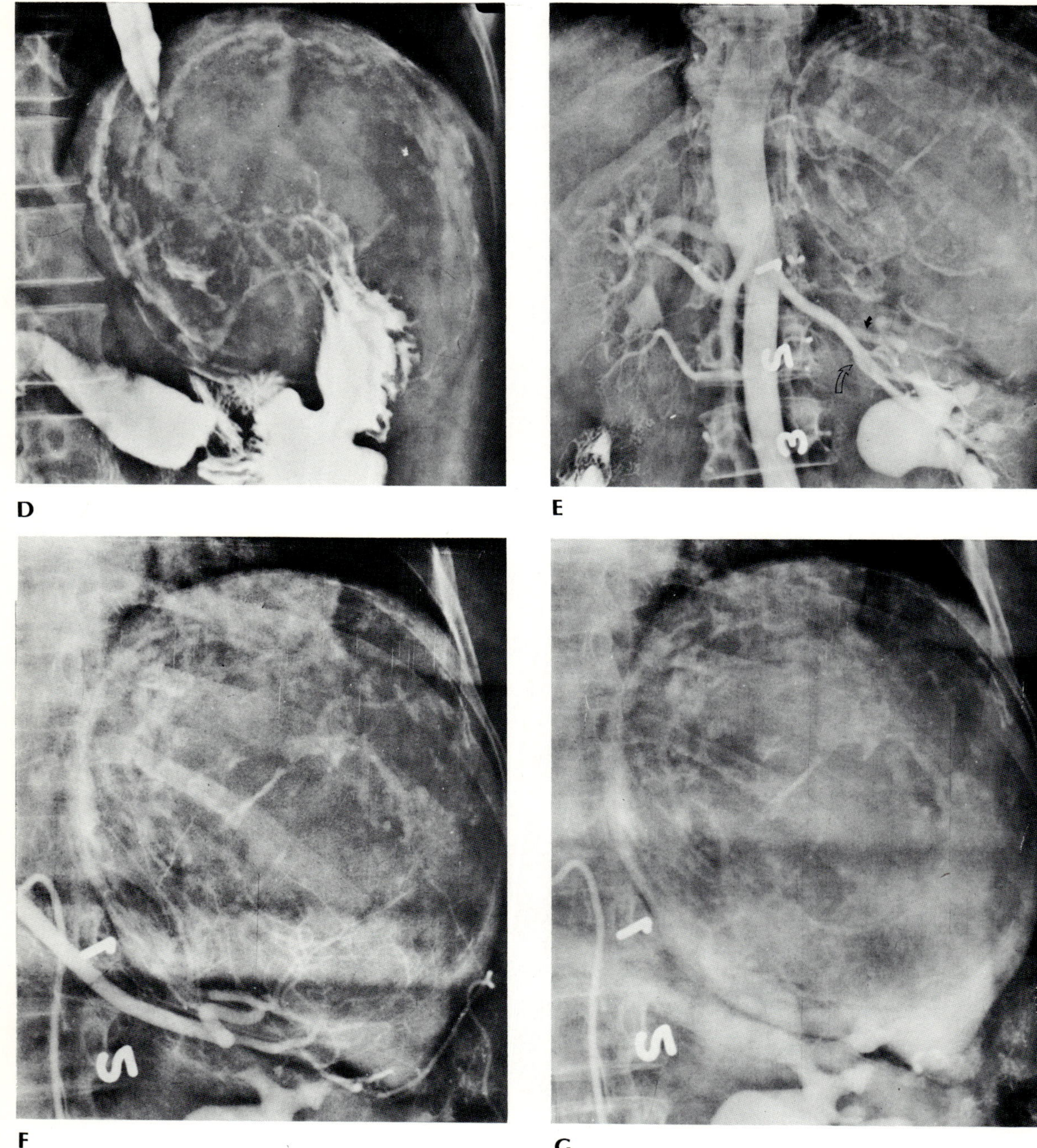

FIG. 3.1. ***(cont.).*** An **(D)** oblique view from an upper GI series shows partial obstruction of the distal esophagus and irregularity but not destruction of the mucosal pattern of the cardia and fundus of the stomach. The (E) arterial phase from a flush aortogram reveals a large avascular LUQ mass that is producing rightward displacement of the proximal abdominal aorta and inferior displacement of the splenic artery *(curved solid arrow),* left renal artery *(curved open arrow),* and left kidney. The **(F)** arterial and **(G)** venous phases from a selective splenic angiogram reveal a large, avascular, intrasplenic mass with inferior compression of the remaining normal splenic tissue. At exploration, a large spleen weighing 1400 g and measuring 15 × 16 × 15 cm was found. When the spleen was opened, a huge fibrotic, partially calcified, monolocular pseudocyst containing brown turbid fluid was found. There was no evidence of current or previous parasitic disease.

Careful inquiry regarding all medications will sometimes alert the physician to the patient's unique drug-related vulnerability. Of course, the routine inquiry about allergy and idiosyncratic drug reactions is most important in all medical workups and must not be ignored in the evaluation of the trauma patient.

The examining physician can be misled by the history presented by a trauma victim. The "contracoup" injury patient may describe the injuring object as striking one side or area of the body, but the organ injury may be on the opposite side owing to the mobility of some of the intrathoracic and intraabdominal organs. The examiner must also consider the possibilities of injury based on the type of accident despite symptoms relating to a single area. An injury "set" is sometimes seen with accidents: the "battered child" and the "battered alcoholic" are examples [45,89]. Often there is craniocerebral injury in addition to trauma to other parts of the body that is not remembered by the patient because the fracture of an extremity or some more obvious injury produces so much pain and deformity. Commonly, pedestrians struck by automobiles are aware of their painful lower-extremity injury and are distracted from the symptoms of abdominal trauma.

The evaluation of the battered child is a special problem in medical history taking. The parents are loath to give an accurate history. In fact, the parents will frequently invent a description of the child's injury. The unfortunate battered youngsters are frightened and will not admit to an injury, particularly in the presence of their parents. Careful questioning of the parents will sometimes elicit contradictions that will alert the examining physician to the special circumstances involved in the battered-child case. Usually it requires evidence of two or three previously occurring traumatic episodes to explain the multitude of physical and roentgenologic findings discovered in these children.

The examining physician must be very alert to the presence of child abuse. The prevalence of this problem is not generally appreciated. Between 2,500,000 and 4,000,000 cases of this type are estimated to occur in the United States each year. Deaths from child abuse number in the thousands [45].

PHYSICAL DIAGNOSIS

The physical examination of the abdomen has traditionally been the most important and sometimes the only procedure determining the therapy of abdominal trauma. This form of evaluation is not as precise as other methods of diagnosis described in this work. However, the universal availability of the physical examination and its application to all patients makes it the most fundamental of diagnostic procedures.

The examination of the traumatized patient is often a hurried procedure. Under pressure to institute immediate therapeutic effort involving intravenous medication, blood transfusion, and respiratory support, the physician may perform the physical examination in a cursory fashion. The failure to look carefully at the patient and to go through the full sequential parts of a proper examination may initiate a sequence of errors that is inexcusable and catastrophic. Although errors of omission in a physical examination are uncommon when well-trained physicians are involved, such errors are frequent under the stress of an emergency situation. The establishment of a "trauma team" approach is a helpful way to deal with the many procedures involved in the initial care of an acutely ill patient. However, the team must be organized in such a way that the responsibility for examining the patient is clearly and specifically delegated.

The initial determination of the vital signs should be made by the best-trained person available. However, the examining physician should also make his own initial confirmatory determination.

The General Examination

The patient's general appearance in the emergency room may reflect the severity of an intraabdominal injury. An unconscious or virtually lifeless patient who presents with an isolated abdominal injury probably has sustained massive blood loss. The possibility of blunt head injury or drug overdose must also be considered. The level of consciousness is not usually impaired by an isolated abdominal injury, and the patient usually will relate the site and character of the pain and the source of injury.

Air hunger is a physical finding requiring immediate evaluation and rapid management. This finding may occur subsequent to massive blood loss and may herald an imminent respiratory arrest. Moreover, any upper thoracic wound associated with air hunger may indicate the presence of hemothorax or pneumothorax. The detection of subcutaneous emphysema can be a helpful sign in this situation. Percussion and auscultation of the thorax may disclose dullness or diminished breath sounds compatible with an intrathoracic injury. If aspiration of the involved thoracic cavity through the fifth or sixth intercostal space with a 21-gauge needle or syringe yields blood, a tube thoracostomy should be performed prior to radiologic examination of the chest.

The dire prognostic implications of hypotension in the trauma patient are well known. The morbidity and mortality related to various levels of hypotension

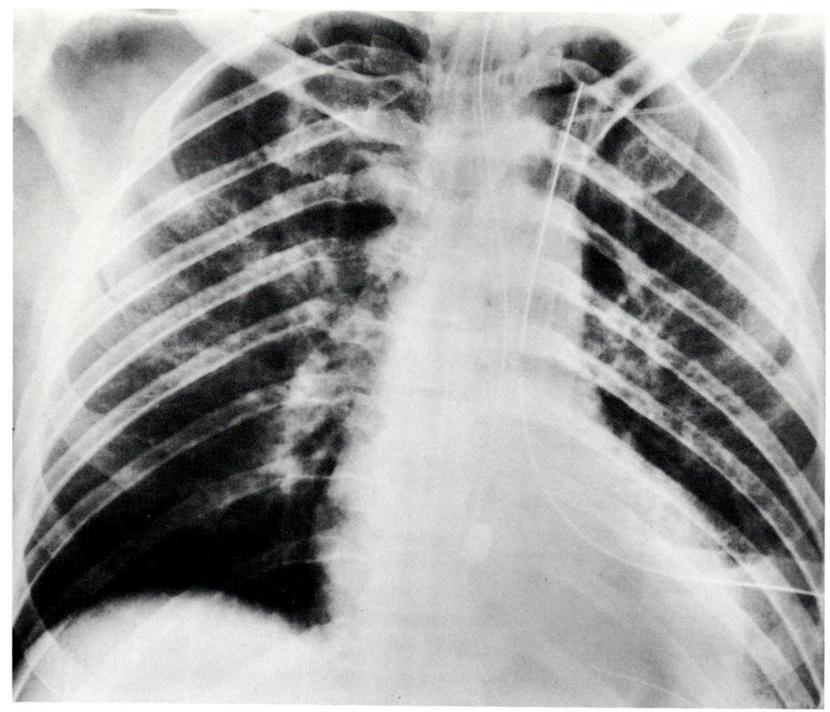

A

B

FIG. 3.2. This 48-year-old male sustained a gunshot wound through the left forearm. After passing through the forearm, the bullet entered the left thoracoabdominal area through the eighth lateral intercostal space. The **(A)** frontal and **(B)** lateral projections of the chest show the bullet to lie in the soft tissues of the lower left chest. The final position of the bullet in relation to the known site of entry suggests at least diaphragmatic injury. At exploration, a laceration of the left diaphragm and two serosal gastric lacerations were found and repaired.

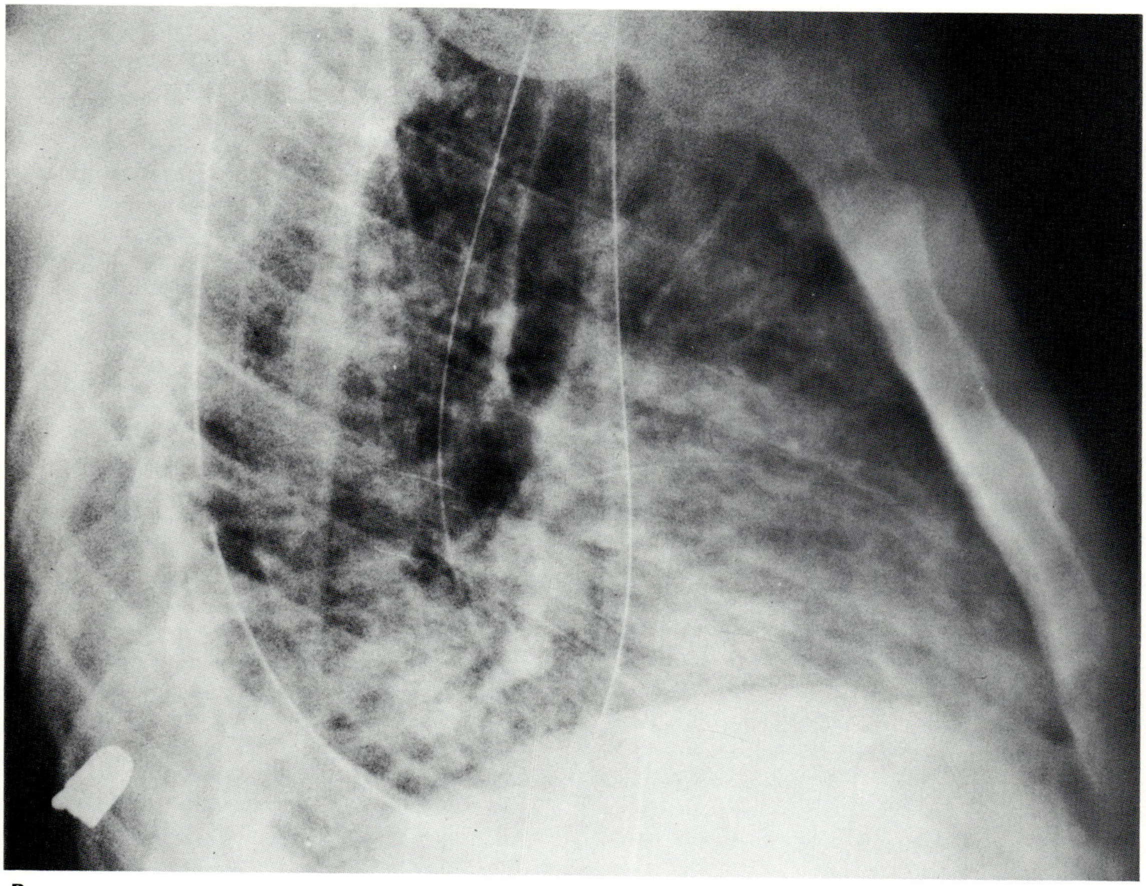

have been reported by a number of authors and are described elsewhere in this work. Alcoholism and drug intoxication are commonly coexisting problems in the urban traumatized patient. Both forms of intoxication may alter levels of consciousness and physical findings. For example, acute alcoholism may reduce the patient's blood pressure and thus suggest traumatic hypovolemia. In such a situation judging the degree of blood loss may be difficult. If the hypotensive traumatized patient has not lost a significant quantity of intravascular volume, an immediate response to 1 liter of crystalloid resuscitation fluid will be apparent.

In the evaluation of the abdomen, inspection, auscultation, palpation, and percussion are recommended. Inspection of the abdomen is the simplest and most informative maneuver, particularly for the patient with penetrating wounds. Most often the patient is conscious and directs the physician to the region of injury. One must be meticulous in the examination of the unconscious patient or the patient with multiple-system injuries, which may divert attention from the abdominal region. All clothing should be removed from the patient before physical examination. It is important to turn the patient carefully to inspect the back for evidence of entrance or exit wounds. Any filth or blood must be wiped away to avoid missing a wound. The suprapubic area or the lower abdominal area in hirsute patients may conceal a nonbleeding, small-caliber gunshot wound. One must also inspect the buttock and intergluteal area for evidence of a penetrating wound.

The examining physician should be constantly aware of the cephalad and caudad reaches of the peritoneal cavity. Our experience indicates that most of the delayed diagnoses of intraabdominal injuries involve patients with thoracoabdominal or pelviabdominal penetrations. The fourth intercostal space or the area of the areola indicates the level of cephalic extension of the diaphragm at the midclavicular line. Penetrating injuries observed to be at or below these levels should be considered to involve the thoracoabdominal space until proved otherwise (Figs. 3.2–3.4). Unfortunately, the abdominal physical examination may be misleading in a patient with a presumed thoracoabdominal wound because of the effects of an ipsilateral hemothorax. Moreover, a tube thoracostomy may produce upper abdominal tenderness. Ancillary diagnostic procedures such as paracentesis with lavage can be of help in such patients (see p. 90 on paracentesis and lavage). If bloody fluid is obtained or if the lavage fluid appears to exit from the chest tube, the presence of diaphragmatic penetration and possible intraabdominal injury should be assumed.

The quadrant of injury and the pathway of the wounding agent must be evaluated. It is often possible to determine whether the wound is superficial (involving the skin and subcutaneous tissue) or whether it involves the deeper structures of the peritoneal cavity. The location of a penetrating injury can to some extent predict the organ injured. However, the combination of organs injured and the severity of the injuries are not easy to predict since some abdominal organs have mobility and may vary in position. A food- and air-filled stomach may extend below the umbilicus and return to its normal position after a puncture injury;

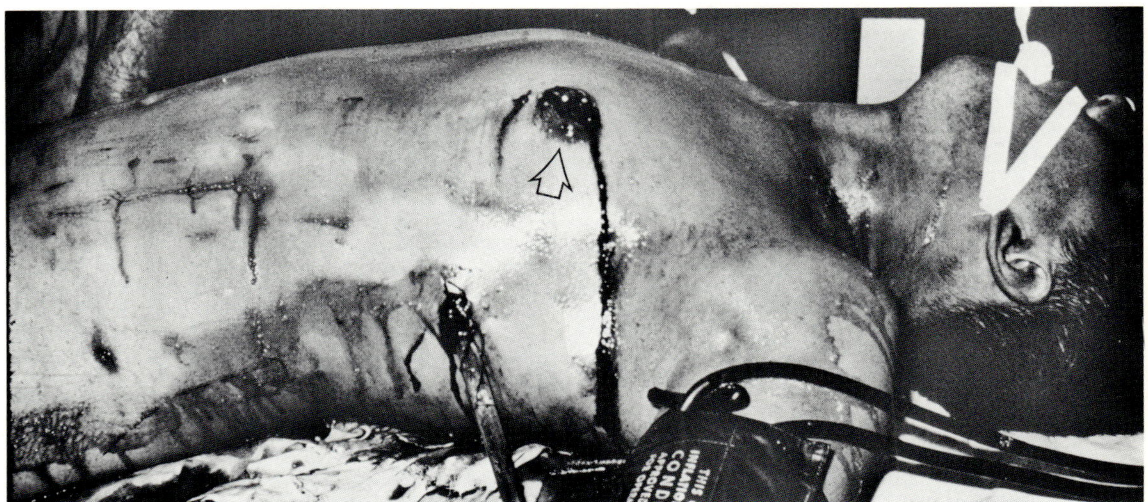

FIG. 3.3. Although the patient sustained a gunshot entrance wound to the left areola, surgical assessment revealed injury to the left lung, diaphragm, liver, and spleen. This pattern of injury can occur despite what may appear to be a primarily thoracic wound. Patients with thoracic injuries must be carefully examined for the possibility of abdominal injuries.

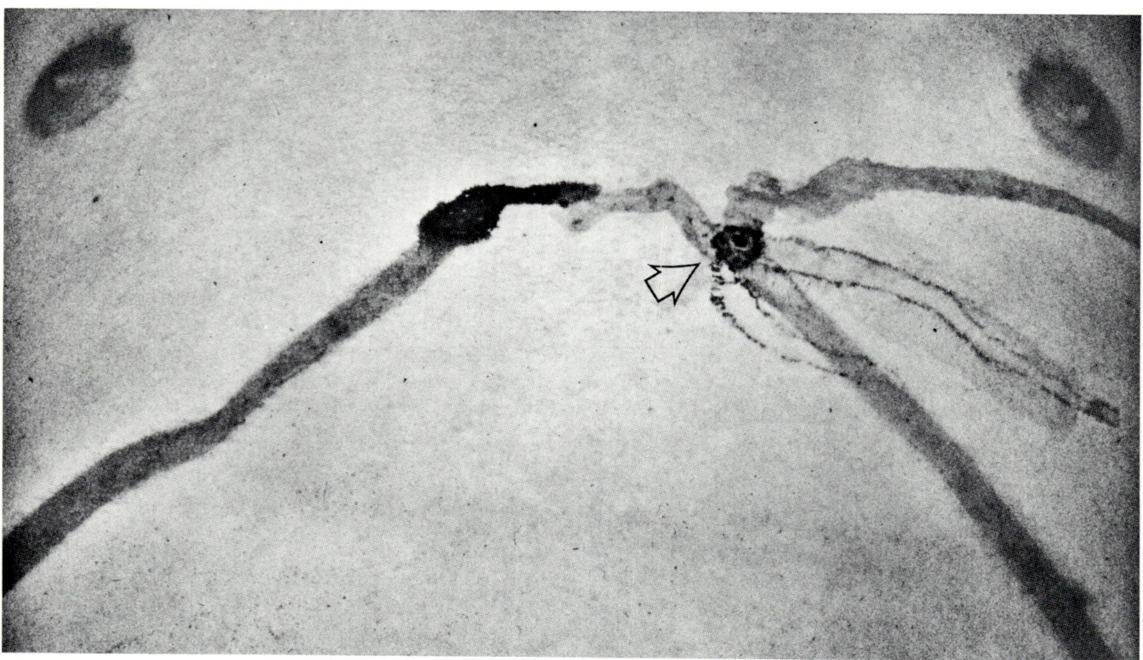

FIG. 3.4. The costal margins of this patient are marked with dye. The bullet entry wound is at the left costal margin. The bullet caused injury to the liver, spleen, and left lung. This represents a typical thoracoabdominal penetrating injury in that the areas of involvement cannot be predicted by the location of the entry wounds.

this is called the "stabbed stuffed stomach syndrome" [78]. Similarly, a mobile transverse or sigmoid colon can sustain injury and move well away from the injury site. In addition, low-velocity gunshot wounds are notorious for changing direction as they pass through the tissues of the body. It is a good idea to draw a diagram of the abdomen and directly indicate the location of the patient's injuries.

The introduction of a nasogastric tube may be a diagnostic procedure relating to injuries of the pharynx, esophagus, and stomach. The return of blood from a nasogastric aspiration can be interpreted as a sign of visceral injury. Severe contusion or penetrating injury involving these upper gastrointestinal tract organs will be signaled by the presence of bright-red blood. A rectal examination must be performed routinely as in a physical examination for any disorder. The presence of blood in the rectum or the palpation of bone spicules or a mass are all significant in the patient with abdominal injury. Blood in the rectum may result from injury to the small bowel or colon, from mesenteric injury with ischemia, or from direct rectal trauma. Similarly, pelvic examinations in women can give valuable information. A careful inspection of the genitalia must be performed. The spontaneous passage of blood from the urethra suggests the possibility of injury to this structure, especially in association with penetrating injuries. Injuries to the membraneous urethra are more common following blunt trauma. The insertion of a Foley catheter, successful or not, is both a therapeutic and diagnostic procedure. A retrograde urethrogram will often confirm the presence of urethral injury.

Examining Stab Wounds

The size, number, or location of abdominal stab wounds will not predict the presence of intraabdominal visceral injury (Fig. 3.5). The size of the knife, its width and length, will often not correlate with the extent of injury even when the penetration is described as deep or superficial. Penetrating injuries can be fairly accurately assessed by physical diagnosis and observation in the majority of patients. The contrast stabogram or digital exploration of the wound under local anesthesia is a poor technique for determining the presence of abdominal penetration and visceral injury. In general, gloved digital examination of the penetrating injury has little to add to the standard careful palpation and auscultation of the abdomen. The finding of penetration of the peritoneal cavity by digital examination is not a universally accepted indication for surgical exploration. Moreover, bleeding and/or pneumoperitoneum may be provoked by this procedure.

The auscultation of the abdomen is an important step in the examination of the patient. Although the presence of bowel sounds does not exclude an intraabdominal injury, absent bowel sounds imply peritoneal inflammation and ileus. Any degree of direct abdominal tenderness and/or rebound tenderness except for the immediate 2–3 cm area surrounding the wound has significance. A wound penetrating the abdominal wall but not injuring viscera will not produce referred tenderness or referred rebound tenderness. Tenderness or rebound elicited in the immediate wound area does not necessarily mandate abdominal exploration. Hourly reexamination should be performed to detect signs of spreading peritoneal inflammation.

The value of physical findings in the assessment of abdominal trauma was described in detail by Shaftan [103]. He reviewed a series of 133 patients treated prior to using selective conservatism to decide whether or not to explore the abdomen and 180 patients treated after instituting the technique. Abdominal injuries of all types were included in the series, and penetrating wounds represented more than one-half of the cases (Table 3.2). The absence of bowel sounds, generalized spasm and/or rigidity, and generalized rebound were the most reliable findings indicative of visceral trauma (Tables 3.3, 3.4).

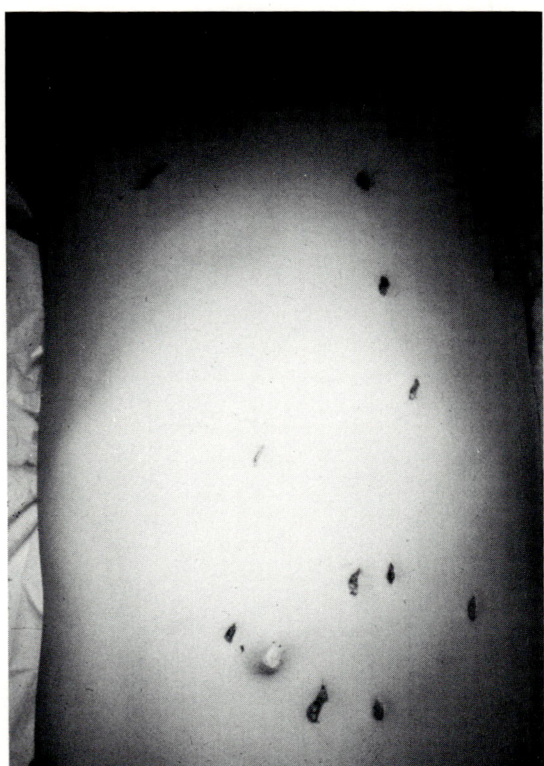

FIG. 3.5. The multiple stab wounds of the patient depicted here are in a pattern expected from a right-handed assailant. When multiple stab wounds are present, a very careful inspection must be made to locate all wounds.

TABLE 3.2. Type of trauma (180 patients, 1956–1958)

Type of trauma	No.	%	% explored
Stab wound	103	57	31
Bullet wound	9	5	55
Auto accident, pedestrian	18	10	28
Auto accident, driver or passenger	16	9	19
Falls	7	4	14
Other blunt	25	14	16
Miscellaneous	3	2	66
Total	182[a]	101	32

Source: Shaftan GW (1960) Indications for operation in abdominal trauma. Am J Surg 99: 657–664

TABLE 3.3. Percentage of patients with physical findings (133 patients, 1952–1954)[a]

	Group		
Findings	A	B	C
Direct tenderness[a]			
None	16	68	29
Local	14	18	50
Regional	30	14	21
Generalized	40	0	0
Rebound tenderness[b]			
None	39	100	86
Local	6	0	0
Regional	20	0	14
Generalized	40	0	0
Spasm and/or rigidity[c]			
None	47	92	79
Local	2	0	7
Regional	20	8	14
Generalized	31	0	0
Bowel sounds[d]			
Normal or hyperactive	36	100	90
Hypoactive	27	0	10
Absent	38	0	0

[a] Not recorded in 20%.
[b] Not recorded in 45%.
[c] Not recorded in 25%.
[d] Not recorded in 32%.

Key: A = Patients found to have visceral injury at operation or autopsy. B = Patients treated but not operated upon. C = Patients with no visceral injury found at operation.

Source: Shaftan GW (1969) Indications for operation in abdominal trauma. Am J Surg 99: 657–664

TABLE 3.4. Percentage of patients with physical findings (180 patients, 1956–1958)

Findings	Group A	Group B	Group C	Findings	Group A	Group B	Group C
Direct tenderness				Spasm and/or rigidity			
Not recorded	0	5	0	Not recorded	10	11	8
None	0	29	25	None	13	64	67
Local	18	40	58	Local	6	11	8
Regional	29	21	0	Regional	29	9	16
Generalized	53	5	16	Generalized	42	1	0
Rebound tenderness				Bowel sounds			
Not recorded	18	20	8	Not recorded	0	6	0
None	18	62	58	Normal	12	69	58
Local	3	8	8	Hyperactive	0	3	8
Regional	18	8	8	Hypoactive	42	8	25
Generalized	42	1	16	Absent	47	0	8

Key: A = Patients found to have visceral injury at operation or autopsy. B = Patients treated but not operated upon. C = Patients with no visceral injury found at operation.

Source: Shaftan GW (1960) Indications for operation in abdominal trauma. Am J Surg 99: 657–664

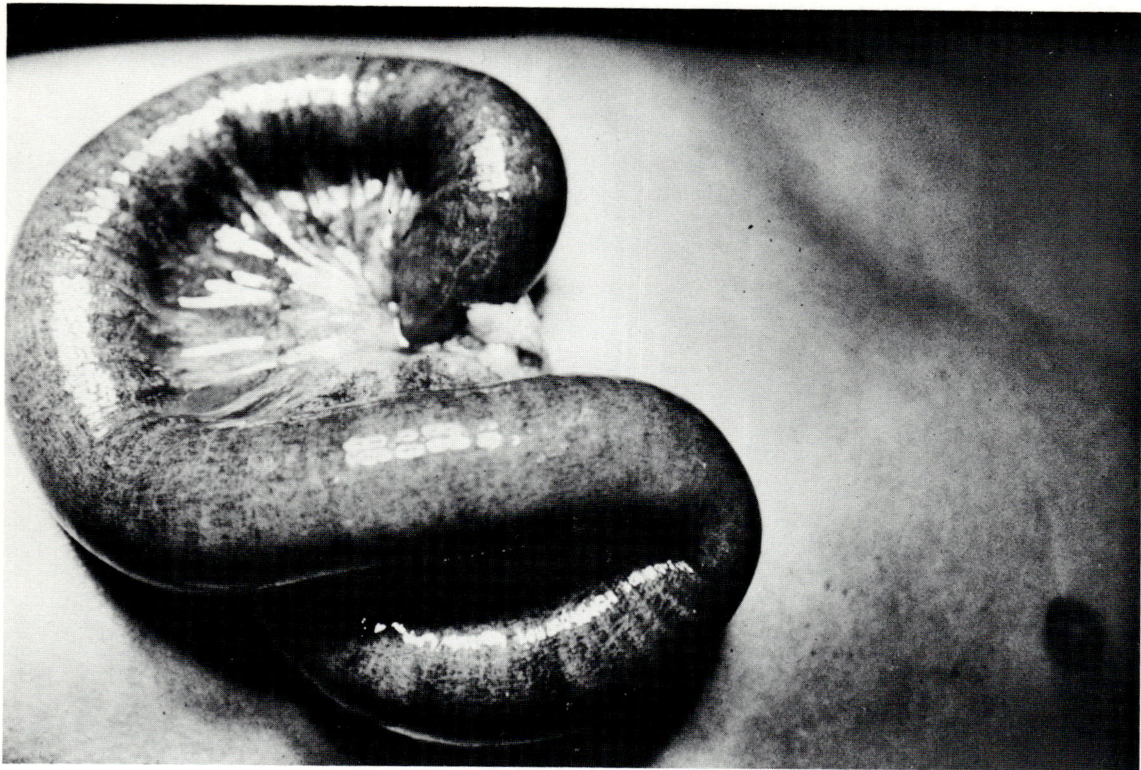

FIG. 3.6. This patient was stabbed in the midline just above the umbilicus. Evisceration of the ileum occurred. The bowel is completely viable and the small-bowel mesentery is intact. Surgical exploration of the abdomen and repair of the abdominal wall were performed.

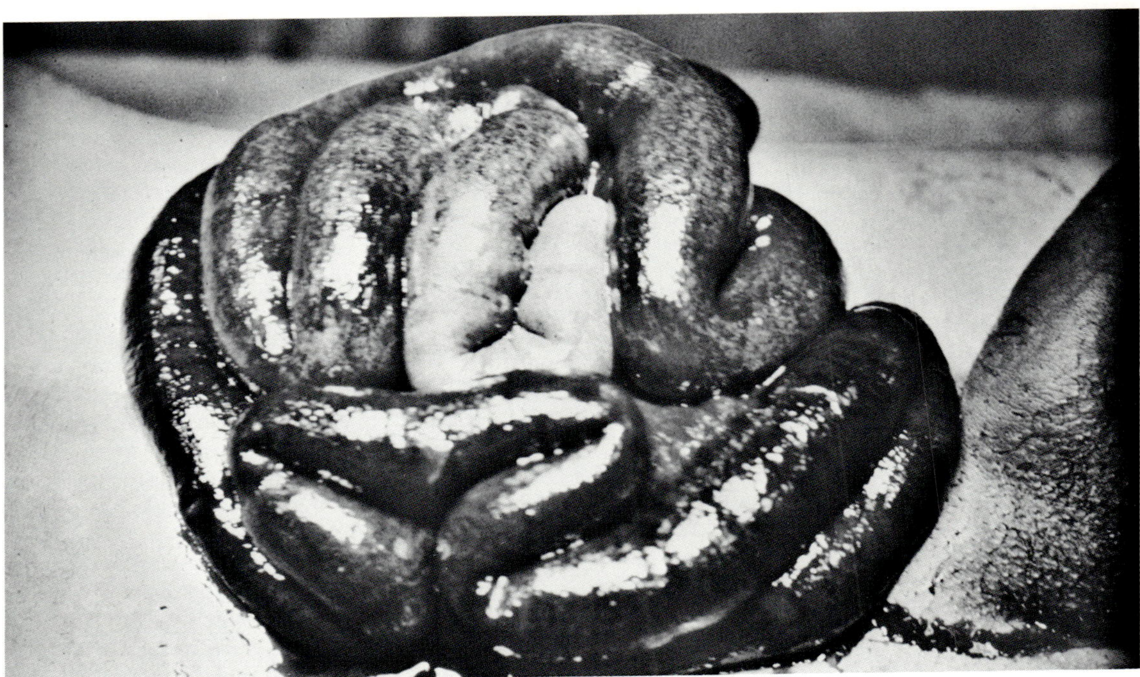

FIG. 3.7. This photograph demonstrates the appearance of a lower abdominal stab wound with evisceration of a greater length of small bowel than was seen in the patient in Figure 3.6. The small intestine is edematous, and there is mesenteric venous occlusion at the evisceration site. A portion of the bowel is gangrenous. Small-bowel resection was required.

In the patient with an eviscerating abdominal injury, the physical examination should proceed as previously described. It is important that the protruding bowel omentum or mesentery should be carefully inspected for abnormal color and bleeding. If fecal material, bile, or large amounts of blood are present, preliminary conclusions can be made as to the extent of injury. The patient's anxiety or abdominal pain may provoke abdominal-wall rigidity and contraction of the stab-wound site. The mesentery of eviscerating bowel will be constricted, and the viability of the eviscerated bowel may be comprised. Bowel strangulation must be avoided in these patients, and prompt surgical intervention is necessary to reduce the bowel and its mesentery (Figs. 3.6–3.8). Once reduction of the eviscerated bowel has been accomplished, the decision for complete abdominal exploration must be made. Despite the presence of evisceration, apparently the presence of signs suggesting peritoneal irritation is still an accurate index of visceral damage. Fear of bowel strangulation is not a concern when a portion of greater omentum is eviscerated. If the results of the remainder of the abdominal examination are normal, ligation and excision of the protruding greater omentum may be considered. Further therapy and exploration would depend on the patient's course and initial physical findings (see p. 15 on selective management of stab wounds).

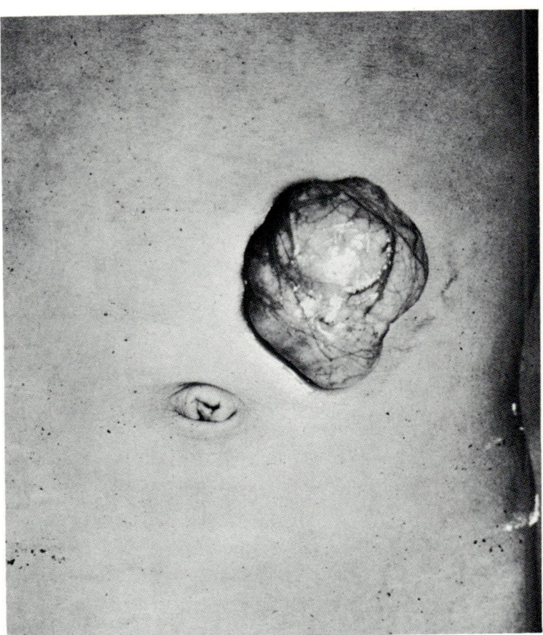

FIG. 3.8. This patient was stabbed in the left upper abdomen. There is evisceration of the transverse colon. The appearance of the colon evisceration differs from small-bowel evisceration in that the colon will often have omental protrusions as well.

Examining Gunshot Wounds

The presence of a gunshot wound in the vicinity of the patient's abdomen will prompt the surgeon to prepare the patient for an exploratory surgical procedure. This approach usually minimizes the value of physical examination and diagnosis. However, gunshot wounds, as do stab wounds, require careful assessment. The entry and exit wounds should be identified if possible. The presence of powder burns and shreds of clothing, bleeding, and local vs generalized abdominal findings should be determined. The location of the gunshot wound is most important, and if an exit wound is present the course of the bullet can be appreciated. The concept of structural damage produced by bullet-blast effect is most applicable to military injuries. In the civilian setting, the low-caliber weapons that are used rarely produce extensive tissue destruction. With low-velocity handgun injuries, the criteria for intervention that apply to stab wounds may be used in the assessment of gunshot wounds. When there is doubt as to course of the bullet and its involvement of the peritoneal cavity, clinical observation, tap and lavage, or a direct exploration of the abdomen can be carried out. The interpretation of the lavage procedure in this situation is discussed in the section on paracentesis and lavage (see p. 91).

Examining the Patient Subjected to Blunt Trauma

The victim of blunt trauma is the most difficult trauma patient to evaluate. Not only are physical signs and symptoms frequently inaccurate as a measure of intra-abdominal injury, but also the common involvement of other body systems compounds the problem. The high incidence of error in the abdominal examination of the patient suffering blunt injury is attributable not just to physician inexperience but also to the unpredictable nature of blunt organ injury and its manifestations. False-positive diagnoses may be a consequence of direct abdominal-wall contusion only. False-negative physical findings are not uncommonly observed in patients with gross hemoperitoneum, primarily because blood alone in the peritoneal cavity may not elicit a dramatic peritoneal reaction. The widespread clinical application of paracentesis and lavage to assess intraabdominal injuries developed because of the well-known pitfalls inherent in the physical examination of the blunt-injury patient.

The presence of shoulder pain (Kehr's sign) can result from subdiaphragmatic irritation secondary to splenic trauma. When shoulder pain is not described by the patient, the Kehr sign can be elicited by deep left-upper-quadrant palpation with the patient in a Trendelenburg position. Ballance's sign can also help in detecting the presence of a ruptured spleen. A positive sign consists of dullness to percussion in the flanks. The dullness is constant on the left regardless of the patient's position. The dullness on the right changes with position, since it is due to intraperitoneal blood. A search should be made for other signs of intraperitoneal or retroperitoneal blood; ecchymosis in the flanks can occur from retroperitoneal hemorrhage. Similarly, periumbilical discoloration can be secondary to intraperitoneal bleeding (Cullen's sign). Ecchymosis and discoloration commonly occur around the pubis, inguinal areas, and genitalia after fracture of an innominate bone. Continuing intraperitoneal or retroperitoneal hemorrhage from trauma is often manifest by progressive abdominal distension. Any significant increase in abdominal girth while the patient is under observation is cause for alarm and necessitates aggressive diagnostic and therapeutic measures. Abdominal distension resulting from blunt trauma in the hypotensive, hypovolemic patient is considered a strong indication for laparotomy. Abdominal-wall abrasions or contusions may be associated with regional areas of tenderness, and it may be difficult to differentiate local regional involvement from significant intraabdominal abnormalities. At the time of abdominal palpation one can clinically check for the possible presence of pelvic fractures by the application of bilateral medial pressure with the palms of the hands on the iliac crests. If this maneuver fails to elicit pain, serious pelvic fractures are excluded. In a similar manner one can exclude rib fractures by gentle simultaneous medial compression of both lower lateral thoracic areas. During this evaluation one may detect subcutaneous emphysema, which can be a consequence of rib fracture. Rib fractures are often accompanied by splenic or hepatic injury. Of course, one should examine carefully to detect the presence of intraabdominal masses. Since, on occasion, a subcapsular hematoma of the spleen or a perihepatic or perisplenic hematoma may be manifest as a palpable abdominal mass (Fig. 3.9), this feature should be considered in the physical examination.

The physical examination is still most important despite its lack of precision. When the question arises whether to rely on physical findings or other diagnostic techniques, one must carefully weigh the accuracy of the diagnostic procedures contemplated. Specific diagnostic tests give information about individual structures or areas and do not cover the multitude of possibilities presented by the traumatized victim. Unless one is confident that all possibilities have been covered by the tests available, physical findings consistent with a serious abdominal injury mandate an aggressive therapeutic effort and ultimately, exploratory laparotomy.

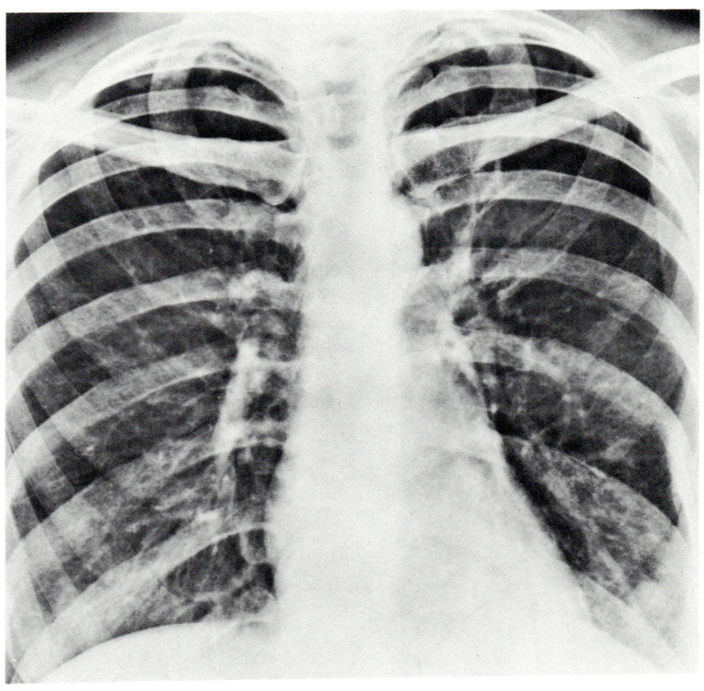

A

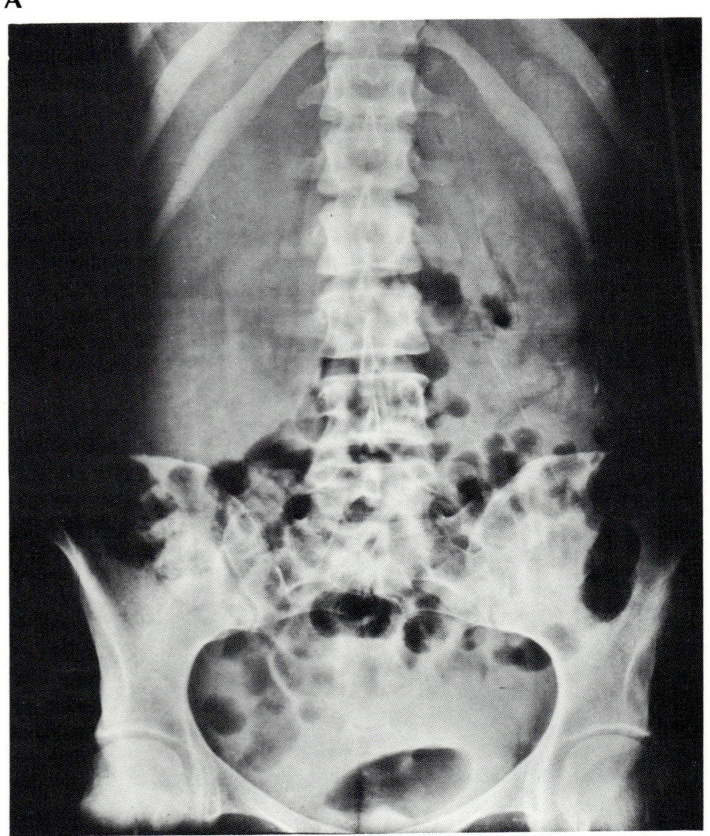

B

FIG. 3.9. This 33-year-old female was admitted through the emergency room with a 5-day history of pain in the back and left flank. She stated that 6 days prior to admission she had fallen at home, striking her left back against the side of a doorway. Since then she had had pain in the left-costovertebral-angle area that radiated down the left flank and around it into the left epigastrium. Deep inspiration worsened the pain and caused radiation of it into the left shoulder. For several days prior to admission, she had felt weak and had noticed ringing in the ears. Both findings were aggravated by her constantly assuming an erect position. The **(A)** chest examination reveals a fracture of the posterior left eighth rib and suggests the presence of a left-lower-lobe retrocardiac infiltration. The **(B)** AP supine view of the abdomen demonstrates hepatomegaly and the presence of a large, soft-tissue mass in the LUQ. Linear soft-tissue densities (not clearly seen on this reproduction) are present in the bilateral paracolic gutters. There is a soft-tissue density in the pelvis with a scalloped upper border that is elevating bowel loops from the pelvis. These findings are consistent with a splenic laceration and intraperitoneal bleeding. At exploration, large amounts of intraperitoneal blood and a lacerated spleen were found.

LABORATORY EVALUATION

The traditional emergency room evaluation of the acutely injured patient includes a rapid clinical examination by a physician and a minimal number of laboratory studies. The extent of further efforts to establish a definitive diagnosis will depend on the condition of the patient and the threat to the patient's life that will result from a delay in initiating surgical therapy. In the acutely traumatized patient laboratory testing has generally been limited to hematocrits, blood counts, stools for blood, amylase determination, and typing and cross-matching of blood. The decision whether or not a surgical procedure should be performed does not usually depend on laboratory studies except when there is a falling hematocrit or an elevated serum amylase. The diagnostic studies used in a large state-wide study of abdominal trauma reported by Strauch are shown in Table 3.5 [106]. The increasing use and appreciation of peritoneal lavage, peritoneal fluid and serum enzymes will introduce more indices for definitive diagnosis of visceral injury. The combination of paracentesis and lavage with careful microscopic and chemical analysis of peritoneal-cavity contents may give information that is of considerable clinical value.

TABLE 3.5. Preoperative diagnostic studies

Studies	No.	%
Hemoglobin-hematocrit	331	96.5
White blood cell count	322	93.9
Type, cross match	311	90.7
Plain roentgenograms	281	61.9
Urinalysis	270	78.7
Bladder catheterization	148	43.1
Diagnostic paracentesis	122	35.6
Blood urea nitrogen	86	25.1
Amylase	79	23.0
Electrolytes	78	22.7
Contrast roentgenograms	59	17.2
Central venous pressure	55	16.0
Electrocardiogram	51	14.9
Blood gases	27	7.9
Other	24	7.0
Thoracentesis	16	4.7
Angiography	8	2.3

Source: Strauch GO (1973) Major abdominal trauma in 1971: A study of Connecticut by the Connecticut Society of American Board Surgeons and the Yale Trauma Program. Am J Surg 125: 413–418

Hematocrits

The initial evaluation of the hematocrit in acute abdominal injury is of very limited aid in determining the hemodynamic status of a patient or in determining the severity of the patient's injury. Significant changes in the hematocrit are primarily a reflection of the hemodilution process. The acutely injured patient may be in a state of profound hypovolemia due to sudden massive arterial or venous blood loss without manifesting significant changes in the peripheral concentration of red blood cells. Measurable and significant changes in the hematocrit in response to hemorrhage occur in response to major body-fluid shifts. This fact is not always appreciated, so that serious errors can be made in the assessment of the injured patient shortly after hospital admission. The lack of diagnostic specificity of serum hemoglobin determinations is described by Perry in 74 abdominal trauma cases. More than one-half of the patients had hemoglobin levels above 12.1 g, and only three patients had less than 10 g [92].

Sequential hematocrit determinations are quite helpful. The negative value of this test in the immediate evaluation of the victim of abdominal trauma is balanced by the help gained in its use over a period of observation. A regularly repeated hematocrit that is falling is diagnostic of blood loss in the traumatized patient and represents an important clue when the clinical findings and history are equivocal. Hepatic, splenic, retroperitoneal, and intraperitoneal bleeding that is progressive over several hours or days will be directly reflected in the hematocrit changes. Many authors have documented the value of the changing hematocrit in the diagnosis of delayed splenic rupture and hepatic bleeding. A falling hematocrit was noted in 83.3% of children with a delayed diagnosis of splenic rupture as reported by Miller and Kelly in a retrospective study of 56 patients (Tables 3.6, 3.7). The intrasplenic or intrahepatic hematoma and retroperitoneal bleeding from the splenic injury may produce a relatively benign clinical pattern, but a fall in the hematocrit or hemoglobin will provide an important clue in establishing the diagnosis.

In the fluid replacement of the hypotensive acutely injured and bleeding patient, the "taking up" phenomenon occurs. This refers to the requirement for the transfusion of volumes of blood in excess of losses to maintain a functional blood volume related to the measured vital signs and venous pressure. The hypotensive, hypovolemic patient after abdominal trauma with associated intraperitoneal-organ fluid leakage and acute peritonitis should be assessed by using the vital signs and venous pressure to determine the clinical hemodynamic status.

TABLE 3.6. Diagnostic factors (56 cases): Splenic trauma in children

	Immediate diagnosis (38 cases)		Delayed diagnosis (18 cases)	
Diagnostic factors	No.	%	No.	%
Abdominal pain	35	92.1	14	77.7
Shoulder pain	22	57.8	9	50
Mild or absent abdominal tenderness	6	15.8	6	33.3
Initial hct <35%	15	39.5	1	5.5
Falling hct on observation	—	—	15	83.3
WBC >15.000	28	73.7	10	55.5
Abdominal x-ray film	7	18.4	4	22.2
Hematuria	12	31.6	7	38.8

Source: Miller DW Jr, Kelley DL (1972) Splenic trauma in children. Arch Surg 105: 561–563

TABLE 3.7. Change in hct observed; delayed diagnosis in 16 cases (8 to 48 h)[a]

Initial hct (%)	No. cases	Hct change at diagnosis	No. cases
Above 38	3	No change	3
35.38	12	Dropped 3–5	6
31.34	1	Dropped 6–11	7

[a] Two additional patients had no hct reading done on initial evaluation, although both had hct values <30% 24 h after injury.

Source: Miller DW Jr., Kelley DL (1972) Splenic trauma in children. Arch Surg 105: 561–563

Leukocyte Count

The value of the leukocyte count in the diagnosis of primary inflammatory and vascular disorders of the intestine does not extend to management of the acute traumatic abdominal injury. In the assessment of patients with blunt or penetrating abdominal trauma, the initial leukocyte count is of value only in splenic and hepatic injuries. In a series of patients with abdominal injuries and visceral rupture reported by Perry, the leukocyte count varied from normal to greater than 20,000 WBC/mm^3. Of 93 patients, 22 had fewer than 10,000 WBC/mm^3, 22 had between 10,000 and 15,000, and 21 had between 15,000 and 20,000. Twenty-eight patients had white blood cell counts over 20,000 [92].

The leukocyte count is specific for hepatic and splenic injury. Ninety-five percent of the patients with hepatic injury had an initial white blood cell count higher than 15,000. Seventy-nine percent of patients with splenic injury had white blood cell counts higher than 15,000. Although this level of correlation does not apply to other abdominal-organ injury, some leukocyte response may occur with intestinal, colonic, or renal injury. Only two of eight cases of intestinal injury had leukocytosis over 10,000 in the series reported by Berman et al. [10]. The severity of hepatic and splenic rupture does influence the degree of leukocyte response. Massive rupture secondary to a blunt injury will give a higher white blood cell count than will a simple knife wound [10].

The presence of leukocytosis is therefore helpful in the diagnosis of splenic and hepatic injury only when injury to these organs is strongly suspected. Although the results reported by Berman et al. are quite convincing, other authors are less certain of the value of the leukocyte count, reporting less correlation with hepatic and splenic injury.

Serum Enzymes

With the exception of the amylase content of serum and peritoneal fluid, amylase enzyme levels have not been clinically utilized as a routine in the evaluation of the acutely injured patient either for diagnosis or for prognosis. The time necessary to obtain the tests and their frequent unavailability have mitigated against the widespread use of these indices other than to assess the postoperative condition of the patient's hepatic, myocardial, and pulmonary function. Reports in the literature indicate that changes do occur in the glutamic oxaloacetic transaminase (GOT), lactic dehydrogenase (LDH), alkaline phosphatase (AP), creatine phosphokinase (CPK), and amylase with varying degrees of clinical and experimental trauma. However, the preoperative use of these tests has not reached the level of a practical working tool. Their potential as a means of predicting organ injury, severity of injury, and prognosis needs extensive study.

Serum Amylase

The serum amylase is a most valuable test in the evaluation of abdominal disorders. Its elevation usually reflects inflammation or injury to the pancreas. However, nonpancreatic abdominal disorders can produce dramatic amylase elevation by the release of amylase into the peritoneal cavity or by the secondary involvement of the pancreas (Table 3.8).

The significance of serum amylase elevation in the patient with abdominal trauma must be appreciated primarily because of the complicated and subtle nature of injury to the pancreas. Retroperitoneal injury can produce a deceptive clinical picture on initial physical examination. The combination of a retroperitoneal duodenal injury and a pancreatic injury may exist without impressive initial physical findings or a positive peritoneal lavage. Careful routine clinical evaluation and contrast studies are an aid in the assessment of the traumatized patient for retroperitoneal injury. In addition, repeated studies of peritoneal-fluid cell count and amylase as well as serum amylase should be performed. The serum amylase is one of the few enzymes which will specifically reflect injury to an intraabdominal organ. Its specificity is in question, however, and its value must be thoroughly understood.

The serum amylase has been used in evaluation of abdominal trauma for many years. Elman et al. described its value as early as 1929 [24]. Interest in the serum amylase as a reflection of pancreatic injury has continued and increased with the incidence of abdominal trauma. Although some authors favor surgical intervention for blunt abdominal trauma based on amylase elevation alone and in the absence of clinical signs of organ injury, others feel the clinical evidence of intraabdominal injury should be present as well. An elevation of the serum amylase is known to occur with injury to organs other than the pancreas. Serum amylase elevation can also occur in the absence of a significant organ injury and the serum amylase level can be normal in the presence of severe pancreatic and intestinal injury. A review of the findings from a clinical report by Olsen is of interest [85]. In 179 patients with blunt trauma, 3 of the 4 patients with pancreatic injuries had elevated serum amylase values. However, 12 of 92 patients with no signs of pancreatic injury also had amylase elevation (Tables 3.9–3.11). The test is more consistent for pancreatic injury resulting from blunt trauma than in patients with penetrating trauma. Trauma to the head and body of the pancreas was more prone to produce amylase elevation than injury to the tail.

The persistent or late elevation of serum amylase value has greater accuracy than initial determinations in predicting pancreatic injury according to Olsen [85].

TABLE 3.9. Incidence of hyperamylasemia with specific intraabdominal injuries

	No. of patients	Patients with hyperamylasemia
Pancreatic injuries	4	3 (75%)
Small-bowel injuries	7	2 (29%)
Patients with other significant abdominal injuries	76	19 (25%)
Patients with no significant abdominal injuries	92	12 (13%)
Total	179	36 (20%)

Source: Olsen WR (1973) The serum amylase in blunt abdominal trauma. J Trauma 13: 200–204

TABLE 3.8. Correlation of highest amylase with diagnosis

		Highest serum amylase (Somogyi units)		
Diagnosis	No. patients	Over 1000	500–1000	200–500
Biliary disease	86	60	17	9
Idiopathic pancreatitis	38	1	6	31
Traumatic pancreatitis	14	9	4	1
Pseudocyst of pancreas	7	2	3	2
Perforated duodenal ulcer	4	1	1	2
Mesenteric thrombosis	3	0	1	2
Acute hepatitis	2	0	0	2
Totals	154	73	32	49

Source: Adams JT, Libertino JA, Schwartz SI (1968) Significance of an elevated serum amylase. Surgery 63: 877–884

TABLE 3.10. Patients with hyperamylasemia but no significant intraabdominal injuries

Patient	Age	Sex	Mechanism of injury	Abdominal signs of injury	Selective visceral angiography	Peritoneal lavage	WBC	Amylase	SGOT	Hematuria	Celiotomy	Follow-up (months)
1	10	F	Auto-pedestrian	Equivocal	No	Negative	10,800	131	175	No	No	14.5
2	22	M	Auto-pedestrian	Unconscious	No	Negative	9,900	130	243	No	No	9.0
3	10	F	Auto accident	Equivocal	Yes	Weakly positive	18,400	150	—	No	No	0.5
4	21	M	Auto accident	Equivocal	Yes	Weakly positive	12,700	130	128	No	No	14.0
5	19	F	Auto accident	Unconscious	Yes	Weakly positive	16,100	173	804	Yes	No	15.0
6	25	M	Auto accident	Equivocal	No	Negative	6,000	174	273	No	No	1.5
7	15	M	Fall	Equivocal	No	Negative	7,900	127	205	Gross	No	12.0
8	36	M	Auto accident	"Obvious"	Yes	Strongly positive	8,900	272	303	Gross	Yes	7.0
9	40	M	Auto accident	Unconscious	No	Negative	6,700	167	167	No	No	12.0
10	30	M	Auto-pedestrian	Absent	No	Negative	6,110	132	50	No	No	7.0
11	16	M	Auto accident	Equivocal	No	Negative	8,000	132	28	No	No	7.0
12	32	M	Auto accident	Equivocal	No	Weakly positive	9,700	180	—	No	Yes	2.5

Source: Olsen WR (1973) The serum amylase in blunt abdominal trauma. J Trauma 13: 200–204

TABLE 3.11. Amylase levels correlated with intraabdominal injuries

Significant intraabdominal injuries	Admission serum amylase levels (Somogyi units)						
	Not determined	0–40	40–120 (normal)	120–150	150–200	>200	Total
Spleen	9	8	16	4	3		40
Spleen + kidney	2		2				4
Spleen + mesentery	1			1			2
Spleen + bladder		1	1				2
Spleen + diaphragm				1			1
Spleen + stomach	1						1
Spleen + liver + mesentery						1	1
Spleen + liver	2	1	3		1		7
Liver	2	1	16	1	1		21
Liver + mesentery		1			1		2
Liver + kidney			1				1
Liver + bladder					1		1
Pancreas + liver			1	1			2
Pancreas				1		1	2
Small bowel	2	4	1	1		1	9
Mesentery		1	1	2	1		5
Bladder			3				3
Hepatic artery	1						1
Massive pelvic injury						1	1
Diaphragm + bladder			1				1
None	26	11	69	7	4	1	118
Total	46	28	115	19	12	5	225

Source: Olsen WR (1973) The serum amylase in blunt abdominal trauma. J Trauma 13: 200–204

A similar statement is made by Bach and Frey in a review of 44 patients suffering pancreatic injury [4]. They emphasize the importance of repeated serum amylase determinations. Seven of nineteen patients in their series had amylase values which were normal within 5 h of injury. Cleveland et al. described three cases with initially normal amylase levels that subsequently became elevated [19]. Although early surgical intervention is strongly advocated by White and Benfield and others based primarily on serum amylase level in the traumatized patient, other authors feel that the amylase level is too nonspecific to rely on in any absolute way [112]. It seems reasonable to combine sequential serum amylase determinations with peritoneal-fluid or lavage analysis and radiologic evaluation. A combination of diagnostic studies will probably establish the diagnosis prior to any irreversible progression of the effects of the injury. The number of missed retroperitoneal injuries involving the pancreas and duodenum will be small using this combination of modalities.

Amylase determination of peritoneal fluid is important in the assessment of abdominal trauma. Several authors have shown that the amylase values in peritoneal fluid will rise more quickly than the serum amylase. Clearly the determination of amylase values in peritoneal fluid is important among the several tests performed to evaluate the nature and extent of intraabdominal trauma. The peritoneal amylase level has been used with considerably more frequency than the erythrocyte count or other peritoneal-fluid enzyme levels. Peritoneal lavage fluid levels that are greater than 100 Somogyi units/100 cc strongly suggest the presence of pancreatic or intestinal injury [26]. The leakage of bowel content into the peritoneal cavity will contaminate the peritoneal fluid with amylase; thus a nonpancreatic visceral injury will often produce a high peritoneal-fluid amylase. The urinary amylase secretion is also of value in the assessment of the traumatized patient. Gambill and Mason report that a 2-h urine amylase is more reliable and sensitive than serum amylase in pancreatic injury [33]. Unfortunately, a delay is necessary to make a time collection of urine for amylase determination.

Creatine Phosphokinase

The enzyme creatine phosphokinase (CPK) is a very sensitive indicator of changes in skeletal muscle tissue. The serum CPK enzyme response is so sensitive that subcutaneous intramuscular injections and minor trauma elicit an elevation. Nevins et al. described elevation of the serum CPK in response to simple exertion and intramuscular injection [82]. Indeed, this high degree of sensitivity of CPK lends value to its use in establishing the diagnosis of myocardial infarction. Unfortunately, the CPK response is nonspecific for abdominal trauma. Operative procedures and the trauma of amputation will produce a rise in serum CPK [47, 83]. Experimental ballistic injury to animal extremities produces a trauma preparation that gives some index of the CPK enzyme response. The CPK in such instances rises consistently [54]. Matsumoto et al. reviewed the enzyme changes in combat victims, and the wide range and sensitivity of the CPK was observed in this setting as well [61].

In view of the sensitivity of the test, the CPK could indicate only whether or not trauma occurred—information already obtained. If severity of trauma correlated with this enzyme change, then the CPK could be used as an index to prognosis or for trauma classification. However, the sensitivity and wide variability of the CPK changes after trauma do not correlate with any single variable.

Glutamic Oxaloacetic Transaminase

Glutamic oxaloacetic transaminase (GOT) has become an important enzyme in the diagnosis of parenchymal hepatic disorders. It is also of value in the diagnosis of myocardial infarction. There is elevation of the serum GOT in response to trauma of various types. Lawson et al. described GOT elevation as a result of experimental ballistic injury to an extremity [54]. Nickell and Albritten [83] and Rudolph et al. [99] have reported GOT elevation after routine surgical procedures and trauma. This nonspecific pattern of response to trauma by the serum GOT is similar to that of CPK. The degree of elevation of GOT, however, is not so variable as that of CPK. In the Morrisania studies of abdominal trauma, the serum GOT had an appreciably high mean level in cases of isolated hepatic injury [20].

Lactic Dehydrogenase

Peripheral blood lactic dehydrogenase (LDH) elevation has not correlated with injury to a specific abdominal organ. In a clinical study, Calman et al. reported four cases of hemoperitoneum with slight peripheral serum LDH elevation [11]. A significant postoperative LDH elevation occurred in patients with fractures and intestinal strangulation. The experimental study reported by Lawson et al. describes the serum-CPK–level elevation in experimental ballistic injury to extremities and a minimal response of the serum LDH and alkaline phosphatase despite the presence of massive skeletal muscle trauma [54].

Alkaline Phosphatase

Although the serum alkaline phosphatase (AP) blood levels have been demonstrated to rise in the course of management of severely injured patients, it is not an enzyme that rises as an immediate response to nonspecific surgical trauma. The elevations of the peripheral blood alkaline phosphatase observed several days after trauma may occur as a result of healing of a long-bone fracture. However, this late posttrauma rise needs further study.

Peritoneal-Fluid Enzymes

Although it is possible that each organ leaves its unique imprint in the form of a peritoneal-fluid chemical identity, the peripheral blood response to trauma noted with some enzymes complicates the interpretation of peritoneal values. The simultaneous evaluation of fluid from the peritoneal cavity and of blood from the peripheral circulation will assess differential changes and establish relative diagnostic criteria of value. The clinical value of peritoneal-fluid analysis in the trauma patient would potentially allow the determination of whether or not laparotomy was indicated and the kind of surgery to be performed.

Peritoneal-fluid analysis could serve as an adjunct to such diagnostic procedures as laparoscopy, arteriography, and endoscopy. Patients with minor liver laceration and contusions, mesenteric lacerations, serosal bowel injuries, and small, controlled retroperitoneal hematomas may manifest significant hemoperitoneum with minimal or no abdominal physical findings. Not all patients of this type require laparotomy, and the analysis of peritoneal blood specimens via paracentesis might help in rendering judgment for or against surgical intervention.

In 1975 our group reported a clinical study of peritoneal and peripheral blood determination in abdominal trauma cases [20]. The study was designed to evaluate the peritoneal blood changes and enzyme levels relative to peripheral blood for various organ injuries.

Seventy-five patients with abdominal injuries and gross hemoperitoneum admitted to the Morrisania City Hospital were studied for peritoneal-blood enzyme content. All of the patients required emergency laparotomy, usually within 1–4 h after hospital admission. There were 28 stab wounds, 29 gunshot wounds, and 13 blunt abdominal injuries. Blood samples were obtained from the peritoneal cavity at the time of the surgical procedure prior to irrigation or manipulation of the injured abdomlnal viscera. Peripheral blood specimens were also obtained during the operation and as close to the time of peritoneal blood sampling as possible. Enzyme analysis was performed using the 12-channel sequential multiple-analysis system. The values of peritoneal and peripheral blood GOT, AP, CPK, and LDH were studied. Mean values, standard deviation, and standard error of the mean were determined for each group.

The findings were categorized according to the type of organ injuries and five extravisceral injuries. The patients with multiple injuries were analyzed with regard to the presence or absence of intestinal injury. The extravisceral category of injury included two patients with simple abdominal-wall and peritoneal laceration, two patients with isolated mesenteric tears, and one patient with a retroperitoneal hematoma without an organ injury.

The findings in the study indicated that isolated liver injuries were associated with significant elevation of peritoneal blood LDH and peritoneal and peripheral blood GOT levels. A multiplicity of abdominal organ injuries results in elevation of peritoneal blood LDH and GOT level. The occurrence of isolated small-intestinal injury and small-intestinal injury combined with other organ injuries produces a significant elevation of peritoneal-blood enzyme levels of GOT, LDH, and AP. Peritoneal-blood alkaline phosphatase elevation is associated with normal mean peripheral blood levels. Therefore, combined peritoneal- and peripheral-blood AP analysis is of potential use in identification of small-intestinal injury in patients with hemoperitoneum of traumatic origin (Table 3.12, Figs. 3.10, 3.11).

In patients with small-intestinal trauma, three of the four enzymes studied had elevations of their mean values in the peritoneal blood relative to peripheral blood. This finding may reflect a release of enzyme-containing fluid into the peritoneal cavity in very high concentration in comparison to simultaneously drawn peripheral blood. The occurrence of peritoneal-blood alkaline phosphatase elevation with injuries of the small intestine represents the only enzyme change that identifies a specific intraabdominal organ injury. There is spillage of alkaline-phosphatase–containing intestinal content and the release of intestinal alkaline phosphatase and other enzymes from the traumatically injured intestinal wall. The findings of elevated peritoneal-blood alkaline phosphatase level with normal peripheral-serum alkaline phosphatase suggest that the peritoneal-fluid levels can be used as a diagnostic test of small-bowel injury. Further studies will be required to establish whether or not the peritoneal-fluid alkaline phosphatase determination is a useful clinical test.

In a subsequent experimental study, Moss et al. produced a visceral-trauma preparation in dogs and studied the isoenzyme profile of the peritoneal-fluid alkaline phosphatase [76]. The results demonstrated a preponderance of intestinal alkaline phosphatase in the blood shed by the injured viscera into the peritoneal cavity. A clinical study of enzyme patterns including amylase and isoenzymes of LDH and alkaline phosphatase in abdominal trauma, both for peripheral blood and peritoneal blood, is needed to ascertain whether differential enzyme and isoenzyme analysis has diagnostic or prognostic value in the management of the traumatized patient.

TABLE 3.12. Mean difference between peritoneal blood and peripheral blood

Organ injury	No.	Alkaline phosphatase Mean difference	Alkaline phosphatase p value	Lactic dehydrogenase Mean difference	Lactic dehydrogenase p value	Glutamic oxaloacetic transaminase Mean difference	Glutamic oxaloacetic transaminase p value	Creatinine phosphokinase Mean difference	Creatinine phosphokinase p value
All small intestine	22	216.09 ± 46.2	<0.001	312.13 ± 31.7	<0.001	178.90 ± 53.6	<0.005	659.54 ± 363.6	NS
Small intestine only	10	257.70 ± 50.9	<0.001	325.10 ± 41.9	<0.001	213.40 ± 116.5	<0.001	280.70 ± 48.6	NS
Multiple with small intestine	12	181.41 ± 74.0	<0.05	301.33 ± 47.7	<0.001	154.72 ± 22.7	<0.001	1021.58 ± 561.2	NS
Multiple without small intestine	9	39.00 ± 20.3	NS	240.66 ± 71.9	<0.01	136.28 ± 56.7	<0.05	710.77 ± 339.6	NS
Liver	18	−0.72 ± 6.0	NS	158.58 ± 54.2	<0.01	225.50 ± 122.9	NS	−140.88 ± 172.3	NS
Colon	5	14.60 ± 10.77	NS	981.00 ± 469.8	NS	81.20 ± 23.4	<0.025	1026.00 ± 736.5	NS
Spleen	5	11.40 ± 8.6	NS	136.00 ± 37.8	<0.025	117.60 ± 125.9	NS	−384.16 ± 277.3	NS
Extravisceral	5	−14.40 ± 14.8	NS	633.40 ± 468.3	NS	106.20 ± 56.6	NS	1555.80 ± 911.7	NS
Stomach	2	2.50	—	952.50	—	53.50	—	15.00	—
Pancreas	2	−12.50	—	981.40	—	482.00	—	1772.50	—
Kidney	1	−1.50	—	−30.00	—	4.00	—	250.00	—

[a] ±1 SEM.

Source: Delany HM, Moss CM, Carnevale N (1976) The use of enzyme analysis of peritoneal blood in the clinical assessment of abdominal organ injury. Surg Gynecol Obstet 142: 162–167

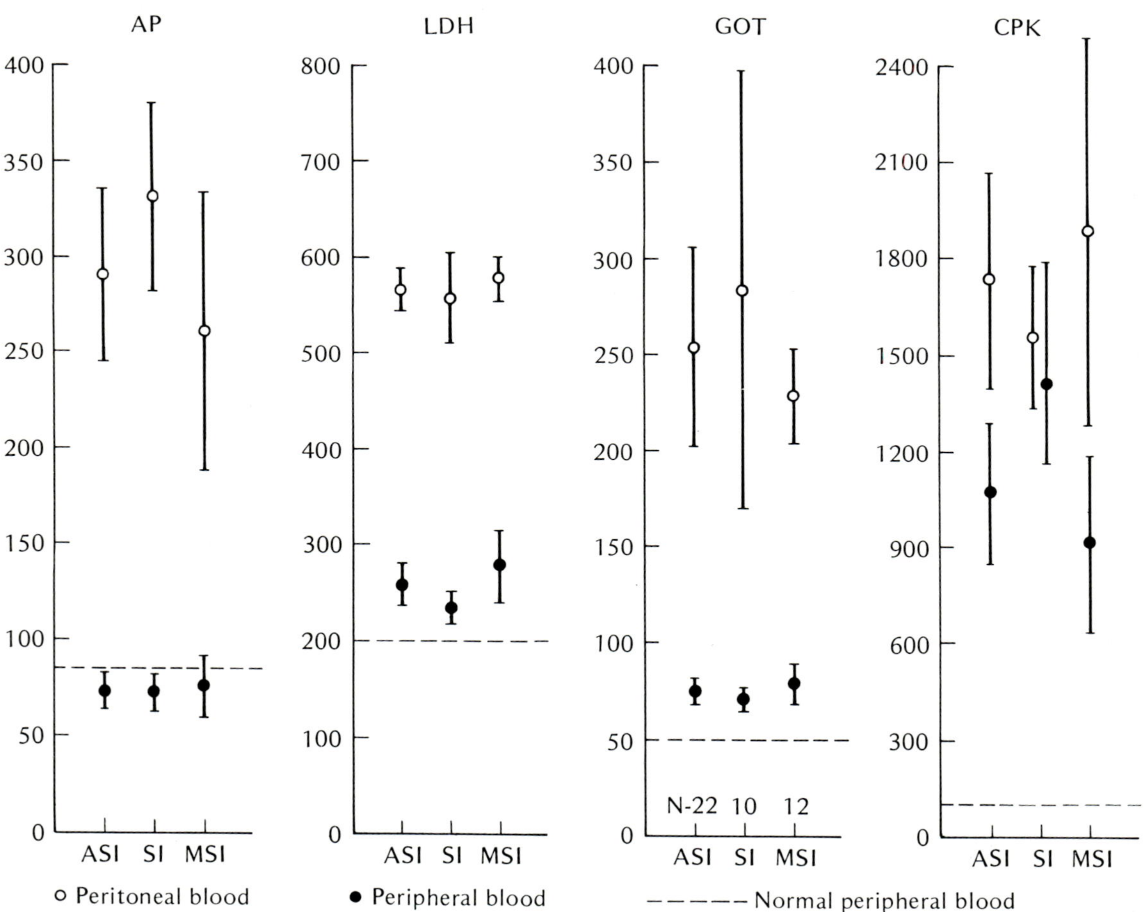

FIG. 3.10. The mean values (±1 SEM) of the peritoneal-blood enzymes and peripheral-blood enzymes are shown for all small-intestinal injuries, ASI; small-intestinal injury only, SI; and multiple injuries including small intestine, MSI. The mean levels of alkaline phosphatase in the peripheral blood were in the normal range. There was significant elevation of peritoneal-blood enzyme levels relative to peripheral-blood levels for alkaline phosphatase, lactic dehydrogenase, and glutamic oxaloacetic acid. All enzyme levels are expressed in international units, milliunits per milliliter. From Delany HM, Moss CM, Carnevale N (1976) The use of enzyme analysis of peritoneal blood in the clinical assessment of abdominal organ injury. Surg Gynecol Obstet 142: 161–167

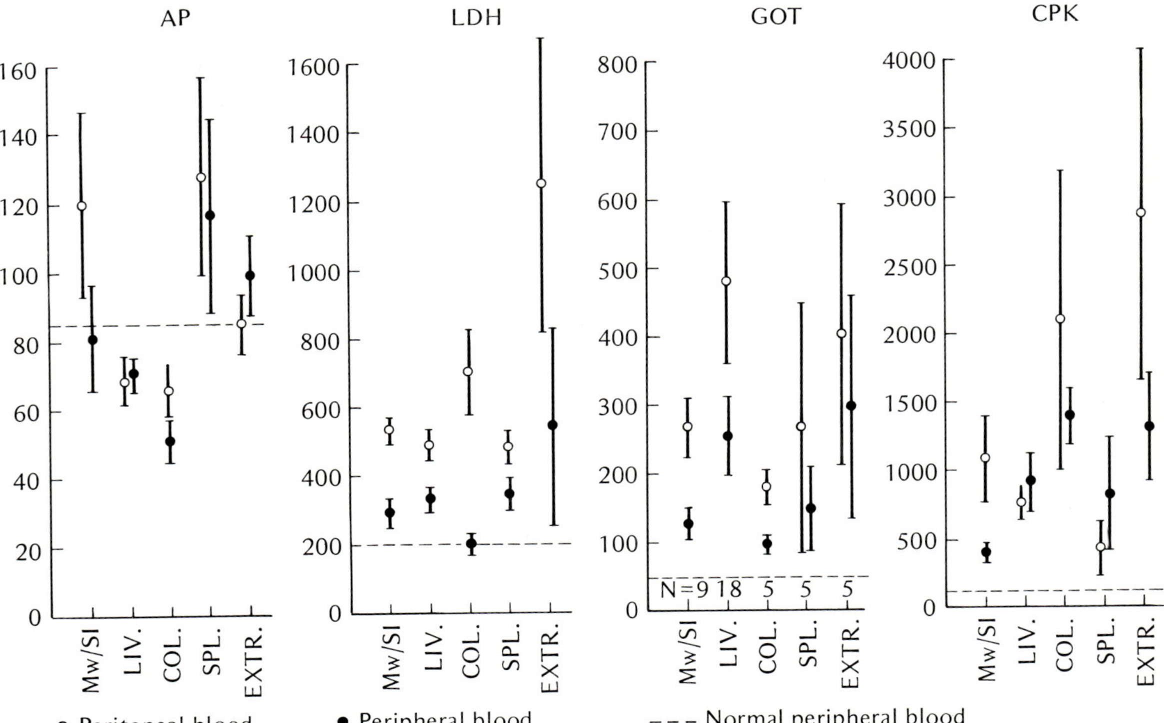

FIG. 3.11. The mean values (±1 SEM) of the peritoneal blood and peripheral blood are shown for multiple injuries excluding small intestine, Mw/SI; liver, LIV.; colon, COL.; spleen, SPL.; and extravisceral injury, EXTR. A wide range of values are seen both in the peritoneal blood and peripheral blood. The elevations of alkaline phosphatase levels were minimal relative to the values shown in Figure 3.10. Mean values for injuries to the stomach, pancreas, and kidneys are not shown because of the small numbers—2, 2, and 1, respectively—involved. From Delany HM, Moss CM, Carnevale N (1976) The use of enzyme analysis of peritoneal blood in the clinical assessment of abdominal organ injury. Surg Gynecol Obstet 142: 161–167

RADIOLOGIC EVALUATION

The high morbidity and mortality of the abdominally traumatized patient has led some to feel that, "due to the definite limitation of roentgenographic examinations, it may be wiser to omit routine studies in order to gain promptness in treatment" [43]. This viewpoint is certainly justified for the patient in severe shock who does not respond to therapy, or who is deteriorating rapidly; but it is not a reasonable approach for those patients whose more stable condition allows a stepwise diagnostic workup.

Radiologic examination is one of the important diagnostic tools in the armamentarium of the physician. The appropriate utilization of this tool can provide pertinent information leading to a speedy and accurate diagnosis, followed by the appropriate therapy. Although the radiologist brings a statistical approach to his analysis of a radiologic study, it must always be kept in mind that each patient, and his response to injury, are unique. In order to gain the most information from any diagnostic tool, that tool must be tailored to fit the needs of the patient. This can only be accomplished through knowledge and experience, coupled with the information derived from a thorough history and physical examination.

Technique of the Radiographic Examination

The patient with abdominal trauma presents a technical as well as a diagnostic problem. Although speed and thoroughness are essential, extreme care must be taken so that additional injury is not produced by the technique of the examination. There is probably no other setting which tests so thoroughly the efficiency and efficacy of the radiologic team as does the examination of the traumatized patient. Strauch [106] found that while 64.2% of traumatized patients arrived in the emergency room in a conscious and alert condition, 26.9% demonstrated some alteration of consciousness and 8.9% were unconscious. In addition, 44.0% were in shock, and 64.6% had associated extra-abdominal injury, of which 51% were of a major nature. Certainly, these are not the best conditions in which to examine any patient, but these are the conditions that represent the reality with which we must deal.

Two essential evaluations of the patient must be performed: plain-film examinations of the chest and abdomen [30,43,73].

Chest Examination

Ideally, the most information is derived from posteroanterior (PA) and lateral projections of the chest, in the erect position, with the X-ray tube 6 ft away from the patient. However, a chest examination, whether posteroanterior (PA) or anteroposterior (AP), supine or erect, is essential since it is not uncommon to find abdominal injuries associated with chest injuries or the reverse. This initial evaluation will establish a baseline appearance of the diaphragm, which may show significant change at a later time as a reflection of either intrathoracic or intraabdominal abnormality. Radiologic examination of the chest will rule out primary chest disease, which presents as abdominal disease; demonstrate sympathetic response within the chest to abdominal disease; and/or reveal concomitant chest and abdominal abnormalities [31] (Fig. 3.12).

Abdominal Examination

The abdomen contains all four degrees of radiographic density: bone, water, fat, and air. The best radiographic technique to bring out the contrast between these densities is to use 55–70 kVp, 300 or higher mA, the shortest time possible, a 12:1 or higher grid ratio, par-

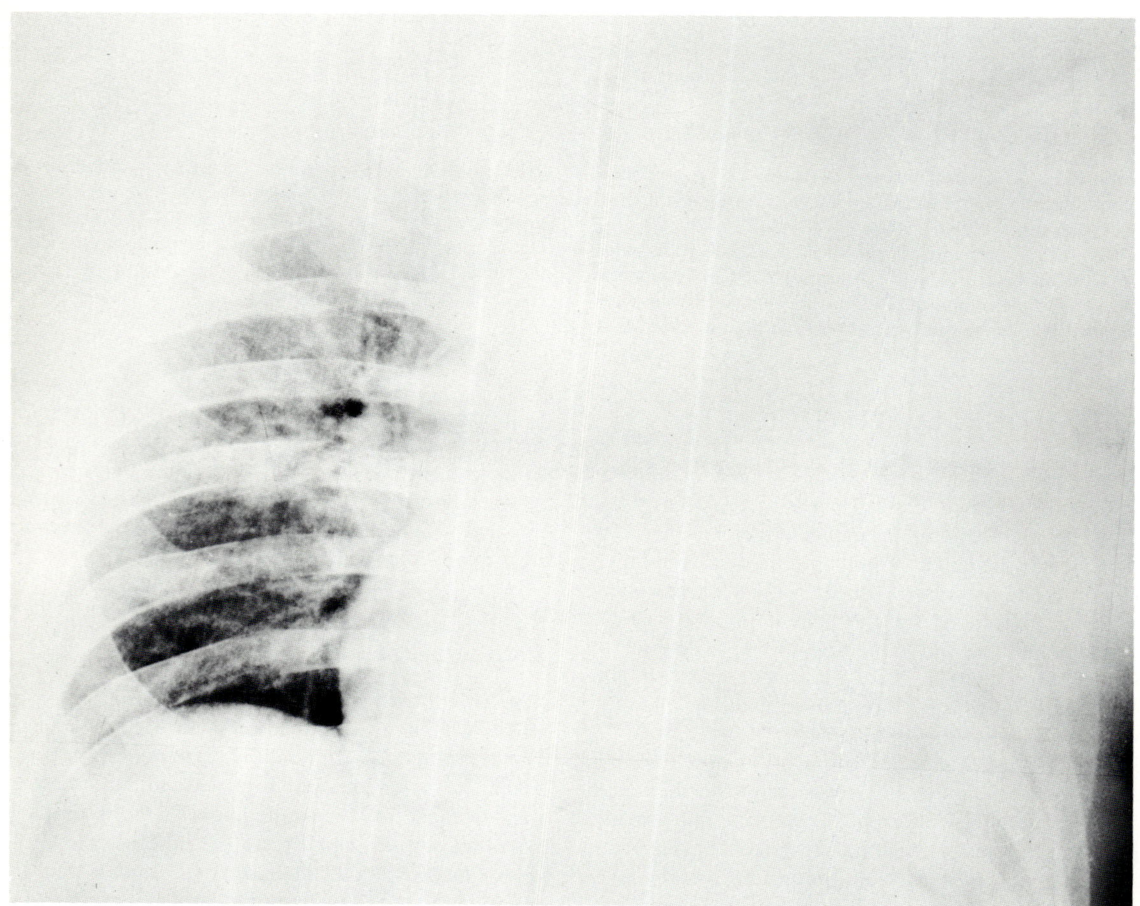

FIG. 3.12. This male was admitted with multiple gunshot wounds. Although multiple views of the abdomen were obtained, they failed to suggest any chest abnormality. A single AP view of the chest reveals opacification of the left hemithorax. A chest tube was inserted and free blood, which eventually cleared, was drained from the left hemithorax.

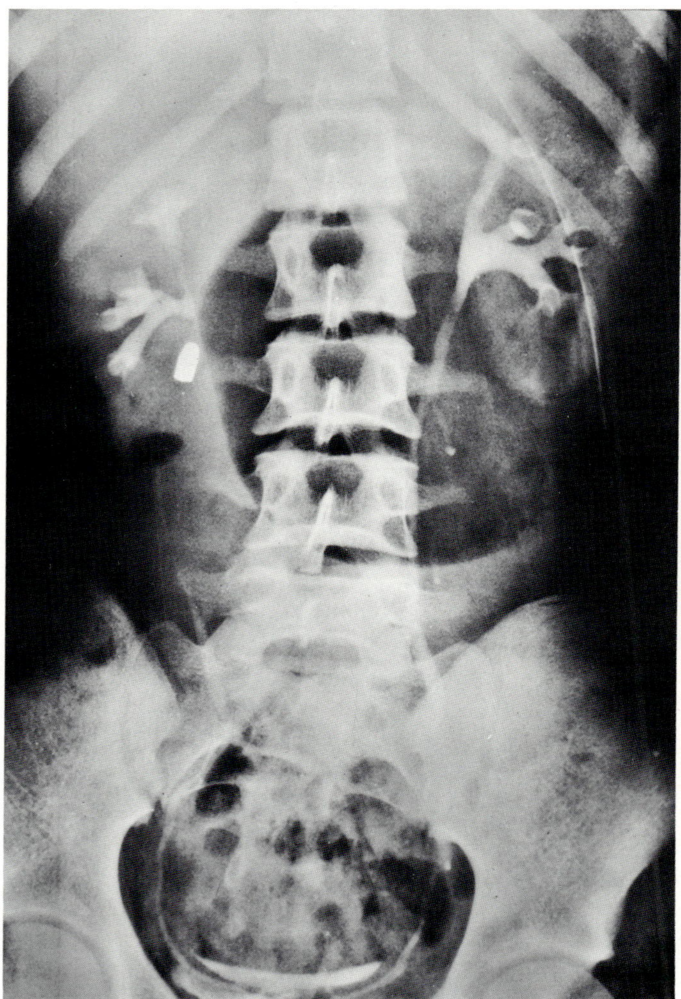

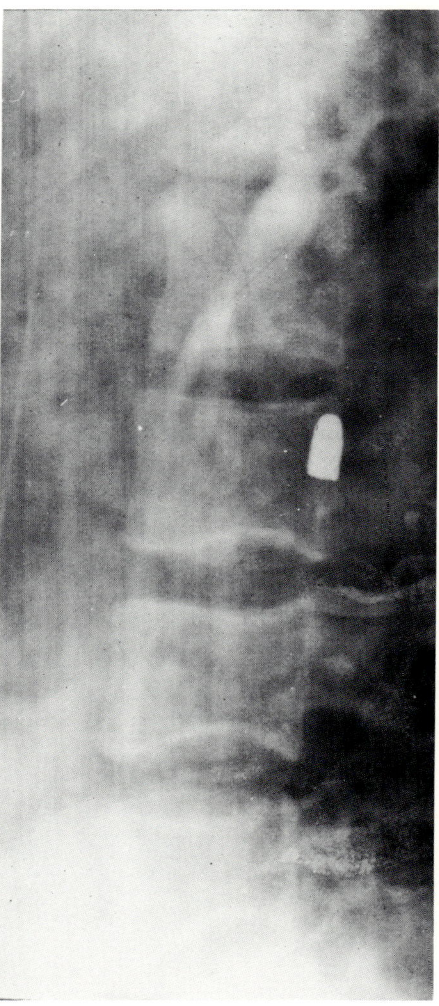

A B

FIG. 3.13. This male patient sustained an abdominal gunshot wound which entered just to the right of the umbilicus; no exit wound was found. The intravenous pyelogram with **(A)** frontal and **(B)** lateral projections reveals a large right retroperitoneal mass displacing the right ureter anteriorly and laterally. The course of the bullet (entrance to final position) suggests inferior vena cava (IVC) injury. Exploration revealed penetration of IVC, duodenum, antrum of stomach, and head of pancreas.

speed screens, and high-speed film [65]. If possible, at least three views of the abdomen should be obtained: AP supine, AP erect, and a left lateral decubitus view [56,65,73,103]. The field size, particularly on the AP views, should be wide enough to include the properitoneal fat lines and the soft-tissue plains of the abdominal boundaries. If the patient's condition is so unstable that this type of evaluation cannot be performed, then AP and transtable lateral supine views of the abdomen may be sufficient.

Whatever the technique of chest and abdominal evaluation, it is important to maintain the patient in the position of examination for at least 5–10 min prior to taking the film. This is particularly important for erect and horizontal films in the detection of free air in the peritoneal cavity.

Love [56] and others advocate the intravenous infusion of 300 ml of 25% urographic contrast medium in order to produce a "bodygram" effect of the abdominal organs. This examination has been found to be beneficial in demonstrating the overall integrity of the liver, spleen, and kidneys; in demonstrating free intraabdominal fluid; and in giving an indication of the integrity and function of the urinary system. This technique not only increases the diagnostic accuracy of the intraabdominal evaluation, but also helps in the evaluation of the retroperitoneal area (Fig. 3.13).

The placement of lead markers at the sites of entrance and exit wounds can suggest the course of the penetrating missile and, thereby, suggest possible organ injury. This technique is far more reliable with stab wounds than with gunshot wounds (bullets may change their trajectories at the interface of tissues of varying densities).

Additional radiologic studies, including contrast examinations, should be performed on the basis of (a) the patient's condition and (b) radiologic, clinical, and other diagnostic indicators of selected organ injury. Although diagnostic pneumoperitoneum had its advocates in the past, Frimann-Dahl [31] feels that it has no particular value in the study of patients with acute abdominal disorders.

Plain-Film Evaluation

Diagnostic radiologic evaluation of the patient with abdominal trauma begins with interpretation of chest and abdominal plain-film examination. According to Cantor [13], 11% of survey films of the abdomen will permit accurate assessment of abdominal injury and 40% of survey films will arouse suspicion that intraabdominal injury has occurred. Williams and Zollinger [113] have reported that films of the chest and abdomen were a diagnostic aid in 34% of patients with abdominal injury, being most helpful in evaluating urinary-tract injuries and least helpful in splenic, pancreatic, and hepatic injuries. Wilson and Sherman [114] reported that survey evaluations of the abdomen were of no diagnostic value in 89.6% of patients with perforating abdominal injuries. These figures clearly demonstrate the difficulty in plain-film diagnosis and suggest that in the patient with abdominal trauma, plain-film examination should be used primarily to direct the attention of the clinician and radiologist to additional areas of investigation.

A systematic approach should be used in the evaluation of all survey studies. This approach includes: (a) evaluation of supporting structures; (b) recognition and localization of foreign bodies; (c) evaluation of organ size, position, and contour; (d) search for any evidence of mass; (e) evaluation for the presence of free or loculated extraluminal gas; (f) search for free or loculated fluid; and (g) recognition of any alteration in the normal pattern of intraluminal gas in the gastrointestinal pattern (Fig. 3.14).

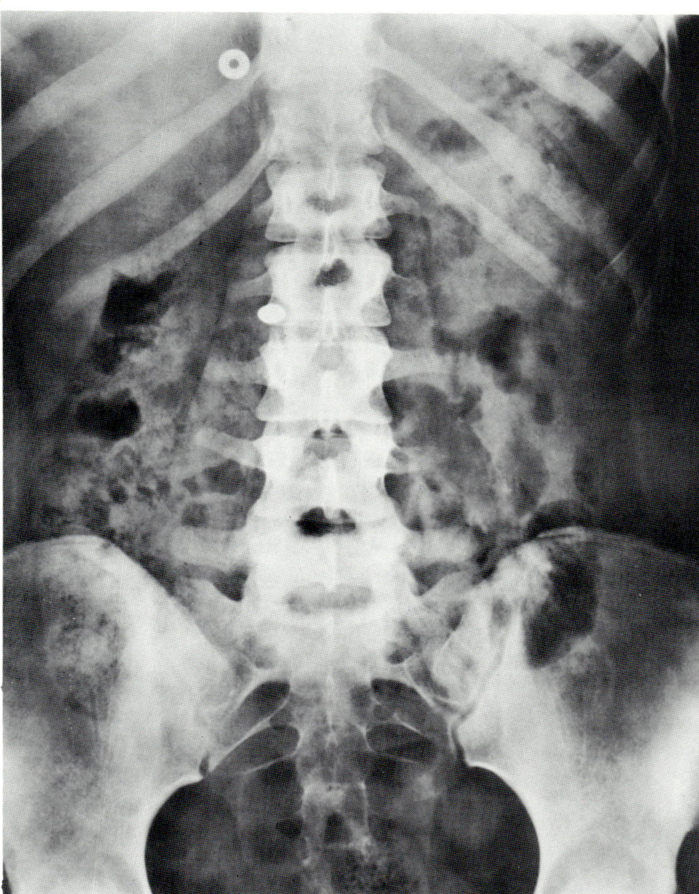

FIG. 3.14. This female patient was seen in the emergency room following blunt abdominal trauma sustained in an automobile accident. The abdominal examination is normal; the abdominal gas pattern is nonspecific; the soft tissue and osseous supporting structures are intact; the paracolic gutters and pelvis are free of fluid; there is no evidence of intraperitoneal or retroperitoneal gas; the inferior hepatic and splenic angles are sharp and distinct; and the psoas and renal silhouettes are unremarkable.

EVALUATION OF SUPPORTING STRUCTURES

A useful finding suggesting significant intraabdominal injury is the presence of fracture. The number and distribution of fractures may not only indicate the site of applied force, but also suggest whether the force was circumscribed or diffuse. In addition, a high association exists between certain types of fractures and specific organ injury. Diaphragmatic rupture and hollow viscus rupture or perforation are frequently observed in the presence of fractures of the lower thoracic and upper lumbar spine—particularly flexion-type fractures [27]. There is also a high association between chance fractures (a transverse, horizontal fracture through the body, pedicle, and lamina of the lumbar vertebral body with no decrease in vertebral body height) and other lumbar-spine fractures and bowel perforations [27,63]. Fifty percent of patients with hepatic or splenic injury have fractures of the lower right or left ribs, respectively [64] (Fig. 3.15). Fifteen to twenty percent of patients with fractures of innominate bones have associated urinary bladder injury [95], and small-bowel perforations frequently occur with these same innominate-bone fractures [64].

The evaluation of fractures may also be significant when dealing with penetrating injuries secondary to a bullet wound. The type of fracture (impact vs shatter) and the degree of distraction of fracture fragments can give some indication of the velocity and/or composition of the bullet on entry, and in turn, suggest the degree of cavitational effect the bullet may have produced as it passed through the abdominal tissues. The location of fractures, as well as the presence of bone fragments at some distance from the original fracture site, can indicate the probable course of the bullet through the abdomen (Fig. 3.16).

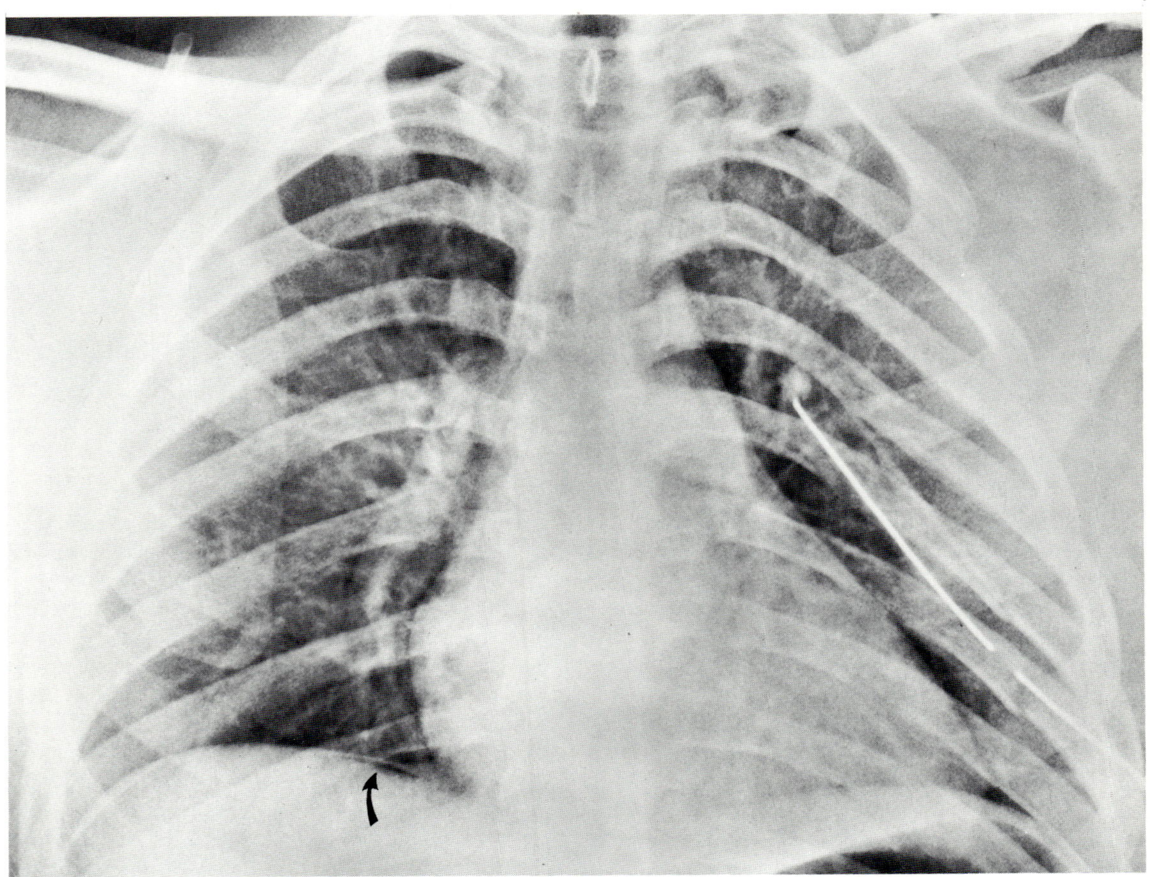

FIG. 3.15. This 22-year-old male was admitted to the hospital after falling down four flights of stairs. A radionuclide scan of the spleen revealed a 4–5 cm defect. The chest examination reveals fracture of the posterior lateral aspects of left ribs 6–10. A chest tube has been inserted for evacuation of a pneumothorax. There is free intraperitoneal air *(curved solid arrow)* that is secondary to an emergency peritoneal lavage and not to hollow viscus rupture. A lacerated spleen was found at exploration.

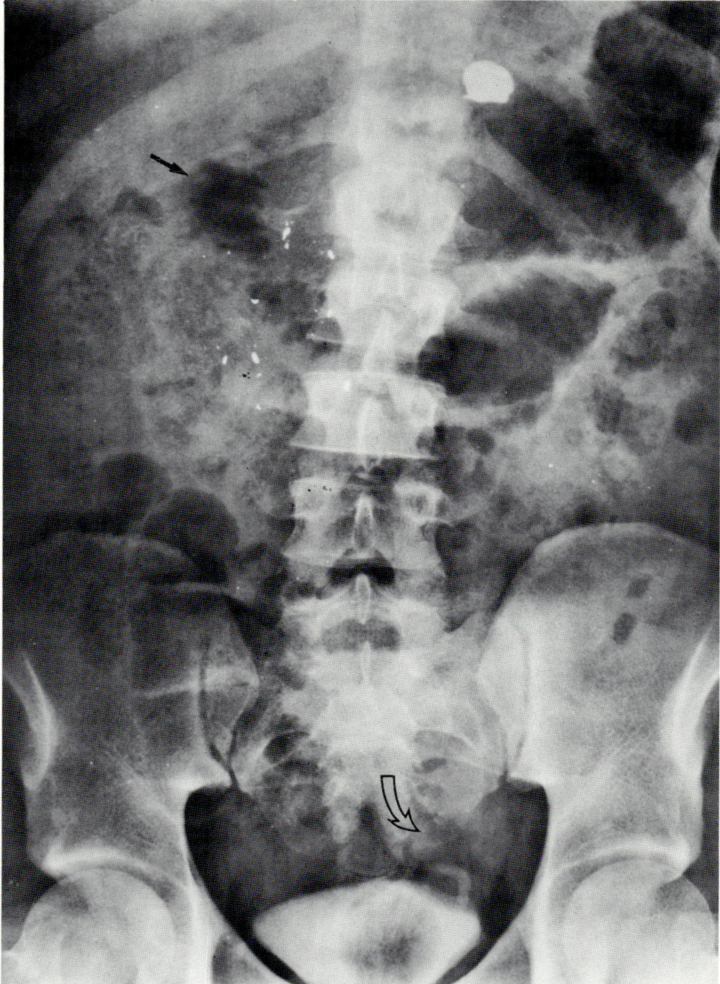

FIG. 3.16. This 22-year-old male was shot in the right back with a rifle. A drip infusion IVP reveals multiple small bullet fragments to the right of L1–3. The major bullet fragment is projected into the medial aspect of the 11th left rib interspace. There is a fracture of the right transverse process of L1 with nonvisualization of the right kidney. The left kidney has a ptotic position in the pelvis *(curved open arrow).* A sentinel duodenal loop *(straight solid arrow)* is present, and multiple bullet fragments are projected over the region of the pancreatic head. Free intraperitoneal air and fluid are present but not clearly seen on this projection. Hepatic, right renal, pancreatic, duodenal, colonic, and/or gastric injuries are suggested by these findings. At exploration, lacerations of the portal vein and liver, pancreas, stomach, transverse colon, and right kidney were found and repaired.

Evaluation of the soft tissues supporting structures can indicate the site of application of the force producing the trauma, the localized effects of that force on the soft tissue, and underlying visceral involvement. The soft tissues of the flanks have a specific structural pattern that is generally concave between the thorax and the iliac crests. Asymmetry of this normal structural pattern may be indicative of localized soft-tissue injury and/or be a reflection of more extensive intraabdominal abnormality. Such asymmetry may be indicated in a unilateral decrease in the distance between the costal arch and the iliac crest and a unilateral increase in the soft-tissue density of the flank due to a shortening and broadening of the muscle mass on that side. There may be ipsilateral broadening and medial curving of the properitoneal fat line in association with the changes in the muscle mass. Caution must be used in such interpretation. Infants, children, the debilitated, and older patients have a relative scarcity of fat, so that properitoneal- and fascial-fat changes may be missed or misinterpreted. Poor positioning of the patient may result in false-positive findings that are unrelated or only incidentally related (such as guarding due to pain) to significant injury. Particular care must be used when evaluating the psoas silhouette radiologically. Elkin and Cohen [25] have reported that changes in the radiologic appearance of the psoas muscles are of questionable diagnostic value. In a review of 200 asymptomatic patients, they found asymmetry of the psoas muscles in 25% of patients on a single study and in 11% of patients on multiple studies. In addition, they found absence of definition of one psoas muscle in 7.5% of patients on a single study and in 2.5% of patients on multiple examinations (Fig. 3.17). They concluded that obliteration of the psoas margin is of significance only when

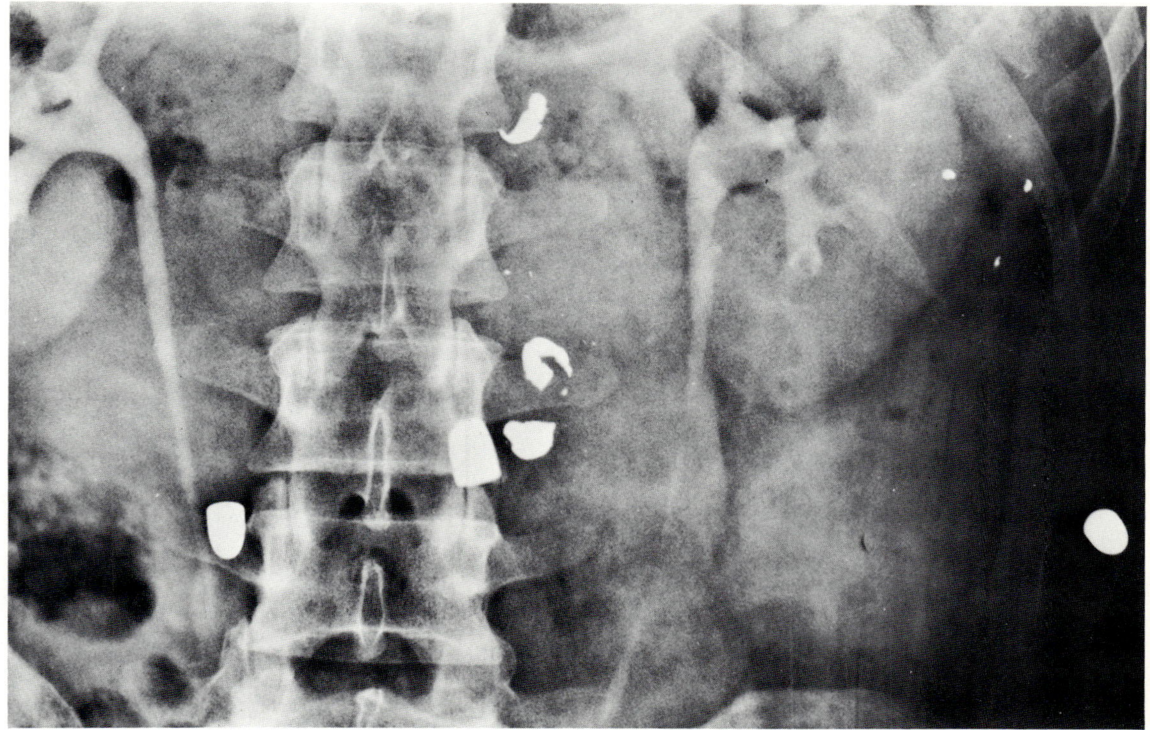

A

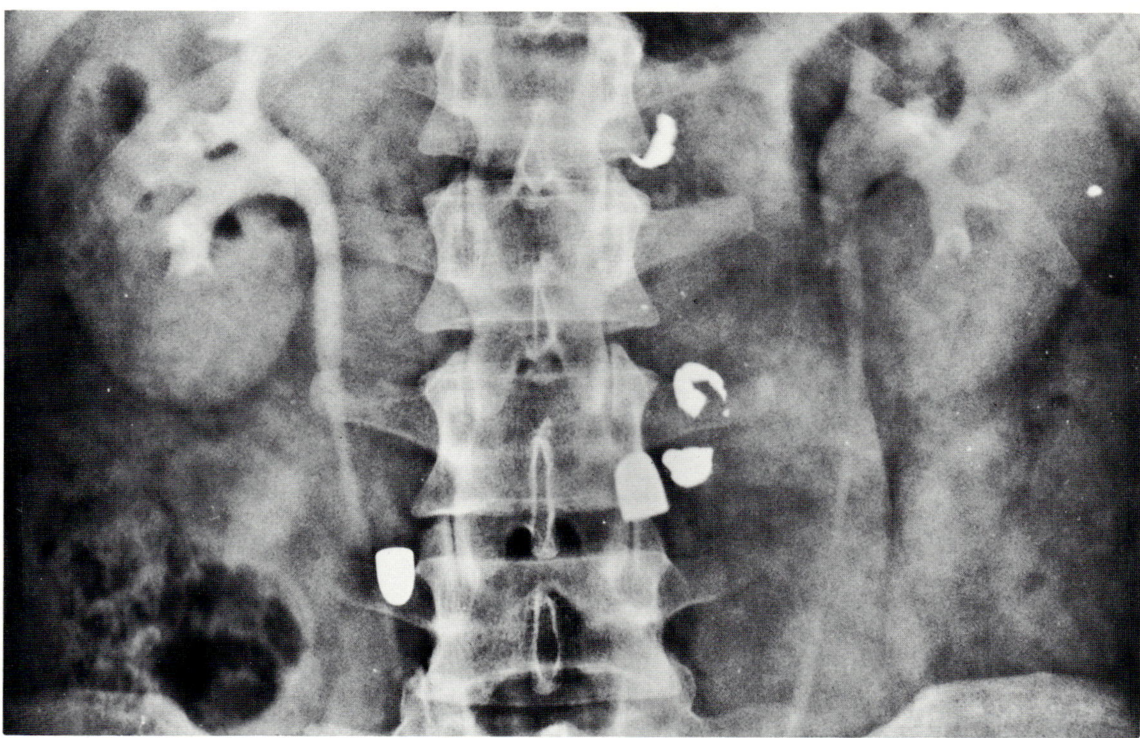

B

FIG. 3.17. This male patient had an infusion pyelogram performed after he sustained multiple gunshot wounds to the abdomen. The examination reveals an intact urinary system. However, the **(A)** 15-min film shows absence of the right psoas silhouette, which is visible on the **(B)** 30-min film of that same study.

it is unilateral and in association with a loss of the ipsilateral renal outline or inferior and medial displacement of the colon.

RECOGNITION OF FOREIGN BODIES AND THEIR LOCATIONS [68]

The presence of an intraperitoneal foreign body is suggestive of peritoneal perforation. For exact localization of such a foreign body at least two views of the abdomen, at 90 degrees to each other, are needed. Even when these views are available, care must be taken in making a definite statement concerning intraperitoneal localization. The reason for this is the cross-sectional geometry of the abdomen. When viewed in cross section from either above or below, the abdomen has the configuration of a cylinder that is flattened anteri-

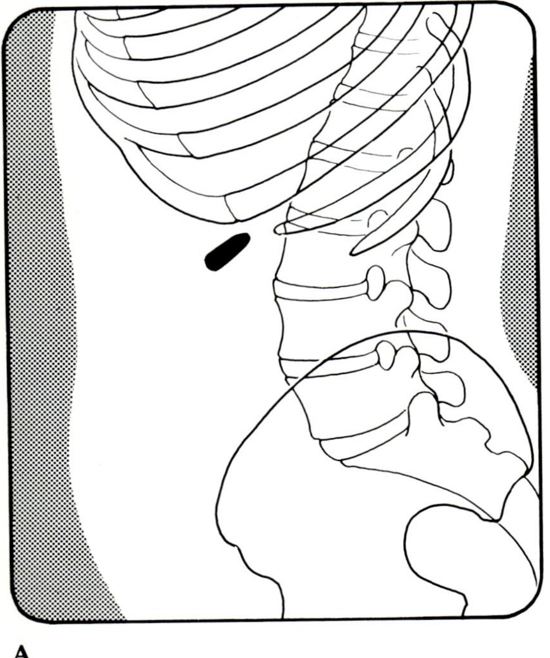

A

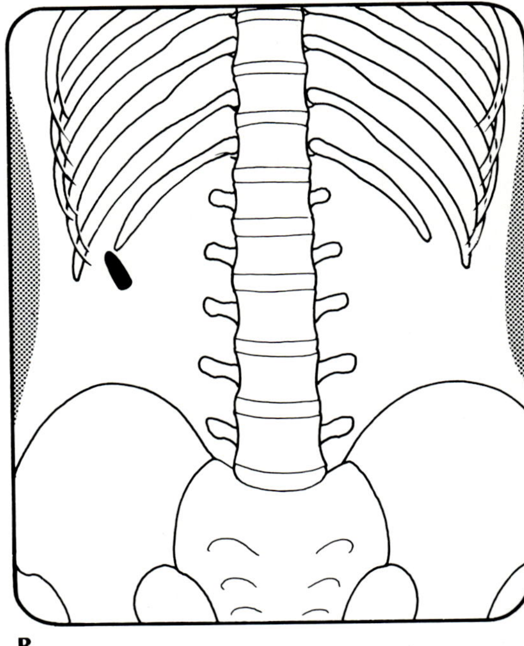

B

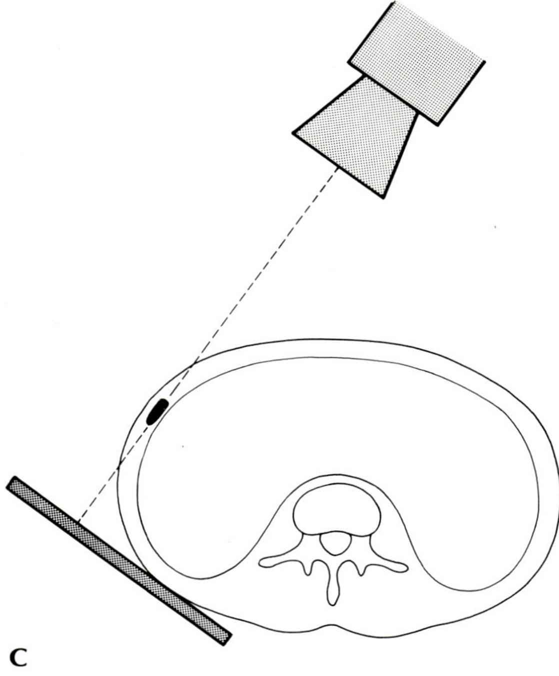

C

FIG. 3.18. Two projections of the abdomen—LAT **(A)** and AP **(B)**—suggest intraperitoneal location of the bullet, which is actually lying in the soft tissues of the right anterolateral abdominal wall. For exact localization, a tangential-beam study **(C)** is necessary.

orly and posteriorly. If a rectangle is constructed by connecting lines that pass at a tangent to the anterior, posterior, and lateral abdominal walls, it can readily be realized that a foreign body lying on or within that portion of the abdominal wall beneath the right angles of the rectangle may appear on the AP and lateral projections to be lying within the abdominal cavity. For exact localization, oblique films, with the patient positioned so that the X-ray beam passes tangentially through the suspected site of the foreign body, are necessary (Figs. 3.18, 3.19).

Although mobility of a foreign body (changes in its position occurring with corresponding changes in the patient's position) is suggestive of intraperitoneal location, this finding (or lack of it) must be analyzed with caution. A foreign body lying within the lumen of the hollow viscus would be mobile but not technically intraperitoneal; a foreign body lying partially or completely within an organizing hematoma on the wall or periphery of an abdominal viscus may be immobile but technically intraperitoneal.

If the site of entrance of a foreign body is labeled with lead markers and if the foreign body is found to be immobile, then a straight line drawn between the entrance wound and the foreign body can suggest its probable course and the structures that may have been injured. However, rapidly moving missiles, such as bullets, may change their trajectory at the interface between tissues of varying density. Therefore, the final position of the foreign body may not bear a straight-line relationship with the entrance wound [21]. The presence of particulate matter, such as bullet fragments or bone spicules, extending from the site of entrance to the final position of the missile may also be used in an effort to determine the probable course and structures injured by the passage of the missile (Figs. 3.20–3.22).

Finally, the presence of an intraabdominal foreign body related to a traumatic lesion is evidence of contamination of the wound and of the peritoneal cavity (Fig. 3.23).

EVALUATION OF ORGAN SIZE, POSITION, AND CONTOUR

In evaluating any traumatized patient, it must be kept in mind that the abnormalities produced by the trauma may be superimposed on preexisting pathologic disorders or alterations. In addition, what is normal for a particular patient may not exactly fit the parameters of normality described in the standard textbook. Because of this, posttraumatic radiologic studies are best analyzed with reference to recent, pretraumatic films, if these are available.

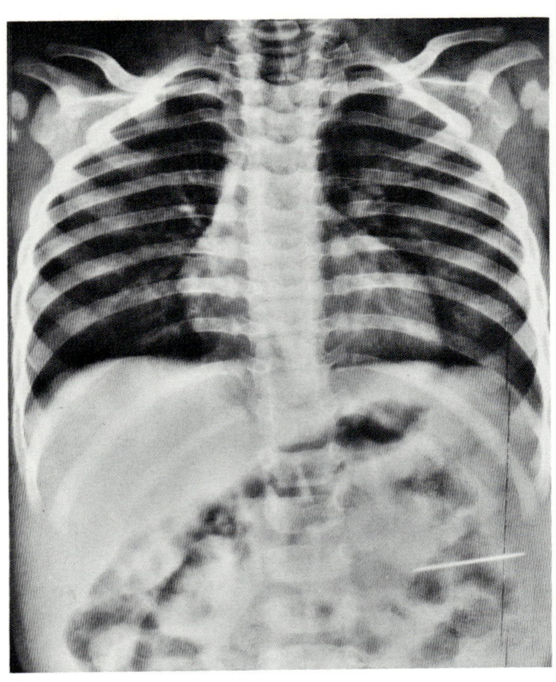

A

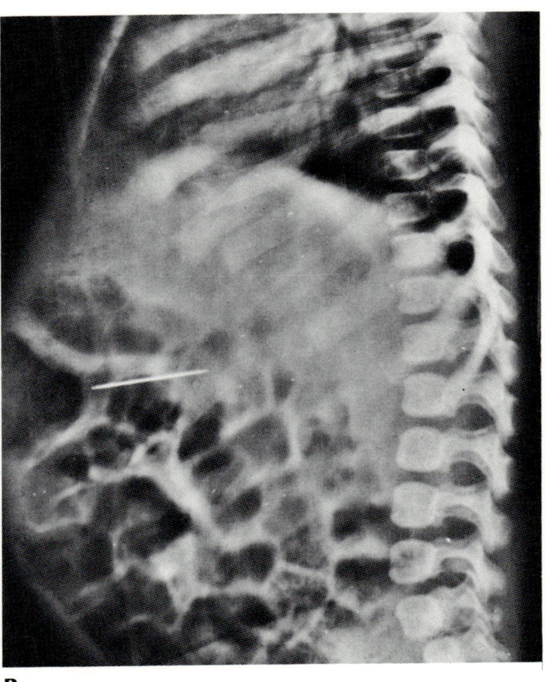

B

FIG. 3.19. The **(A)** frontal and **(B)** lateral projections of this child's abdomen suggest intraperitoneal location of a metallic foreign body (sewing needle). Physical examination revealed that this needle was in the soft tissues of the left anterolateral abdominal wall.

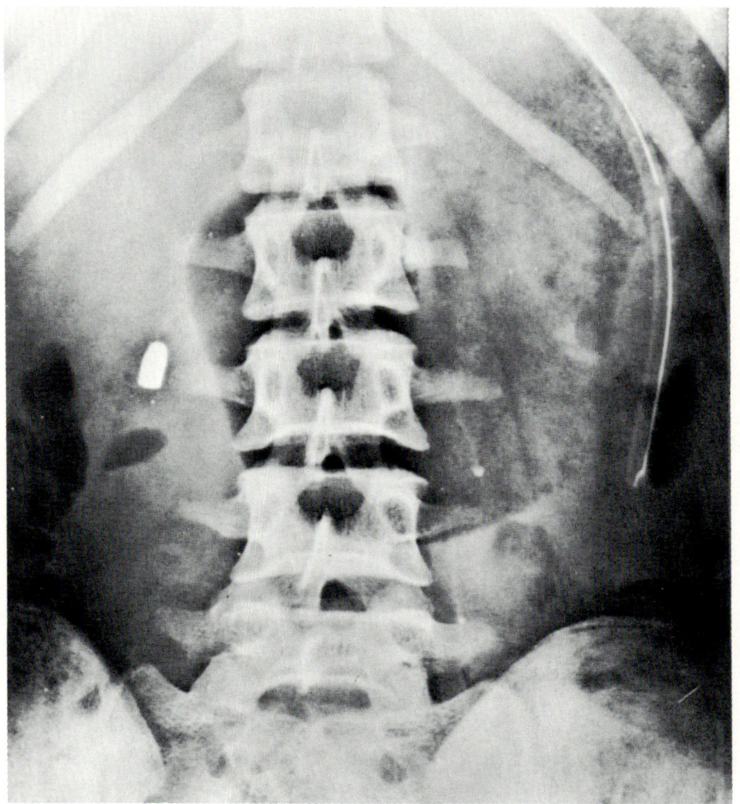

A

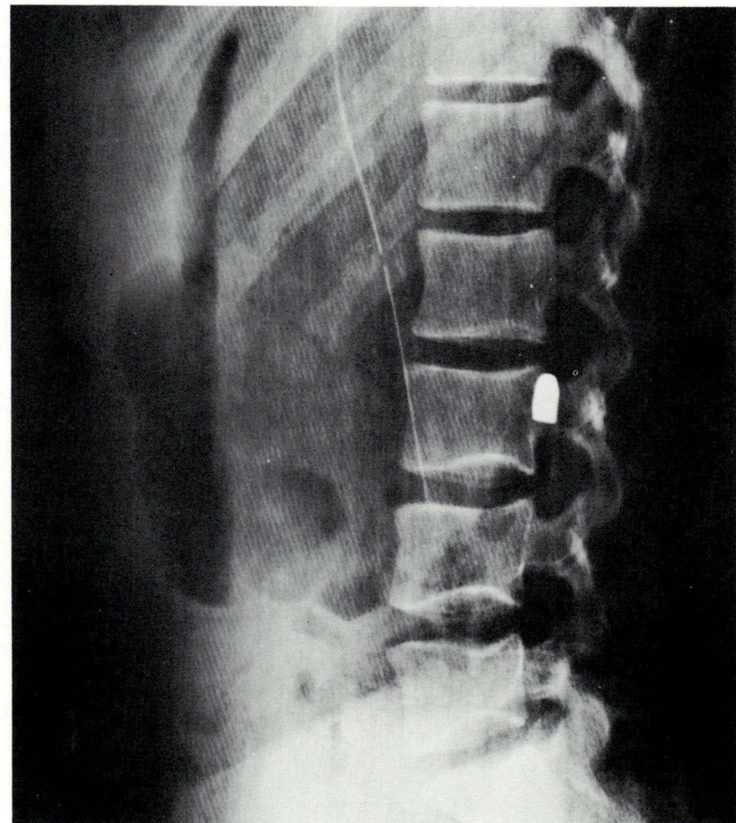

B

FIG. 3.20. (A) Frontal and **(B)** lateral examination of the abdomen of this male patient with a gunshot entrance wound to the right of the umbilicus reveals the bullet lying in the posterior soft tissues of the right side of the abdomen. Loss of the right psoas silhouette and increase in the retrogastric space are consistent with a large retroperitoneal-fluid collection. At exploration, lacerations of the antrum of the stomach and head of the pancreas were found and repaired (same patient as in Figure 3.7.).

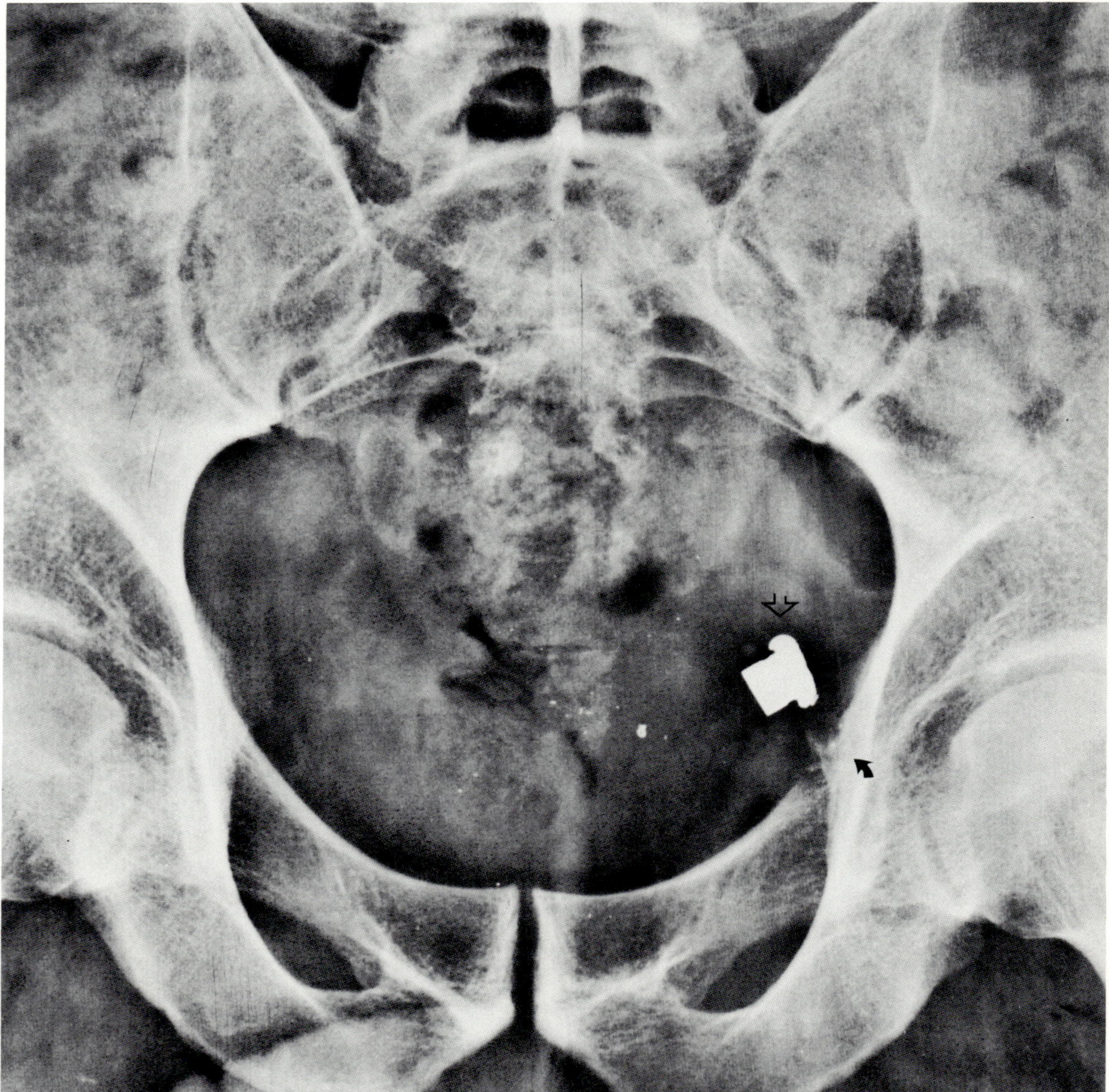

FIG. 3.21. This 41-year-old male sustained a gunshot wound to the right buttock. AP examination of the pelvis reveals an impact fracture of the left superior pubic ramus *(curved solid arrow)* with multiple metallic densities in the pelvic soft tissues. The bulk of the bullet *(open arrow)* lies in the soft tissues of the left hemipelvis. The implied course of the bullet suggests bladder and/or rectal injury. The patient was found to have a laceration of the posterior bladder base.

The plain-film evaluation of the abdomen requires the presence of either fat density or air to outline and define the abdominal viscera. Unfortunately, the properitoneal and extraperitoneal fat layers define posterior structures better than anterior ones. Thus, in evaluating an AP view of the abdomen, the posterior aspects of such organs as the liver and spleen are defined primarily. Therefore, deviations in contour or organ size anteriorly may not be appreciated on these studies. In addition, changes in the patient's position may result in alterations of organ position, contour, and size as a response to gravity.

In spite of these pitfalls, a recognition of abnormalities in size, position, and contour may be of benefit in suspecting the presence of intraabdominal injury. Such suspicion should be confirmed or denied by appropriate, additional diagnostic studies.

SEARCH FOR MASS

Abdominal masses in the acutely traumatized patient appear as soft-tissue densities that displace and separate normal anatomic structures. The recognition of such masses is dependent on the contrast provided by the fat and air densities within the abdomen.

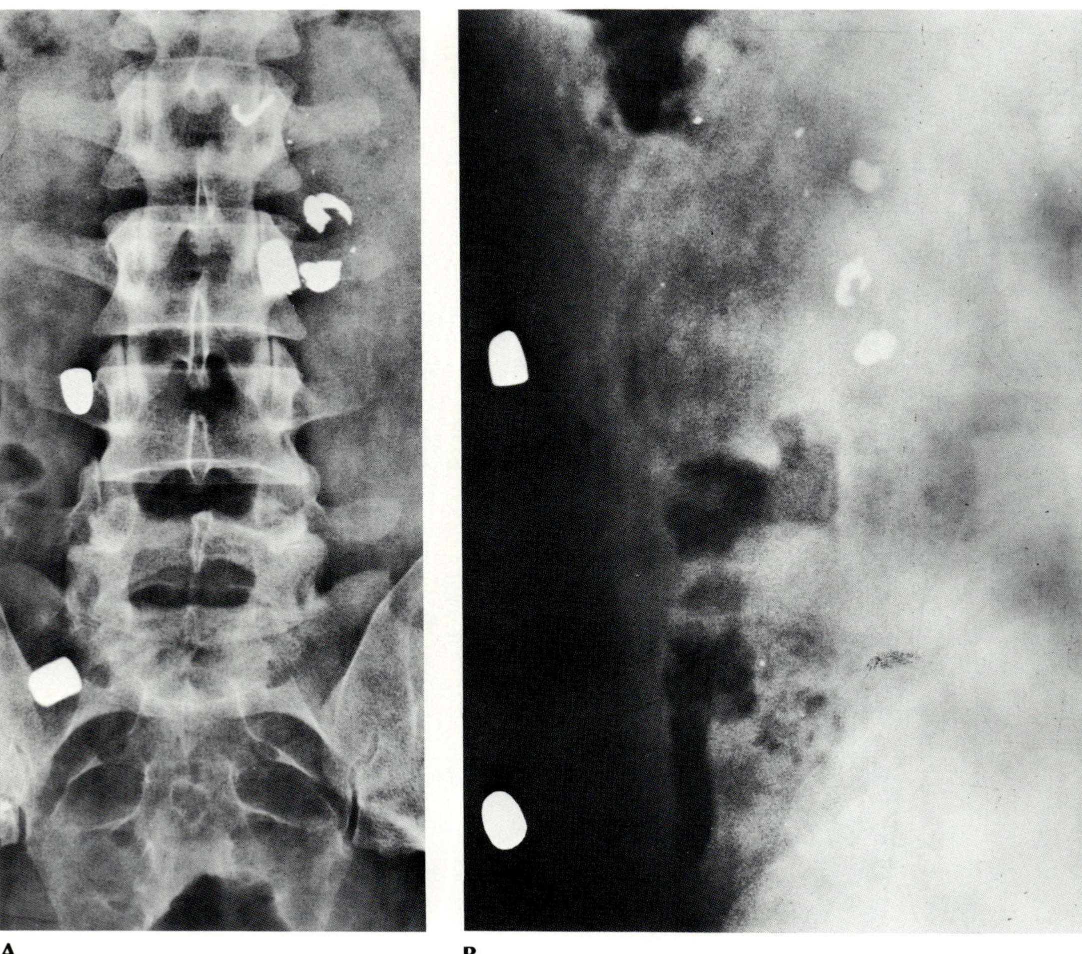

FIG. 3.22. The **(A)** AP abdominal examination of this male patient with multiple gunshot wounds to the chest and abdomen suggests intraperitoneal location of all the bullets. The **(B)** lateral projection reveals that two of the bullets are in the anterior abdominal wall and a third is in the retroperitoneal area.

Splenic and Parasplenic Masses. Normally, only the inferior one-half or one-third of the spleen is visible on plain films of the abdomen [68]. Therefore, contour defects, localized bulges, and significant enlargement of this organ may be difficult to appreciate. However, the effects of these changes may be more obvious and thus diagnostic. There may be elevation of the left hemidiaphragm, medial displacement of the stomach, indentation and distortion of the gastric fundus, and depression of the splenic flexure and left kidney. The presence of such findings indicates the need for more definitive diagnostic studies (Fig. 3.24).

Liver and Parahepatic Masses. The liver represents the largest soft-tissue density present beneath the right hemidiaphragm. The superior and lateral margins of this structure are normally not clearly visible. The lower, posterior border of the liver is usually found under the costal margin on the right side and passes obliquely upward to the eighth or ninth costal cartilage on the left. The quadrate and caudate lobes of the liver are subdivisions of the right lobe and can cause an irregularity on the inferior margin of the liver. The lower liver edge shows a significant change in position and contour when the patient changes from the supine to the erect position. In addition, normal or exaggerated respiration can alter the position of this lower liver edge.

Because of the large area the liver occupies, there are a variety of findings that may be observed on plain-film examinations, indicating diffuse or localized hepatic changes. The right hemidiaphragm may be elevated; there may be a bulging of the right flank, the stomach may be displaced to the left and posteriorly;

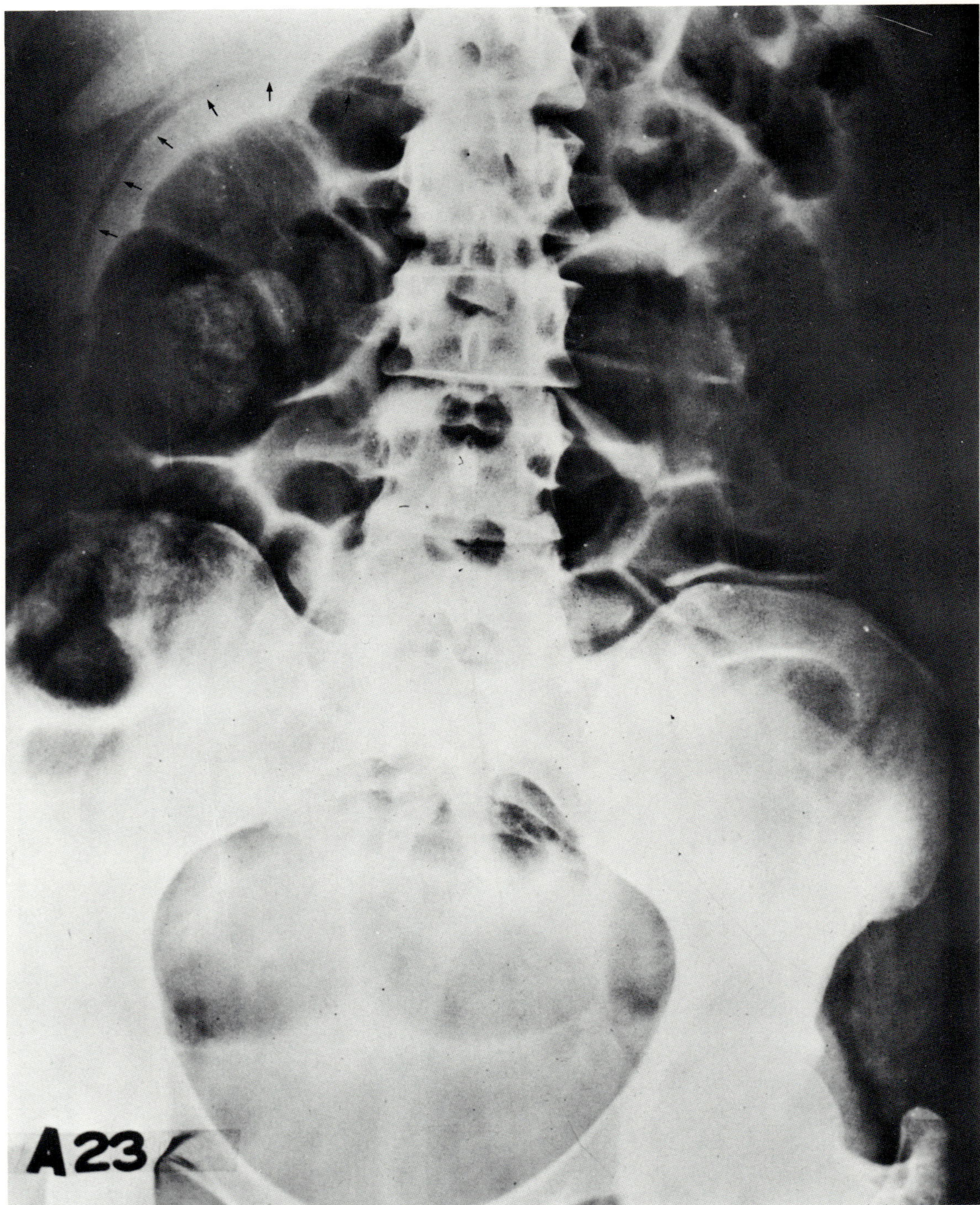

FIG. 3.23. This 33-year-old pregnant female attempted an illegal abortion on herself. Twenty-four hours after the attempt, she developed the signs and symptoms of an acute abdomen. The AP supine examination of her abdomen reveals a curvilinear foreign body *(small arrows)* in the RUQ, representing a catheter that was "lost" in the peritoneal cavity during the attempt. The increased pelvic soft-tissue density and elevation of bowel loops out of the pelvis are due to fluid accumulation and abscess formation following the perforation of the uterus.

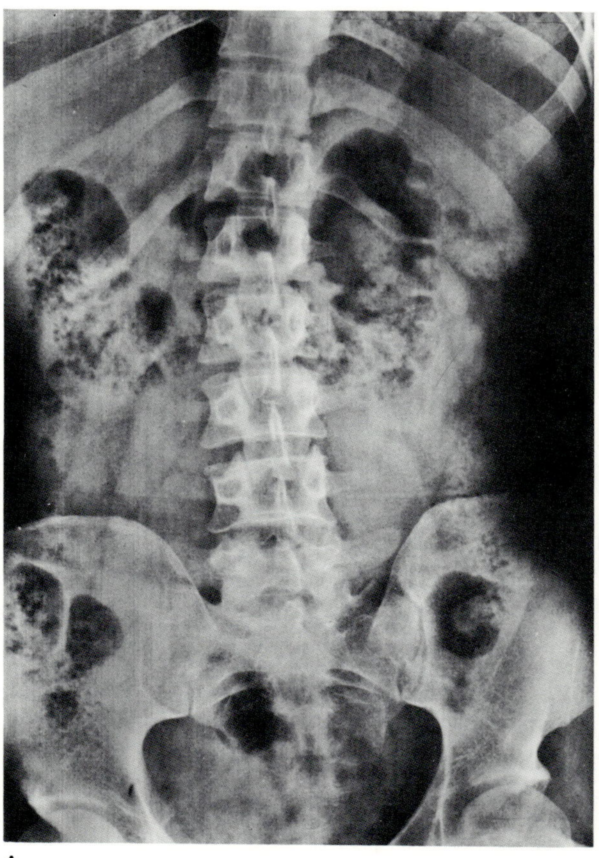

A

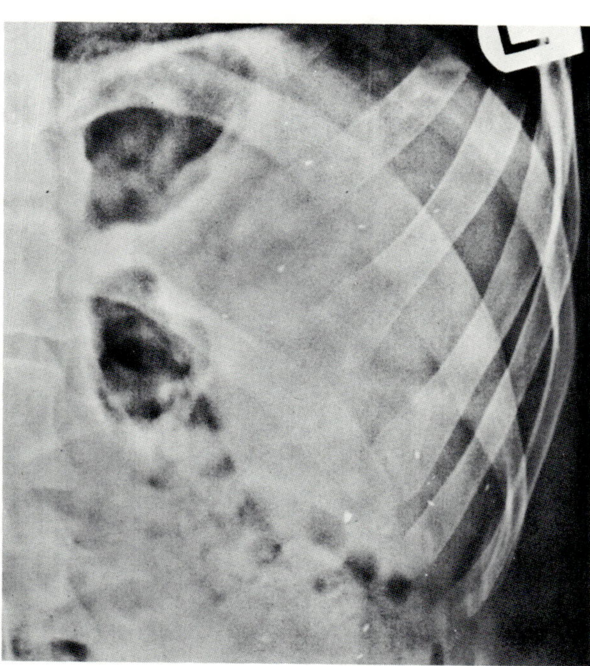

B

FIG. 3.24. This male patient was admitted to the hospital with the history of blunt abdominal trauma—he was beaten. **(A)** AP examination of the abdomen fails to reveal any evidence of lower-rib fractures. However, there is a LUQ soft-tissue mass that is depressing the splenic flexure of the colon and medially deviating the stomach; pelvic soft-tissue findings (dog-ear sign of McCort) suggest the presence of free intraperitoneal fluid. **(B)** Close-up view of the left-upper-abdominal mass. Exploration of the abdomen revealed a large splenic laceration that was confined by an intact capsule; minimal free blood was present in the peritoneal cavity.

the hepatic flexure and transverse colon may be depressed; the right kidney may be depressed and its axis altered; and if the mass effect is extensive enough, there may be downward and leftward displacement of small-bowel loops. Usually, there is no displacement of the second part of the duodeum or the duodenal-jejunal junction.

The two examples of regional masses detailed above indicate that the major radiologic findings of importance to the radiologist are the presence of an area of increased soft-tissue density (mass) with displacement of adjacent structures. Not only may the mass cause displacement, but if the mass is strategically located, it may cause compression of surrounding structures and result in obstruction of the bowel, ureters, blood vessels, ductal systems, or any other structure that normally acts as a transporting conduit. Because of the varied manifestations of mass effect, the radiologist must have a detailed understanding of radiologic anatomy and its variations—normal and abnormal.

EVALUATION FOR THE PRESENCE OF FREE OR LOCULATED GAS

The only reasonable approach to the evaluation of plain film for the presence of free or loculated gas requires close communication between the radiologist and the referring clinician. The radiologist must be informed by the clinician of any therapeutic information (peritoneal lavage, wound synogram examination, excessive probing of a penetrating wound, etc.) that occurred between the time of trauma and the presentation of the patient for radiologic examination. Without adequate information, the diagnosis of free intraperitoneal air secondary to hollow-viscus injury may be in error (Fig. 3.15).

Free Intraabdominal Air. It is possible for air to be introduced into the peritoneal cavity along the course of a penetrating wound, through the vagina–uterus–fallopian-tube pathway in the female as a result of gynecologic procedures (Rubin's test), through variations in sexual activity, or as the result of recent abdominal surgery. However, in the acutely traumatized patient, the presence of free intraabdominal air must be assumed to be due to the rupture of a hollow viscus. Failure to follow this dictum will lead to an increased morbidity and mortality in the traumatized patient.

Jacobson and Carter [50] reported that in 80% of patients with stomach or duodenal-bulb perforations and in 100% of patients with colonic perforations, free air will be demonstrated radiologically. However, less than 50% of patients with small-bowel perforation will show free air and, when present, the air will be demonstrated in unusual locations (Fig. 3.25). This occurs because small-bowel perforations are usually short (0.4–2 cm in length), the interval between injury and radiologic examination is usually brief, the healthy adult has a small bowel that is usually devoid of gas, and the omentum of the transverse mesocolon may form an effective barrier against the escape of air from the small bowel [110]. In spite of these difficulties, with the appropriate technique as little as 1 cc of free intraabdominal air may be demonstrated on plain films [56] (Fig. 3.26). The classic method for demonstrating this finding is the erect chest film. An erect abdominal film may also be beneficial, but frequently the size of the patient precludes the diaphragmatic leaflets being included on the film.

Erect Chest Film. Air, because of gravity, tends to seek the highest level in a closed space. In the erect position, the highest portion of the abdominal cavity is just beneath the diaphragmatic leaflets. However, because of the many peritoneal reflections in the abdominal cavity, air may not be able to move freely. Occasionally, free air becomes trapped behind the transverse mesocolon and may present as a well-defined collection (radiolucent area), just to the left of the body of L2 [50] (Fig. 3.25). If air is able to reach its highest level in the abdominal cavity, small amounts will present as thin radiolucent lines just beneath one or both hemidiaphragms. Larger amounts may form lucent crescents, and still larger amounts may present as lucent hemispheres in the same areas (Fig. 3.27). Characteristically, the radiolucencies change location with changes in the patient's position, usually parallelling the curvature of the diaphragmatic dome at its apex. These lucent areas tend to decrease in size on expiration and increase on inspiration as the result of a relative negative-pressure area beneath the hemidiaphragms due to the algebraic sum of the pressures generated by the downward motion of the hemidiaphragms and upward, outward motion of the ribs on inspiration [69]. Confusion with intraabdominal air may occur in interposition of a loop of gas-filled bowel between the diaphragm and the liver or spleen. Plain-film differentiation is dependent on identifying the valvulae conniventes or haustral markings of the bowel and noting that changes in the patient's position fail to significantly modify the infradiaphramatic findings. If, for some reason, the differential cannot be made on plain films, then contrast evaluation of the upper and/or lower gastrointestinal tract is helpful. Extraperitoneal fat below the diaphragm (irregular diaphragm, or pseudopneumoperitoneum) [74], manifests as a crescentic radiolucency usually observed on the left side. It is the result of accumulation of extraperitoneal fat between the parietal peritoneum covering the inferior aspects of the diaphragm and the diaphragm

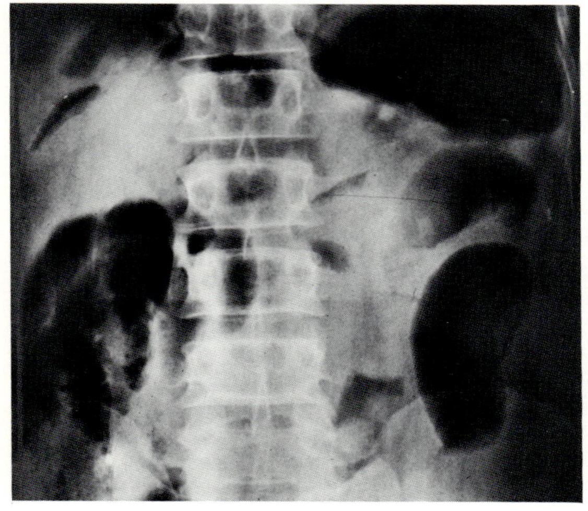

A

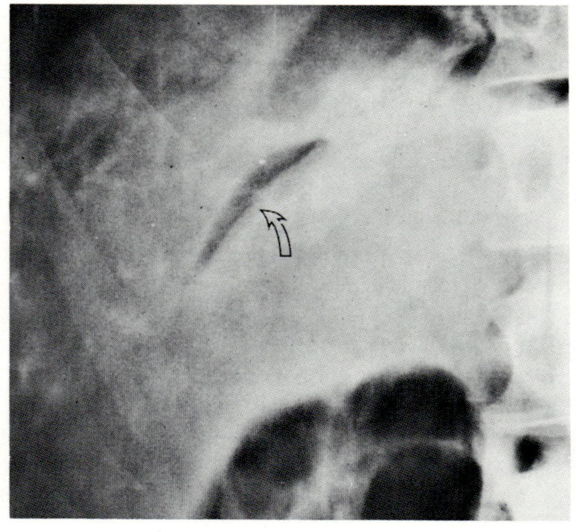

B

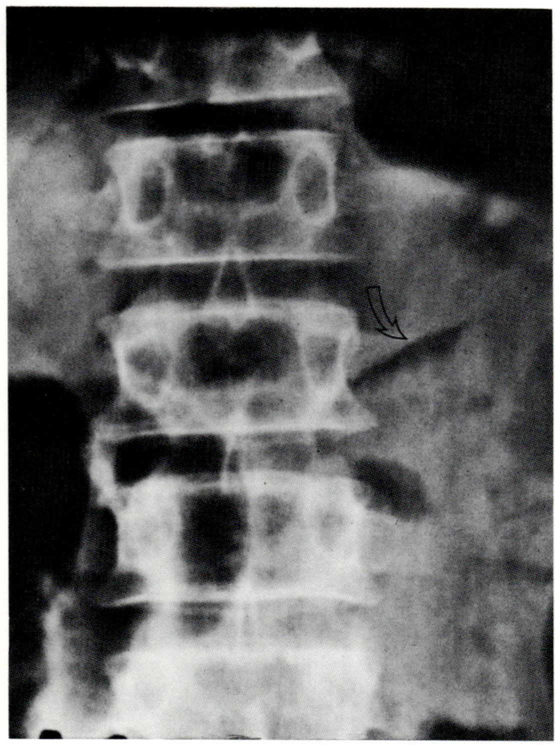

C

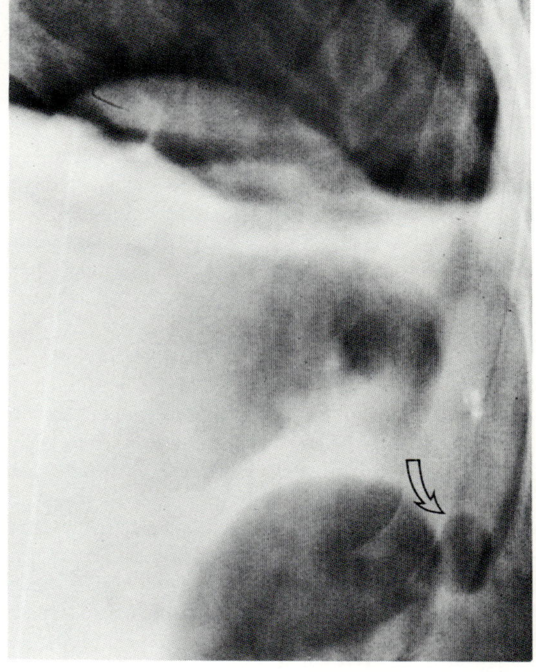

D

FIG. 3.25. This young male patient received multiple stab wounds to the abdomen. The **(A)** erect AP examination of the abdomen reveals the classic collection of radiolucency beneath the left hemidiaphragm indicative of free intraperitoneal air. Closer evaluation of this film shows less typical locations of free air: **(B)** RUQ—free air in Morrison's pouch *(open arrow)*: **(C)** epigastrum—free air beneath the transverse mesocolon *(open arrow)*; and **(D)** LUQ—free air beneath the phrenocolic ligament *(open arrow)*. These atypical locations raise the possibility of small-bowel perforation. Abdominal exploration revealed lacerations of the stomach, small bowel, and colon.

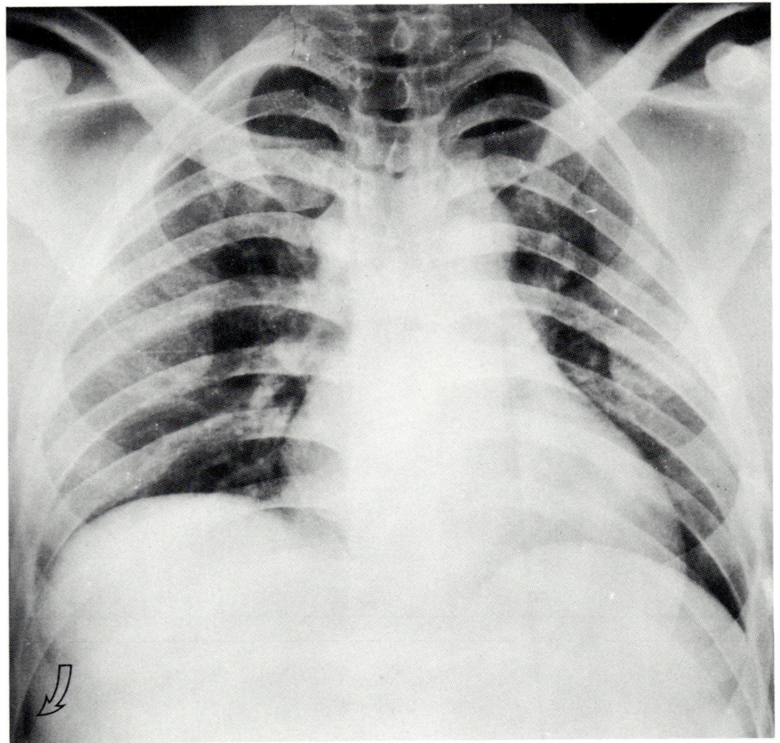

A

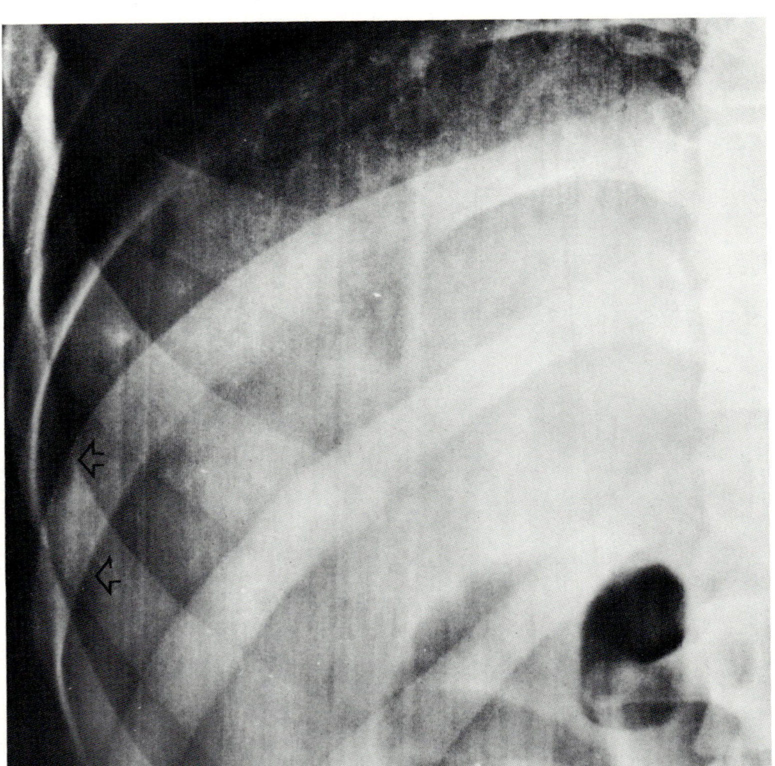

B

FIG. 3.26. This middle-aged male patient was admitted with an abdominal gunshot wound. The **(A)** chest examination reveals an unusual location of free intraperitoneal air between the right lateral abdominal wall and the liver silhouette *(curved open arrow)*. The **(B)** left lateral decubitus view of the abdomen shows a larger collection of free air *(arrowheads)* beneath the lateral abdominal wall.

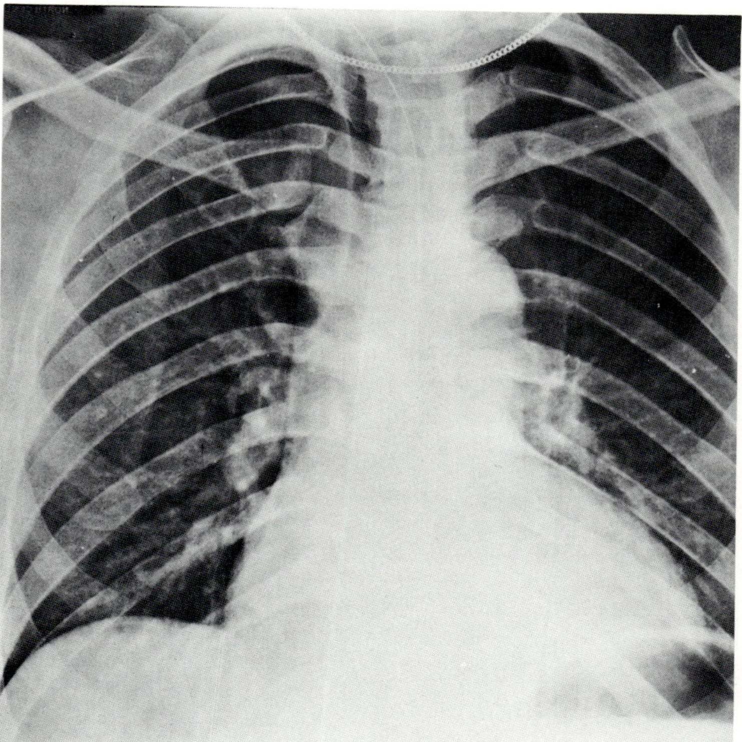

A

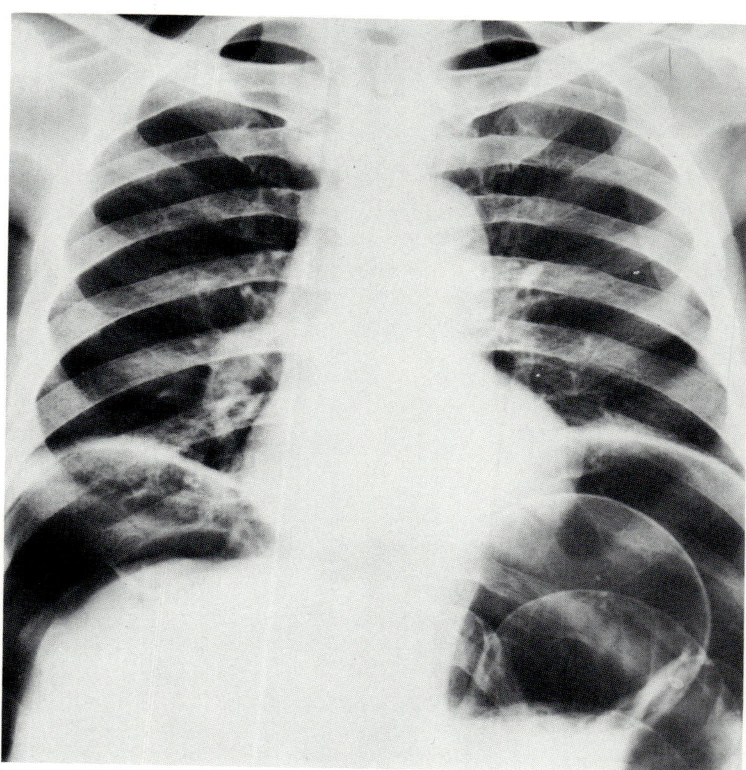

B

FIG. 3.27. These erect chest examinations of traumatized patients show the classic presentation of free intraperitoneal air as lucent collections beneath the diaphragms. In addition, the second **(B)** examination demonstrates Rigler's sign of free air.

itself. It may be recognized and differentiated from free intraperitoneal air by noting that the radiolucency fails to change its relationship to the diaphragm with changes in patient positioning. Contrast studies will fail to show bowel loops in the area of lucency.

Left Lateral Decubitus Views of the Abdomen. With the patient in the left lateral decubitus position, the highest point of the abdominal cavity is either between the lateral border of the right lobe of the liver and right abdominal wall or just above the right iliac crest. In patients with wide transverse pelvic diameters (females), this latter location is frequently the highest portion of the abdominal cavity in the left lateral decubitus position. If time is allowed for the air to gravitate to the most superior portion of the abdominal cavity, it will present as an area of radiolucency (lucent stripe, crescent, or hemisphere) in either of these locations [73] (Fig. 3.26). The right lateral decubitus position is not used because of the frequent problem of confusing free intraperitoneal air with air either in the stomach, descending colon, or small-bowel loops.

Supine Abdominal Films. In the supine position, the highest portion of the peritoneal cavity lies just beneath the anterior abdominal wall. When using the horizontal-beam technique, air may be identified as collections of radiolucency beneath the anterior abdominal wall. These collections will appear as lucent stripes, circular areas, crescents, hemispheres, or spheres and will be devoid of the usual bowel markings (Fig. 3.28).

On the AP supine film, a collection of air beneath the anterior abdominal wall will appear as a circular area of relative lucency on a background of soft-tissue density. The circular margin of the relative lucency represents the circumference of the air–fluid interface. A large collection of air, identified in this projection, has been called the "dome sign." The "dome sign" is converted to the "football sign" when a thin soft-tissue stripe is visualized running through it from the right upper abdomen to the umbilicus. This soft-tissue stripe represents the falciform ligament, which is visualized because of the contrast offered by the air collected on either side of it [64] (Fig. 3.29). On occasion, other linear soft-tissue densities, representing peritoneal reflections, may be demonstrated. Remnants of the omphalomesenteric vessels may appear as an inverted V with the apex of the V at the umbilicus and the legs extending distally below the umbilicus along the anterior abdominal wall. The residual of the urachus with its peritoneal reflection may present as a soft-tissue stripe in the midline, extending distally from the umbilicus [56]. For physiologic as well as pathophysiologic reasons, air within the peritoneal cavity may not be able to seek its highest level in this enclosed space. The previous discussion concerning air trapped beneath the transverse mesocolon and presenting as a lucency to the left of L2 is an excellent example. Air may also find itself trapped between bowel loops. When present in this location, both the inner and outer walls of the bowel may be demonstrated. The ability to identify the inner and outer margins of a segment of bowel wall (Rigler's sign) is pathognomonic for the presence of free intraperitoneal air (Fig. 3.30)

Loculated Intraabdominal Air. The pathologic alterations of tissues resulting from the trauma may trap air escaping from a hollow viscus and result in unusual radiologic presentations (Fig. 3.20). These collections may resemble abscess cavities or have the appearance of fecal material within the colon. Plain-film examinations with the patient in different positions or the use of contrast material introduced into either the large or small bowel may be of benefit in distinguishing such collections from fecal material. These same films may also be helpful in distinguishing intraperitoneal from retroperitoneal air collections.

Air in the Retroperitoneal Compartment. The retroperitoneal space is a totally closed area in both male and female. Therefore, air can enter the space in only one of three ways: (a) artificial introduction; (b) infection by a gas-forming organism; or (c) retroperitoneal rupture of the hollow viscus [105]. Since this area is not a potential space like the peritoneal cavity, air introduced into it is not freely mobile. The radiologic hallmark of retroperitoneal air is the presence of mottled or linear radiolucencies that often lie along established fascial planes and show little change with changes in the patient's position [69]. Air introduced into this space may dissect along a variety of pathways producing a wide variation in radiologic findings. Some of the possible routes of this dissection include: (a) around the kidneys, increasing their degree of definition; (b) upward, to lie beneath the hemidiaphragms or extend into the posterior mediasternum and even to the neck; (c) medially and downward along the margins of the psoas muscles, thereby increasing their degree of definition (and even down into the retroperitoneal pelvic tissues); (d) between the leaves of the transverse mesocolon or small-bowel mesentery; (e) inferior extension below the level of the renal fascia and the limitation of the lateroconal fascia with direct entrance into the properitoneal flank fat; and (f) through the posterior parietal peritoneum to enter directly into the peritoneal cavity [41,69,70,110,29].

Gas in the subphrenic, extraperitoneal tissues invariably has the appearance of a crescent. This crescentic area of radiolucency often parallels the lower plane

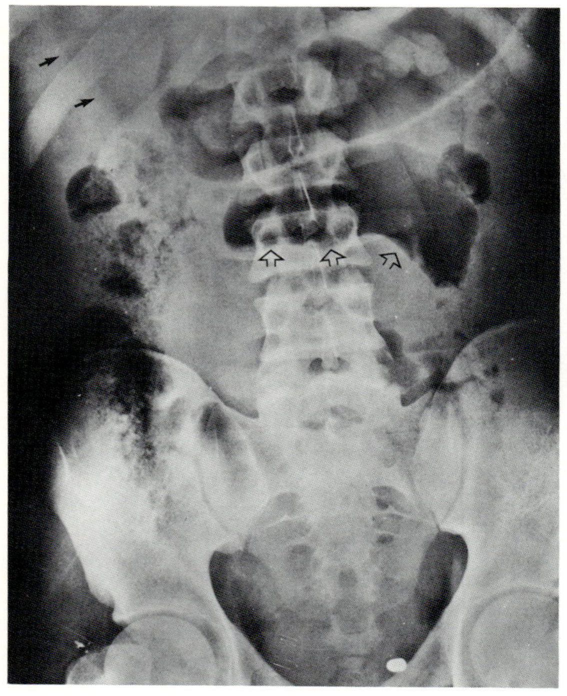

A

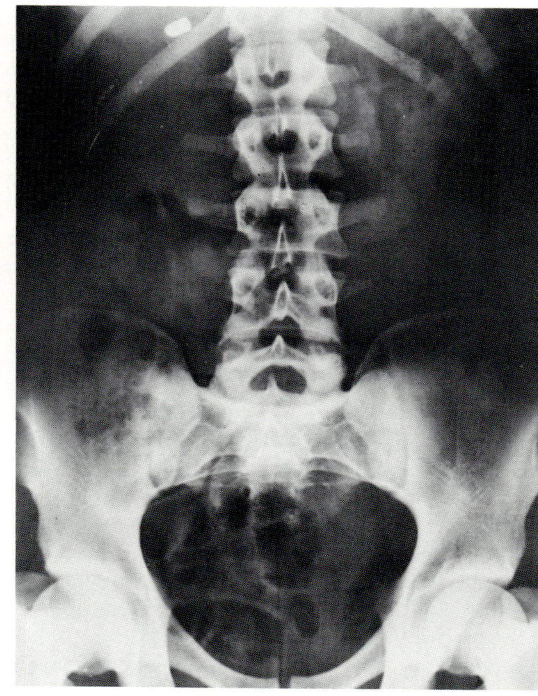

B

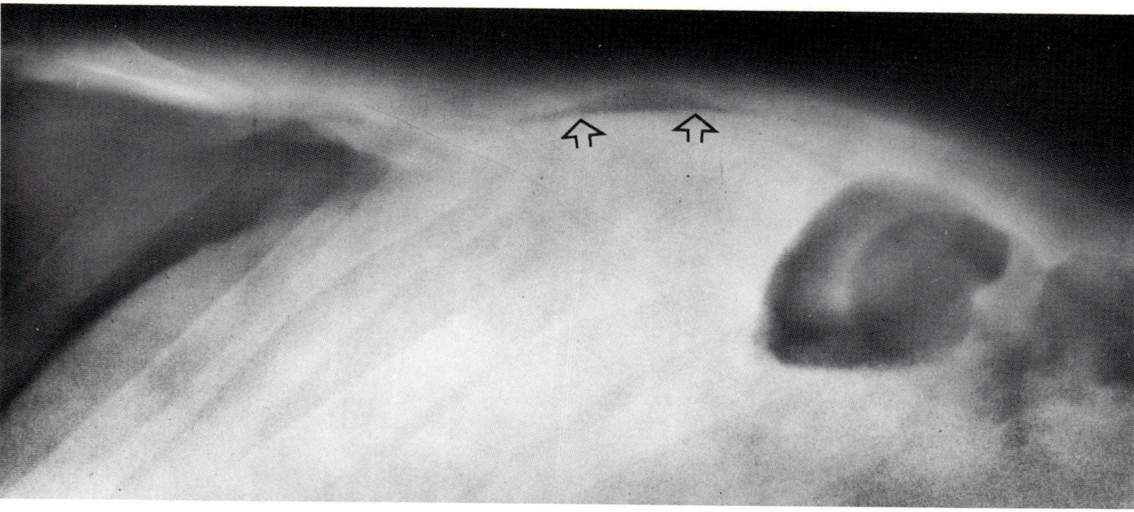

C

FIG. 3.28. This male patient had small-bowel perforation secondary to a gunshot wound to the abdomen. The **(A)** AP supine view of the abdomen reveals a relative lucency over the liver *(short arrows)* and a large, formless lucency beneath the transverse mesocolon *(open arrow)*—both are signs of free intraperitoneal gas. **(B)** This 18-year-old male received multiple gunshot wounds to the chest and abdomen. At exploration, splenic, diaphragmatic, and gastric perforations were found. The AP supine view of the abdomen fails to reveal evidence of free air. **(C)** Free air is clearly demonstrated, however, on the transtable lateral view *(open arrows).*

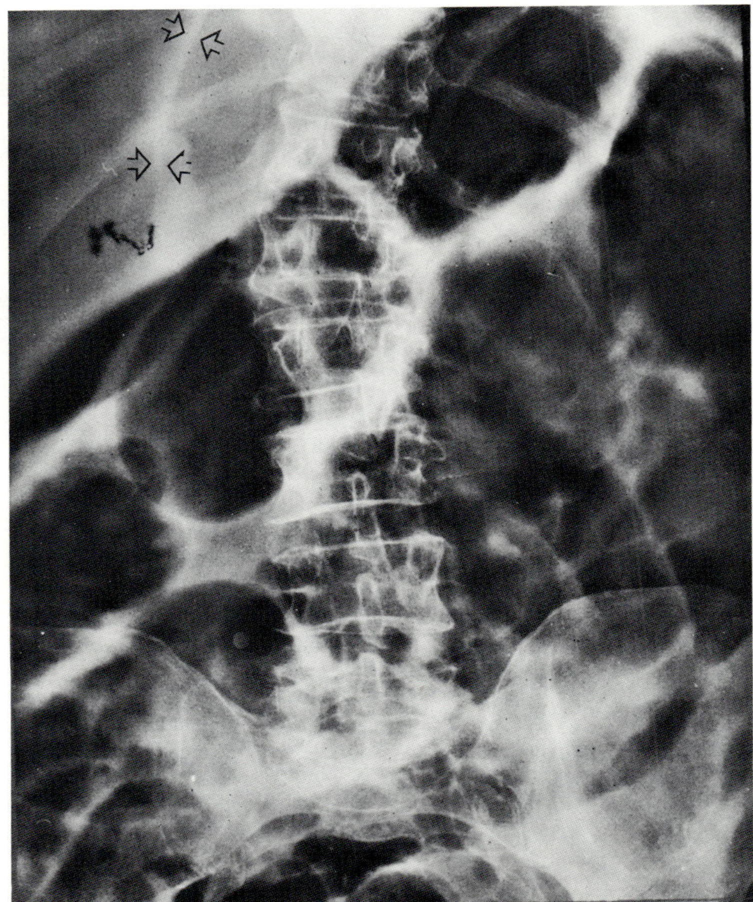

A

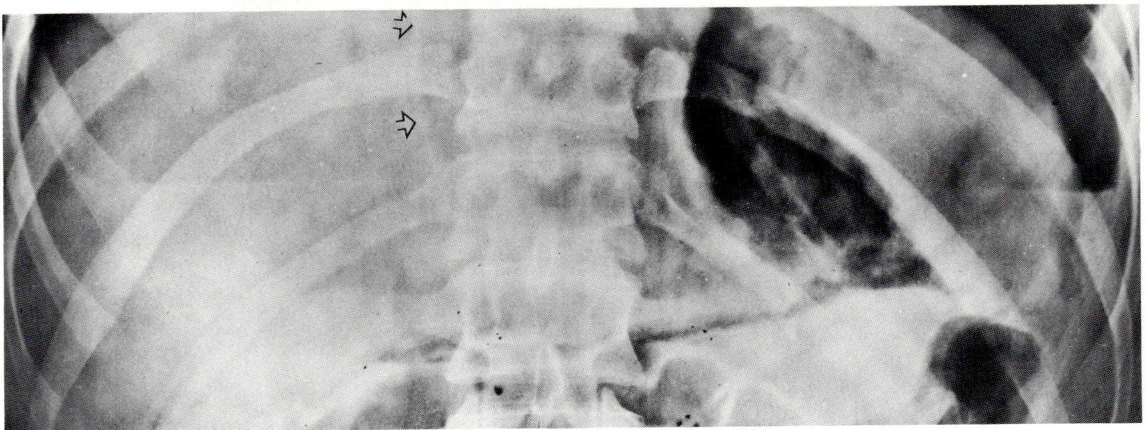

B

FIG. 3.29. In the presence of free air, the falciform ligament may be seen on supine (and occasionally erect) AP abdominal examinations as a curvilinear, vertically oriented, RUQ soft-tissue density. The contrast necessary for its demonstration is provided by the presence of air to either side of the ligament. **(A)** This supine AP abdominal examination of a blunt-trauma patient clearly demonstrates the falciform ligament *(open arrows),* which indicates the presence of free intraperitoneal air following hollow viscus rupture. **(B)** The erect abdominal examination of this victim of multiple abdominal stab wounds with hollow viscus perforation reveals air beneath both hemidiaphragms. In addition, the falciform ligament *(open arrows)* is also seen.

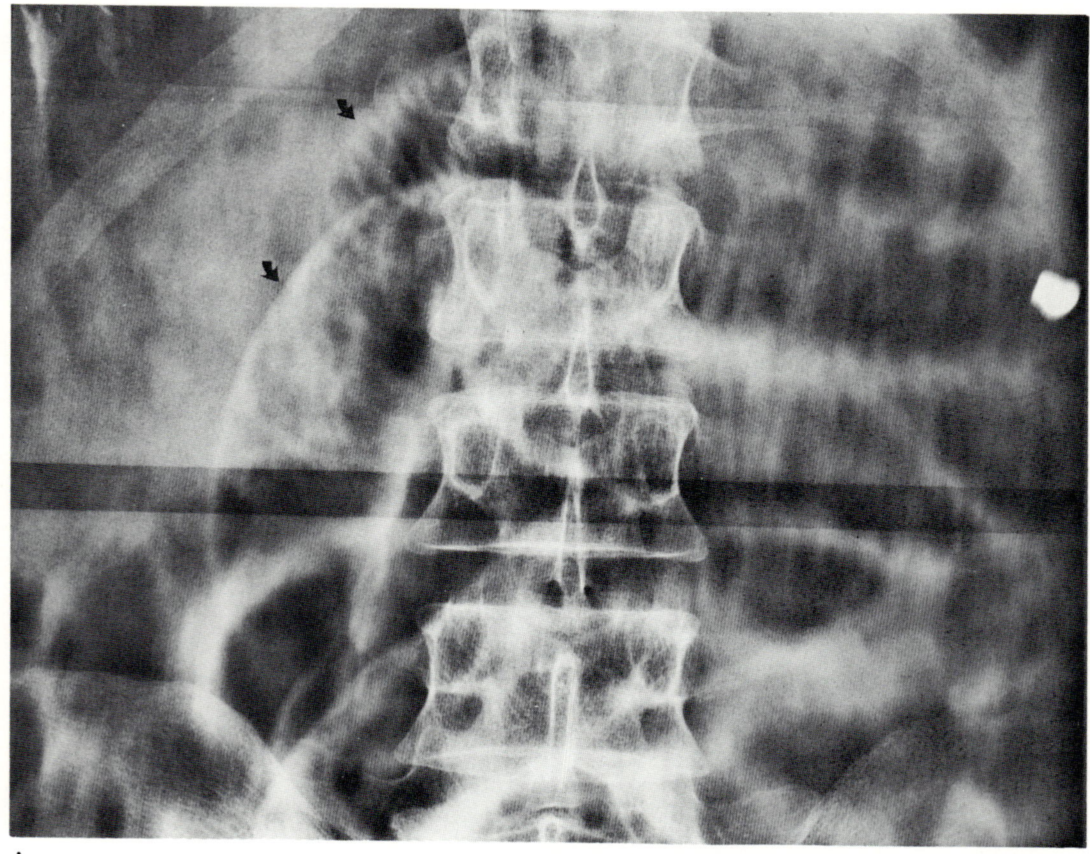

A

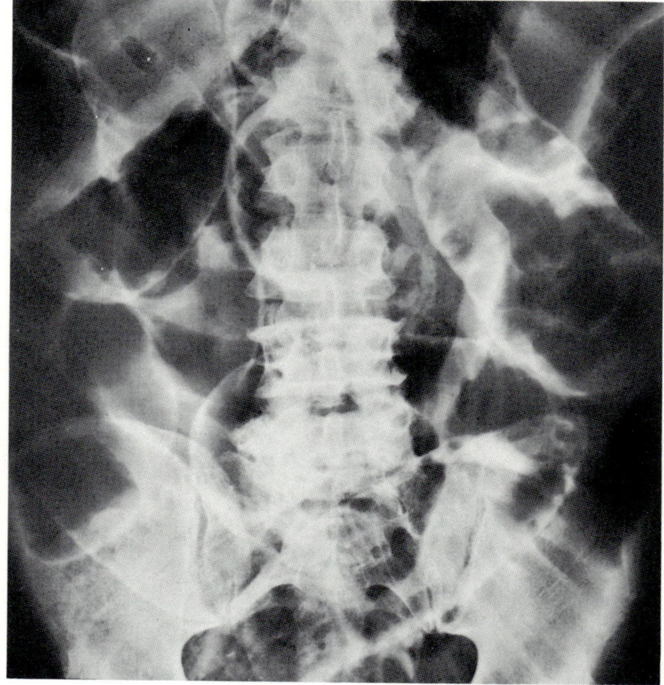

B

FIG. 3.30. The presence of intraluminal bowel gas and free intraperitoneal air may result in the clear and distinct visualization of the full thickness of the wall (or walls) of a bowel loop (or loops). This finding, called "Rigler's sign" is pathognomonic of free intraperitoneal air. **(A)** The AP supine abdominal examination of this 45-year-old gunshot victim with perforations of the stomach and colon reveals the presence of free intraperitoneal air by the clear visualization of the inner and outer bowel wall surfaces in RUQ. **(B)** The supine abdominal examination of a blunt-trauma patient with colonic perforation gives a more dramatic demonstration of the Rigler's sign of free intraperitoneal air.

(not the highest curvature) of the diaphragmatic dome and usually lies medial or lateral to its apex. This collection of gas appears to increase on expiration and decrease on inspiration on erect frontal plain films. This behavior is just the reverse of that observed with free intraperitoneal air [69].

When retroperitoneal air presents as bubbly or mottled lucencies against a soft-tissue background, it may be difficult to differentiate this finding from stool in the colon or from an intraperitoneal or retroperitoneal abscess (Fig. 3.31). The judicious use of additional radiographic plain film, contrast studies, and tomographic and ultrasound evaluations, coupled with pertinent clinical and laboratory data may aid in making this distinction. However, because of the high morbidity and mortality of the unrecognized retroperitoneal traumatic lesions, a thorough diagnostic workup by both the radiologist and the clinician should be obtained.

SEARCH FOR FREE OR LOCULATED FLUID

One of the major results of abdominal trauma is the escape and accumulation of fluid (blood, contents of hollow viscera, lymphatic material, and interstitial fluids) into the peritoneal cavity, the retroperitoneal space, solid organs, the walls of hollow viscera, and the supporting structures of the abdomen. Sonographic evaluation of the traumatized patient is an ideal diagnostic tool for the demonstration and localization of fluid collections. The use of sonography is discussed in the section on renal trauma (p. 184). The plain-film radiologic signs of such accumulations are dependent on whether the fluid is free or loculated.

Loculated Fluid. Compartmentalization of fluid accumulation generally results in a localized increase in the soft-tissue density of the region of fluid accumulation and may produce findings consistent with a mass or result in tumorlike alterations of the contour of the viscus. Diffuse, intraparenchymal accumulation of fluids within a solid organ can result in diffuse enlargement of that organ (Fig. 3.24). However, a subcapsular or subserosal accumulation of fluid will produce a nodular outline of the viscus at the site of this accumulation. Infiltration of fluid into areas normally occupied by fat or between compartments of fat and solid organs (e.g., liver and spleen) will diminish the radiolucency of the fat and thereby produce either a localized or diffuse loss of delineation of an organ (Fig. 3.20A). Fluid infiltrating the wall of a hollow viscus (e.g., bowel) can result in a diffuse nodular thickening of bowel wall, producing "thumb printing," or result in the presence of localized intramural masses. In addition, there may be alterations in the distensibility of the involved viscus. Any one or any combination of these manifestations of infiltration can result in incomplete or complete bowel obstruction with characteristic radiologic changes. Localized accumulation of fluid outside of and contiguous to the wall of the hollow viscus, such as the duodenal sweep, the ascending colon, and the descending colon, can produce, by mass effect, obstructive changes or result in significant deviations of the contour and course of the hollow viscus. Dissection of fluid into the thorax, along the paths of the great vessels, can result in widening of the thoracic perivertebral soft tissues.

Free Intraabdominal Fluid. Fluid accumulates in the abdominally traumatized patient either through rupture of a hollow viscus and the subsequent leakage of contents of that viscus into the peritoneal cavity or through frank bleeding, either associated with rupture of the hollow viscus or with injury to a solid organ. When bleeding occurs, a portion of the blood coagulates at the site of laceration. The remainder is defibrinated, remains liquid, and flows freely within the peritoneal cavity [63]. Thus, whatever the source, the radiologic features are those of free intraabdominal fluid.

Free fluid, like free air, is subject to the laws of gravity, seeking the most dependent portion of the abdominal cavity. With the patient in the supine position, the most dependent portions are the pelvis and the paracolic gutters.

Blood in the Pelvis. The pelvic portion of the peritoneal cavity constitutes approximately one-third of the entire volume of this sac [63]. With the patient in the supine postion, the retrovesical pouch (retrouterine pouch in the female) and the lateral recesses of the pelvis become the most dependent portions to which free fluid will gravitate. Small amounts of fluid filling the pouch of Douglas and the peritoneal recesses to either side of the bladder and rectum will appear as soft-tissue densities above and lateral to the superior aspect of the urinary bladder and separated from the soft-tissue density of the bladder by the extraperitoneal and perivesical fat [56]. McCort [63] has termed this radiologic appearance the "dog-ear sign." The soft-tissue density of the bladder represents the dog's face, and the superior lateral densities of the pelvic fluid represent the dog's ears (Fig. 3.32). Two major conditions may mimic this appearance. The first is the presence of fluid-filled bowel loops within the pelvis. This normal variant may be differentiated from the "dog-ear sign" by noting a sausagelike configuration of the bowel loops that tends to change in succeeding films, by the lack of homogeneity of the soft-tissue densities due to flecks of intraluminal air, and by the visualization of anatomic features consistent with bowel pattern

FIG. 3.31. (A) This 39-year-old male was admitted with multiple abdominal stab wounds. The **(1)** AP supine abdominal examination reveals an area of mottled lucency projected over the right-lower-liver silhouette. This is due to a combination of free intraperitoneal and retroperitoneal air. The loss of the silhouette of the inferior hepatic angle and the soft-tissue density in the right paracolic gutter are due to intraperitoneal and retroperitoneal fluid. The **(2)** left lateral decubitus view shows gravitation of some of the lucency to a position between the liver and lateral abdominal wall, but most of the lucency is unchanged in its position. There is some improved visualization of the inferior hepatic angle. Exploration revealed perforations of the duodenum and small bowel.

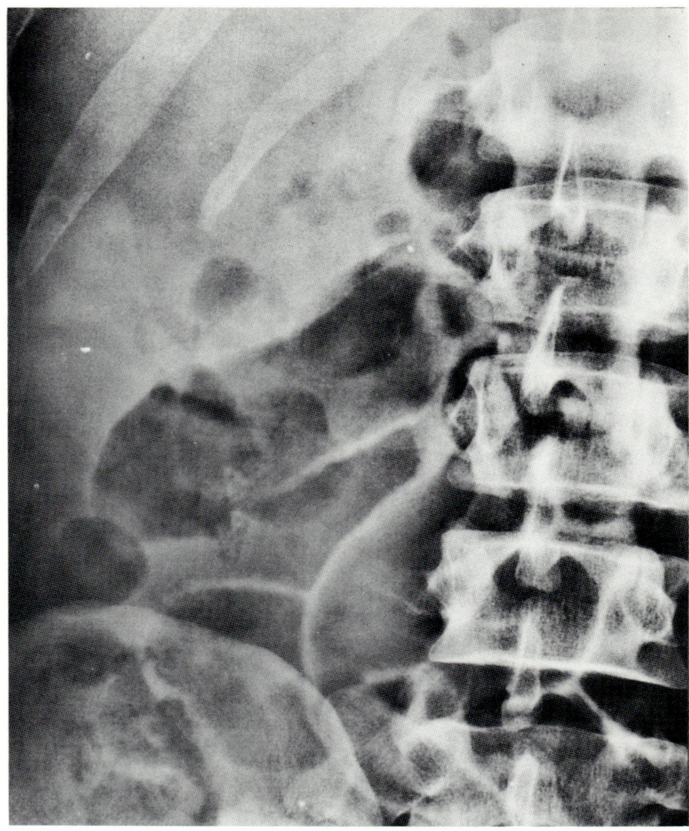

1

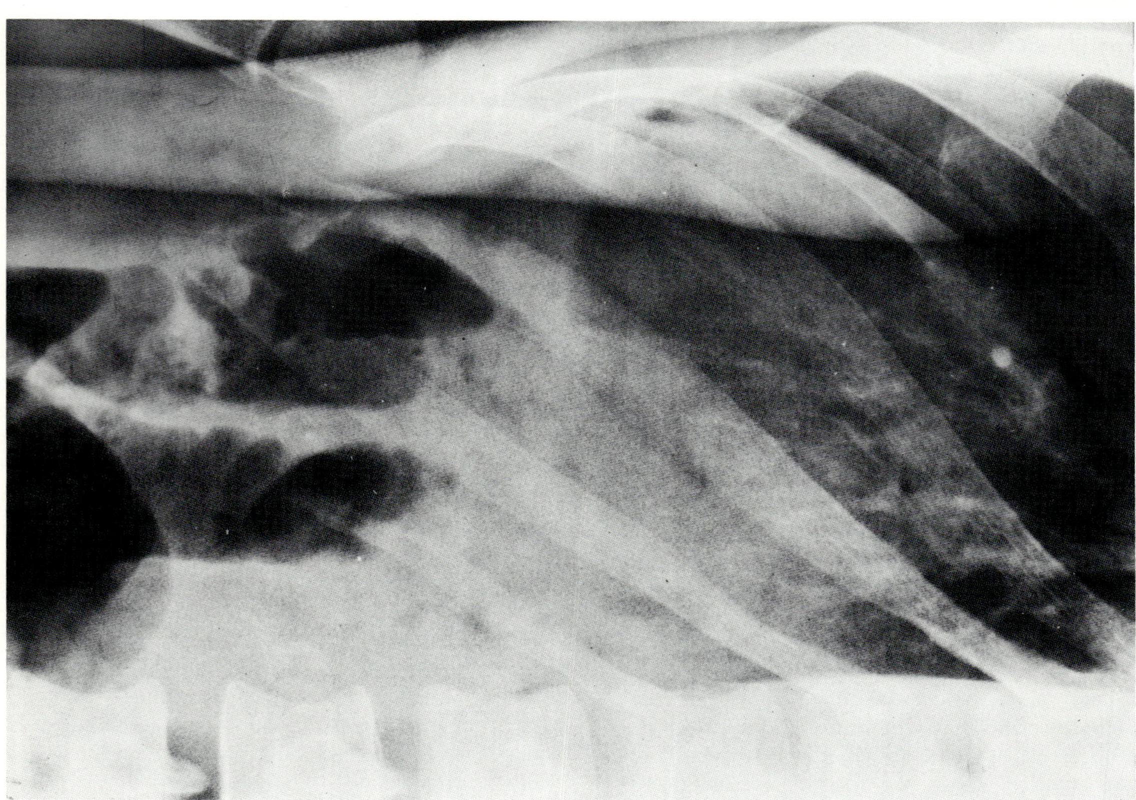

2

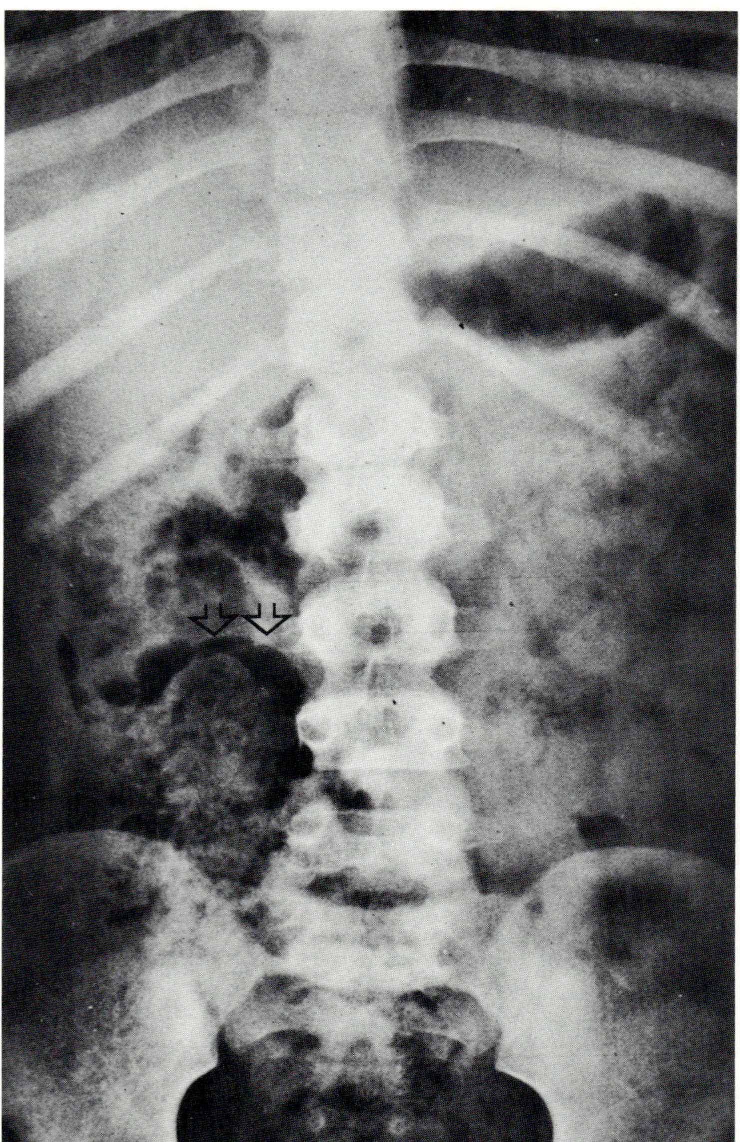

1

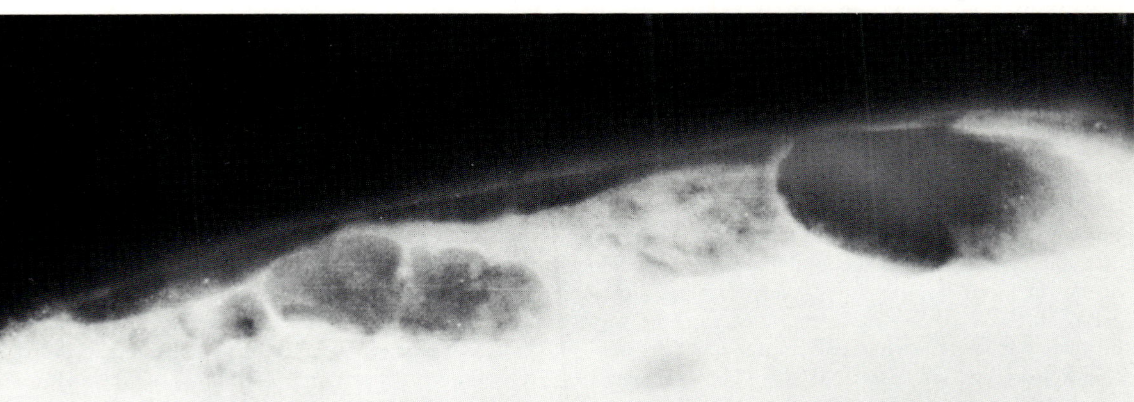

2

FIG. 3.31. ***(cont.)*** **(B)** This middle-aged male sustained blunt abdominal trauma in an automobile accident, resulting in combined retroperitoneal and intraperitoneal rupture of the duodenal sweep. The **(1)** AP supine abdominal examination reveals horizontal radiolucency *(open arrows)* to the right of L3 that represents free air beneath the transverse mesocolon. In addition, there is extensive mottled radiolucency projected over the soft tissues of the right flank, which seems to extend higher than the expected level of the hepatic flexure and is a manifestation of retroperitoneal air. The **(2)** transtable lateral view reveals free air beneath the anterior abdominal wall.

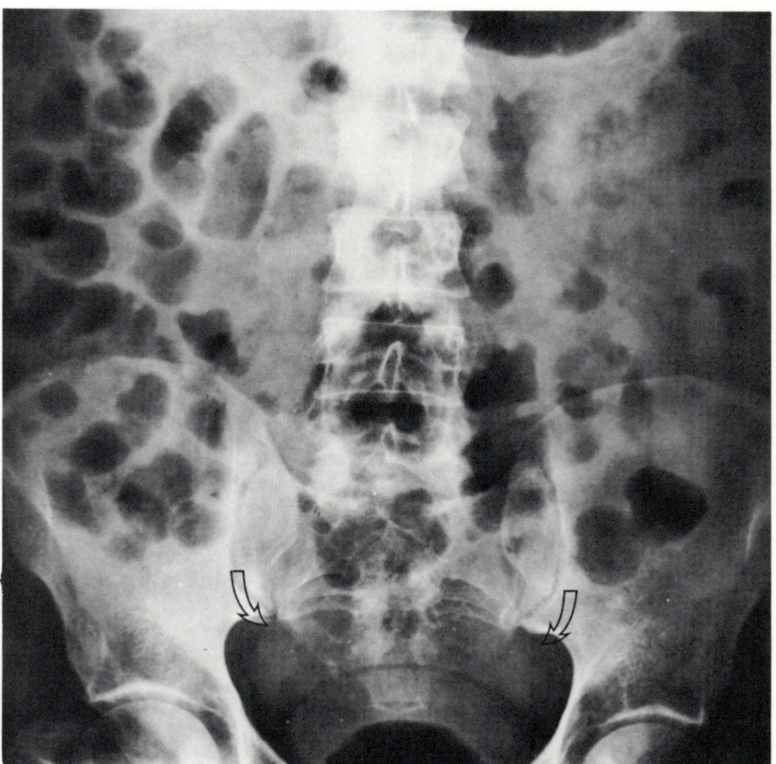

FIG. 3.32. This male patient was admitted with a history of blunt abdominal trauma. The AP supine view of the abdomen reveals two soft-tissue densities *(curved arrows)* superior and lateral to the bladder silhouette. This combination of findings, the "dog-ear" sign of McCort, is consistent with the presence of free pelvic fluid. At exploration, a splenic laceration and the accumulation of blood in the pelvis were found.

(bowel markings) [15,65] (Fig. 3.33). The second differential problem is the presence of a pelvic tumor. Pelvic-tumor masses tend to indent and deform the contour of the bladder, particularly its roof. Free fluid, which is easily displaced, does not usually create this type of indentation [65]. Sonographic evaluation of the abdomen and pelvis usually is diagnostic in confusing cases [40,44,101].

When multiple loops of air-filled bowel are present in the pelvis, demonstration of free fluid may be facilitated [15]. Small collections are visible as regular soft-tissue bands between air-filled bowel loops. As more fluid accumulates, the pelvic contents become obscured by a generalized, hazy density through which can be observed broad, bandlike, triangular or stellate soft-tissue densities between the distended bowel loops. Larger fluid accumulations elevate the bowel loops from the pelvis and replace them with a crescentic (concavity upward) soft-tissue density. The upward concave margin of the density is scalloped, representing the interface between accumulated pelvic fluid and the bowel loops floating on its surface. The lateral apices of this crescent represent fluid tracking into the lower portion of the paracolic gutters. Such a radiologic appearance indicates that there is more than 1 liter of fluid present in the pelvic portion of the peritoneal cavity [68] (Fig. 3.34).

Fluid in the Flank: The Paracolic Gutters. In the supine position, a natural potential space is created on either side of the abdomen by the reflection of the parietal peritoneum of the posterior lateral abdominal wall over the ascending and descending colon. When this space is empty, the parietal peritoneum of the lateral abdominal wall abuts on the visceral peritoneum and conforms to the haustral pattern of the colon. Although the parietal peritoneum is too thin to be identified, its lateral surface is defined by the properitoneal fat. The radiographic evidence of an empty paracolic gutter is a nodular outline of the medial border of the properitoneal fat stripe as this border follows the undulation of the parietal peritoneum [65] (Fig. 3.35).

As small amounts of fluid enter the paracolic gutters to separate the visceral from the parietal peritoneum, the medial border of the properitoneal fat line assumes a straight or slightly curved configuration, indicating a lack of conformity of the peritoneum to the haustral markings of the colon. As still larger amounts of fluid accumulate in this space, the colon is displaced medially by a soft-tissue density that has a smooth lateral border and a comblike medial border, representing projections of fluid into the spaces formed by the haustra [64] (Fig. 3.34A). This appearance is best appreciated when the colon is distended with air,

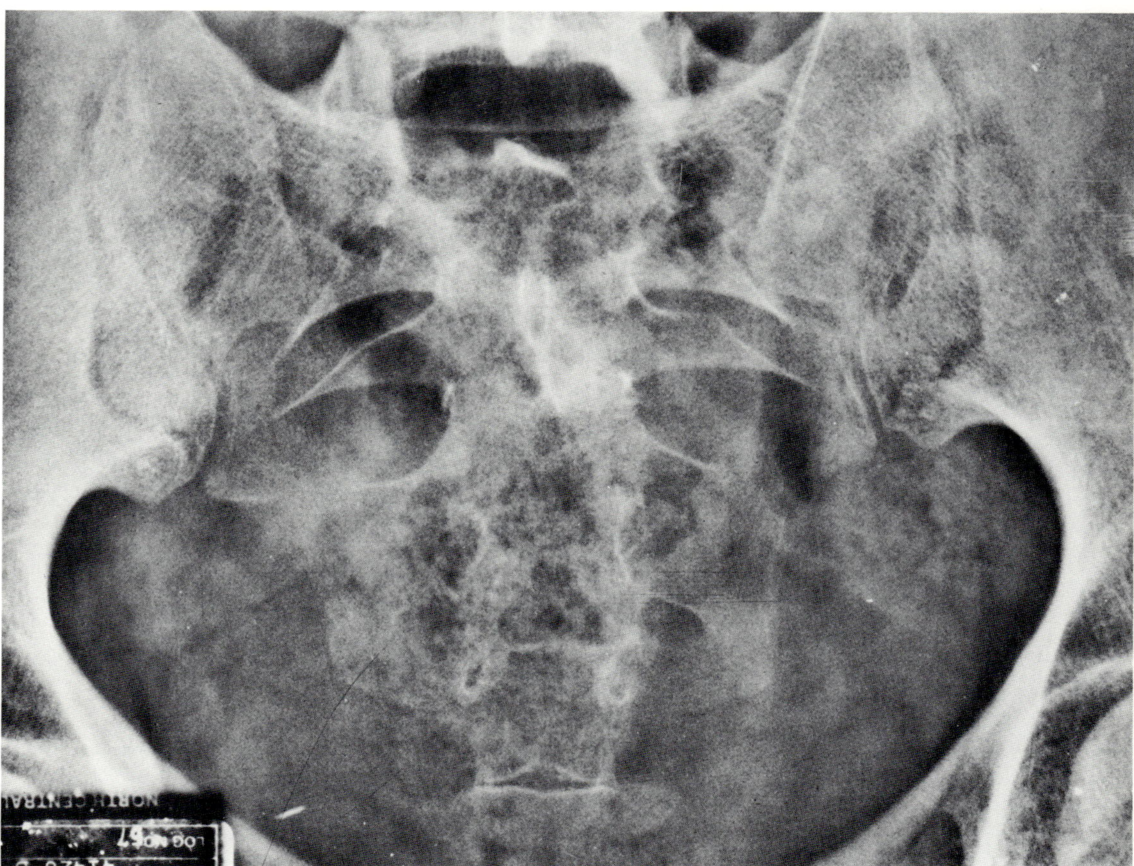

FIG. 3.33. This 33-year-old male was admitted following a stab wound to the lower abdomen. The AP supine examination of the abdomen prior to laparotomy revealed two pelvic soft-tissue densities adjacent to the superior, lateral margins of the urine-filled bladder. The multiple lucencies within them suggested that these masses are fluid-filled loops of small bowel and not collections of intraperitoneal fluid. At exploration, a laceration of the sigmoid colon was found, but there was no significant intraperitoneal fluid.

since a fluid-filled ascending or descending colon can mimic the bandlike soft-tissue density noted in patients with large amounts of fluid in the paracolic gutters.

In addition, there may be interposition of a loop of small bowel in the paracolic gutter. According to Cimmino [15], small-bowel interposition into the left paracolic gutter occurs in 50% of normal individuals. If the small-bowel loop is fluid-filled, it may mimic the bandlike soft-tissue sign of fluid accumulation. Identification of this soft-tissue band as a small-bowel loop can be made by nothing changes in pattern (except expansion) of the soft-tissue density on successive examinations, by the demonstration of flecks of intraluminal gas in the soft-tissue density, by the visualization of the contour of the small-bowel loop, and by the demonstration of a fuzzy contour border to the soft-tissue density that is more suggestive of bowel than of free intraabdominal fluid [15]. If a problem in diagnosis still exists, contrast studies of the upper or lower gastrointestinal tract should be diagnostic. On occasion, and particularly in women, a low liver edge may interpose itself between the ascending colon and the lateral abdominal wall, simulating the accumulation of fluid in the upper right paracolic gutter (Fig. 3.35).

Another important differential problem is due to the presence of retroperitoneal fluid. Dissection of retroperitoneal fluid into the tissues about the peritoneal reflections forming the paracolic gutters can produce similar bandlike areas of soft-tissue density. Lateral decubitus views of the abdomen can be used to identify retroperitoneal accumulation of fluid. With free peritoneal fluid there is widening of the dependent soft-tissue band of paracolic fluid and disappearance of the contralateral (up side) band; with retroperitoneal fluid, no significant change in the configuration of the soft-tissue band will occur.

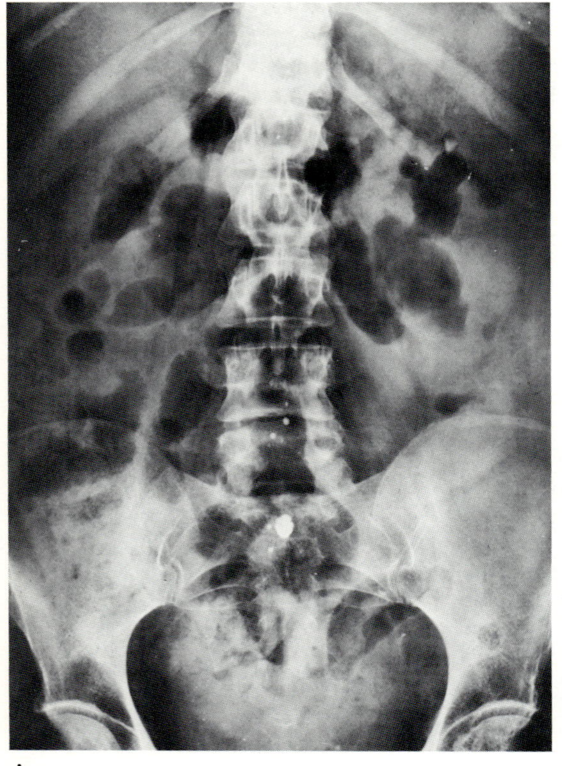

A

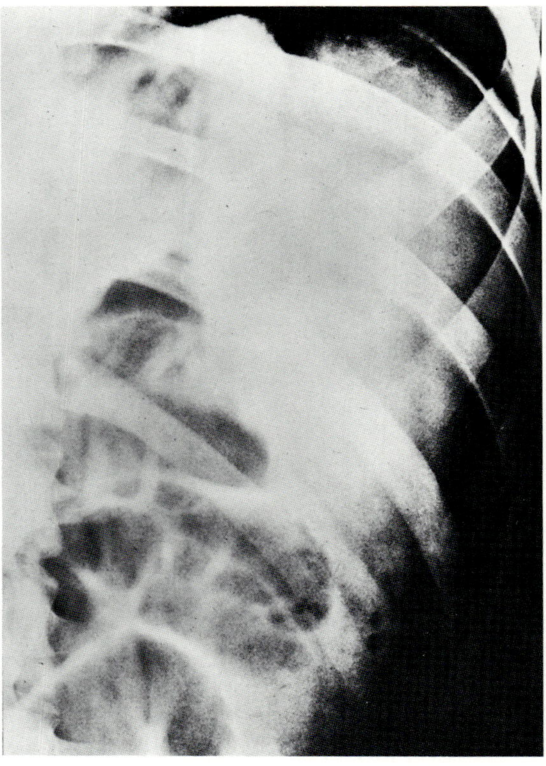

B

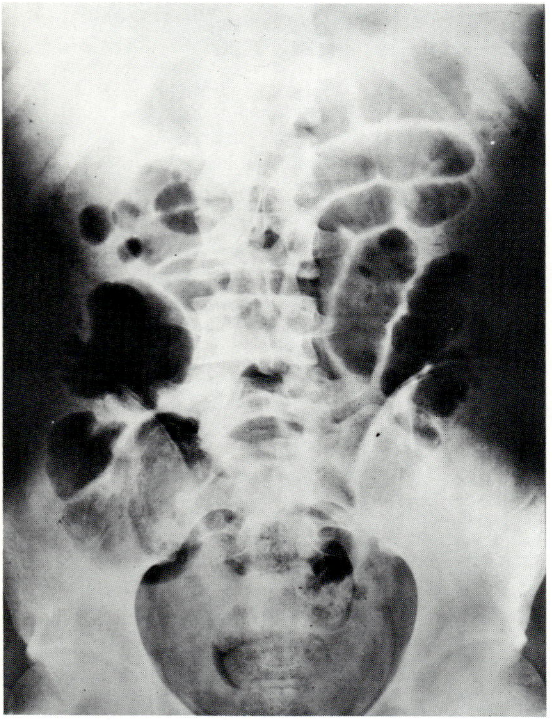

C

FIG. 3.34. The **(A)** AP supine abdominal examination of this victim of blunt abdominal trauma fails to reveal evidence of rib or other osseous fracture. There is a soft-tissue LUQ mass that is displacing the splenic flexure inferiorly and the stomach medially. A "ground glass" haze is over the abdomen, soft-tissue bands are present in the paracolic gutters, and small-bowel loops are elevated out of the pelvis by a soft-tissue density with a concave, scalloped superior border. These are all signs of a large quantity of intraperitoneal fluid. The **(B)** cone down view of the LUQ confirms the presence of a mass and demonstrates its effect on neighboring structures. The diagnosis of a splenic laceration with massive intraperitoneal hemorrhage was confirmed at surgery (courtesy of Dr. L. Barris). **(C)** This 49-year-old female was observed in the emergency room 6 days after being assaulted. Although the patient complained of gross hematuria, an intravenous pyelogram was normal. Fractures of left ribs 7–9 were seen on her admission chest examination. The AP supine evaluation of her abdomen reveals a soft-tissue LUQ mass with elevation of bowel loops from the pelvis by a soft-tissue density. The diagnosis of splenic rupture with intraperitoneal hemorrhage was confirmed at surgery.

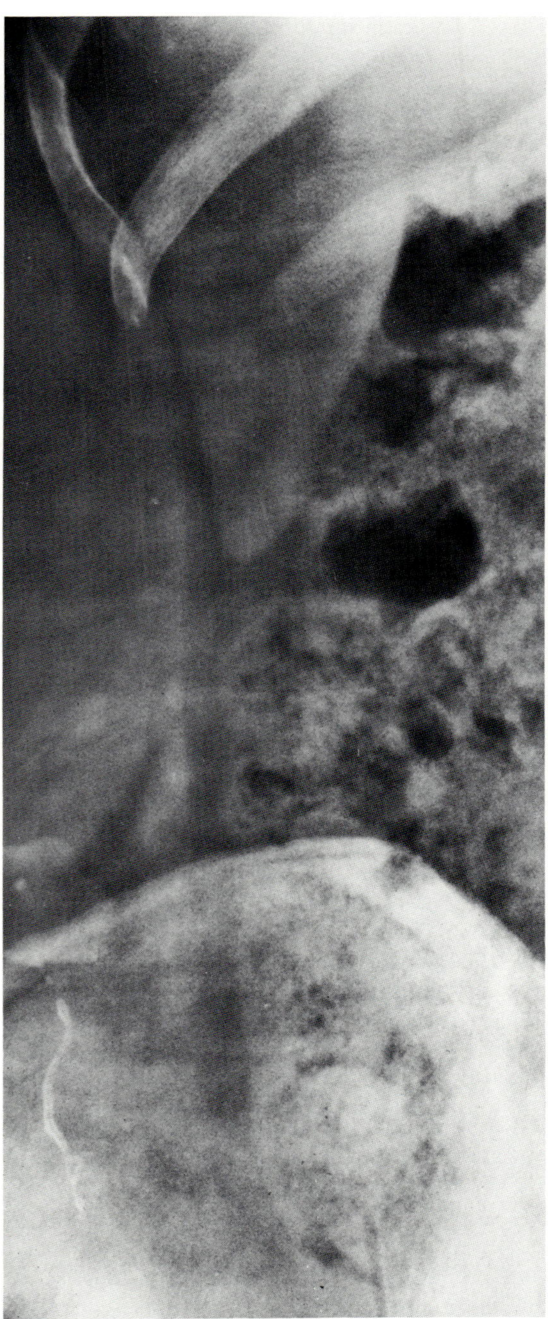

FIG. 3.35. The lateral border of the properitoneal flank fat is smooth, sharp, and slightly concave. The medial border undulates as it follows, along with the parietal and visceral peritoneum, the haustral pattern of the ascending colon. The inferior hepatic angle is sharply outlined by its retroperitoneal fat bed. These findings indicate an empty paracolic gutter and absence of infiltration by fluid of the right retroperitoneal and flank fat.

The Hepatic and Splenic Angles. The inferior angles of the liver and spleen indent the posterior abdominal wall and are normally outlined by the larger amount of surrounding fat (of the properitoneal fat lines and of the para- and perirenal spaces). These areas of fat allow for the exquisite definition of the hepatic and splenic angles, by offering a relatively lucent background on which the soft-tissue density of these structures is superimposed. As fluid accumulates in the peritoneal cavity it separates the inferior hepatic and splenic angles from their fat beds, resulting in the loss of definition of these angles (Figs. 3.34A and 3.35). The most significant differentiation to be made in this circumstance is between free intraabdominal fluid and fluid infiltrating the retroperitoneal fat spaces. The use of decubitus films should be diagnostic. With dissection of fluid into the retroperitoneal and properitoneal fat areas, the fat lucency is converted to soft-tissue density. Decubitus views will not alter this pattern of fluid infiltration and thus, there will be no improved visualization of the angle of the up side viscus. However, with free fluid, the dependent angle remains obscured but the up side angle becomes visible [68] (Fig. 3.31).

Displacement of Abdominal Organs. Free intraabdominal fluid can dissect between the parietal peritoneum of the lateral abdominal walls and the liver and spleen, resulting in medial displacement of both structures. Since there is normally marked variation in the position of the spleen in the LUQ, this finding is less reliable on the left side than on the right. Significant separation of the lateral border of the liver from the lateral abdominal wall is indicative of a mass, and in the patient with a history of abdominal trauma it is most likely due either to free intraperitoneal fluid, loculated intraperitoneal or retroperitoneal fluid, or loculated subcapsular fluid.

Detection of fluid in the midabdomen relies on features similar to those used for the detection of fluid in the pelvis. As in the pelvis, the findings are best demonstrated when air-filled small-bowel loops are present. The soft-tissue bands between contiguous loops of air-filled bowel represent the combined thickness of these contiguous bowel walls and normally measure no more than 2 mm [68]. Increases beyond this limit suggest the accumulation of intraabdominal fluid, obesity, or infiltration of the bowel wall by a variety of disease processes. Small amounts of fluid appear as dense bands between the bowel coils, sometimes producing a netlike pattern. With larger amounts of fluid, several nonspecific findings may be observed: (a) effacement of the posterior abdominal-wall markings due to the large amount of overlying soft-tissue density; (b) medial positioning of small-bowel loops; and (c) shortening and squaring of the configuration of the large bowel. In addition, there may be bulging of the flanks or the demonstration of a "ground glass" appearance or hazy density of the abdominal radiograph (Fig. 3.34).

Generally speaking only two radiologic features suggest accumulation of retroperitoneal fluid: loss of normal visceral- or fascial-plane outline and a mass effect producing organ displacement.

Loss of Normal Visceral- or Fascial-Plane Outline. The dissection of fluid into the retroperitoneal fat converts the fat lucency into soft-tissue density. Such infiltration results in the loss of one of the major contrast factors used in the radiologic differentiation of structures. The result is the disappearance of normal anatomic outlines in the area where the infiltration has occurred. Classic examples of this are loss of the renal and psoas silhouettes (Figs. 3.13 and 3.20).

Displacement of Organs by Mass. Since the retroperitoneal space is not an open compartment, accumulation of fluid has to be localized, resulting in masses that can displace or indent surrounding structures (Fig. 3.13). Although the changes will be greatest on retroperitoneal structures, if the mass becomes large enough its anterior extension behind an intact posterior peritoneal layer may result in displacement of intraperitoneal structures as well. The major problem in radiologic interpretation lies in defining the nature of such masses. Ultrasound, by determining whether the mass is solid or cystic, can help in determining their significance in the acutely traumatized patient [40,44,101].

EVALUATION OF THE INTRAABDOMINAL GAS PATTERN

The air in the gastrointestinal tract provides contrast for defining solid organs and masses but also helps to identify mural and intramural hollow-viscus lesions. Normally, air is present in the stomach and colon, but the duodenal sweep and small bowel are usually devoid of gas. Properly evaluated, the observed gas patterns can be used to indicate and define the sites of trauma as well as the pathologic alterations produced by that trauma. Many authors have noted an increase in serration of the greater curvature of the stomach following splenic trauma. This serration is believed to be due to the infiltration of the gastrolienal ligament by blood (and other fluids) as a result of the splenic injury. This infiltration, either directly or indirectly (via alterations in hemo- or neurodynamics), can result in accumulation of fluid in the wall of the greater curvature of the stomach, accounting for the serrated appearance. However, the reliability of this finding is questionable. Similar findings in other portions of the gastrointestinal tract (e.g., small bowel and colon) have a relatively high diagnostic reliability.

Two major patterns of infiltration can be identified on plain-film evaluations. The first is a localized, intramural mass that may or may not obstruct the bowel in which it is present. The second major pattern is that of diffuse infiltration of the bowel wall, which can result in diffuse thickening or in a nodular pattern in the wall of the bowel ("thumbprinting"). If these soft-tissue densities are due to fluid accumulation in the absence of significant vascular compromise, they will rapidly clear over a period of days to weeks and result in normal posttraumatic plain films and contrast studies. However, if there is significant vascular compromise, the result may be a rigid loop of narrowed bowel, causing partial obstruction.

Another plain-film finding, which may occur in conjunction with the above findings or alone, is irregular distensibility of a segment of bowel. Normally, distension of a portion of bowel by gas is usually uniform, and the usual configuration of the various portions of the gastrointestinal tract is maintained. Alterations in this pattern, with one portion of a loop of bowel appearing larger or smaller than a contiguous or distant portion of that same loop, can occur on the basis of infiltration of the wall of the loop of bowel by fluid, vascular compromise with ischemic change, or compression of that loop of bowel by an intrinsic mass or a collection of fluid, semisolid, or solid material [115]. Another frequent cause of such change is spasm of the segment of bowel secondary to the irritation produced by the trauma, by the escape of blood and other fluid content into the peritoneal cavity and by transient alterations of hemo- and neurodynamics.

Bowel gas patterns are also used to identify and localize soft-tissue masses. These masses may displace bowel segments, alter the configuration of a hollow viscus, or produce partial or complete obstruction.

Most of the changes described above are not pathognomonic in themselves. They suggest the possibility of significant tissue abnormalities or alterations in physiology that need further evaluation for diagnostic clarification. One additional radiologic modality, computerized tomography (CT scan), can be extremely helpful in providing this diagnostic clarification (Fig. 3.36A–C). Although the expense of this examination usually precludes its use in the abdominal trauma patient, it can be extremely helpful in identifying and defining the extent of abdominal masses and fluid accumulations. The authors have used the CT scan in the diagnosis, treatment, and follow-up of at least one patient (Fig. 3.36A) with a severe hepatic injury following blunt abdominal trauma and have found it to be an excellent tool in the management of selected trauma patients.

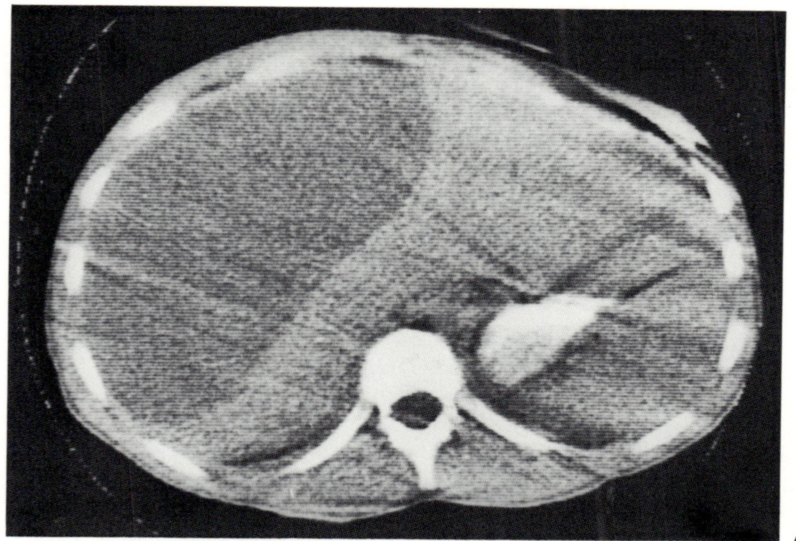

A

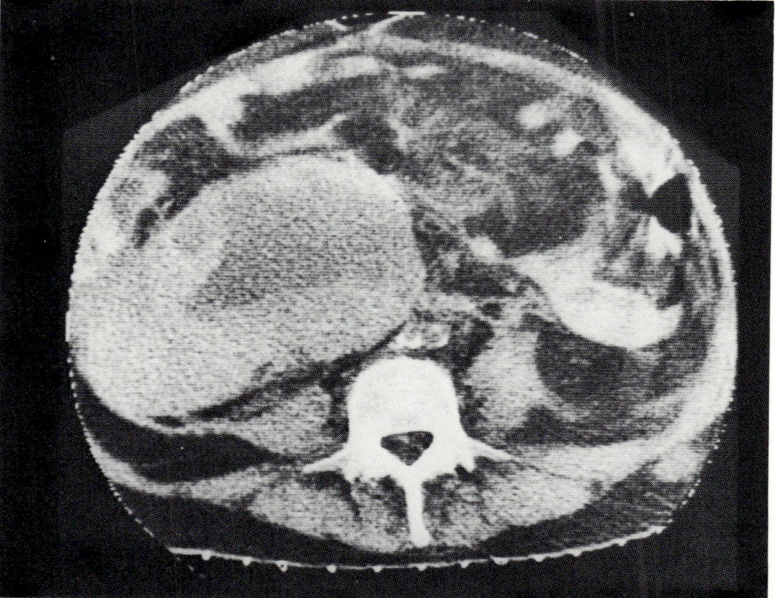

B

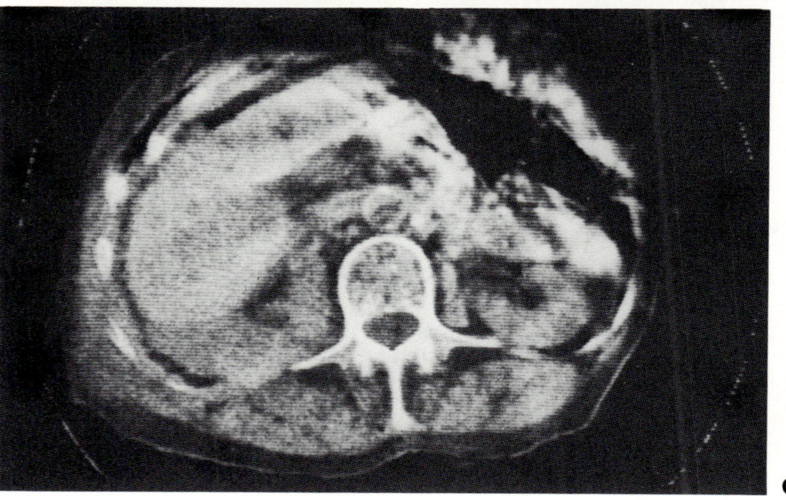

C

FIG. 3.36. (A) This 20-year-old male sustained blunt abdominal trauma with hepatic injury in an automobile accident. The transverse CT scan of the upper abdomen reveals enlargement of the liver with a large intermediate-density lesion filling almost the entire right lobe. Diagnosis: subcapsular hematoma with suggested intrahepatic extension. **(B)** A transverse CT scan of the lower abdomen following abdominal surgery reveals an intermediate-density collection in the right abdomen. Diagnosis: intraabdominal hematoma. **(C)** A transverse CT scan of the abdomen at the level of the kidneys reveals clear definitions of the left kidney and of the perinephric fat. The right renal silhouette is obscured by an intermediate-density lesion that is infiltrating the perinephric fat. Diagnosis: right retroperitoneal, perinephric hematoma.

PARACENTESIS AND PERITONEAL LAVAGE

Paracentesis and peritoneal lavage are used extensively in the diagnosis of abdominal trauma and represent important contributions to the management of abdominal injury. The reported high accuracy in detecting intraperitoneal blood is responsible for their rapidly increasing popularity. The fundamental work of Root et al. [96], Olsen and Hildreth [87], Engrav et al. [26] and others has been of great value in the development of these procedures. Paracentesis and peritoneal lavage are of primary value in the diagnostic management of the patient suffering blunt abdominal injury when an accurate diagnosis cannot be made by clinical examination, radiologic evaluation, and laboratory determination. The use of lavage for patients suffering penetrating injury, pelvic fractures, and thoracoabdominal injuries is currently under study by several authors [3,108].

The most important contribution of the lavage procedure is that it has reduced the number of unnecessary laparotomies performed for abdominal trauma. The accuracy of the clinical impression of an examining physician based on history and clinical examination alone is limited, especially for patients suffering from nonpenetrating injuries. The initial clinical diagnosis was inaccurate in 35% of the Pacey et al. series of 51 patients with blunt trauma [91] and 45% of the patients reported by Olsen and Hildreth [87]. The introduction of paracentesis and lavage to the clinical assessment of the traumatized patient has improved the accuracy of the diagnosis of hemoperitoneum in blunt abdominal trauma to over 90% (Table 3.13).

The first description of needle aspiration of the abdominal cavity is attributed to Solomon in 1906 [104]. Neuhof and Cohen reported the use of this technique for clinical diagnosis and described the relative safety of the procedure in 1926 [81]. Studies by Moretz and Erickson demonstrated the effects of needle abdominal injury in dogs and proved that the procedure was relatively free of complications [75]. When long needles are inserted into the abdomen, they bypass the intestine. When puncture of the intestine does occur, the injury is negligible in its effect. In accord with these earlier studies there is a low overall incidence of complications from the current clinical use of the procedure (Table 3.14).

Needle aspiration of the abdomen without lavage is variable in its success in detecting the presence of intraperitoneal blood. The accuracy of paracentesis alone is reported as above 80% in a number of earlier series (Table 3.15) with a relatively high incidence of false-negative results. The findings with this technique are confirmed in reports by Fitzgerald and Crawford [30] and Giacobine and Siler [36] in 1960. Aspiration of the abdomen using several different sites was popularized as the "four-quadrant tap." This multiple-site approach resulted in a higher level of accuracy with a lower incidence of false-negative results compared with single-site paracentesis. The four-quadrant technique was described in detail and reported by Olsen and Hildreth in 1971 [87]. The false-negative results varied from 10% to 50% with this technique, and therefore multiple-site abdominal aspiration was never widely adopted.

TABLE 3.13. Correct detection of visceral injury or hemoperitoneum with paracentesis and lavage

Author	Year	No. of cases	%
Root	1970	304	96
Olsen	1972	232	90
Engrav	1975	1465	98
Ahmad	1976	315	97

TABLE 3.14. Complications following diagnostic peritoneal lavage in blunt abdominal trauma (15 patients, or 1% of 1465 patients)

Complications	No.
Small-bowel laceration	5
Wound problem	5
No fluid return	4
Evisceration, loop of small bowel	1
Laceration, huge ovarian cyst	1

Source: Engrav LH, Benjamin CI, Strate RG, Perry JF Jr (1975) Diagnostic peritoneal lavage in blunt abdominal trauma. J Trauma 15: 854

TABLE 3.15. Results of peritoneal taps in experimental and clinical reports on abdominal trauma

Report	No. of cases	% accuracy
Giacobine and Siler (1960)	101 patients	82
Williams and Zollinger (1959)	200 patients	79
Baxter and Williams (1960)	80 dogs	90
Economy and associates (1960)	47 patients	83
	80 patients	82

Source: Drapanas T, McDonald J (1967) Peritoneal tap in abdominal trauma. Surgery 50: 742–746

The important experimental work of Canizaro et al. in 1964 demonstrated the value of saline infusion in detecting small amounts of intraperitoneal blood in animals [12]. Their work established that in dogs with small volumes of intraperitoneal blood saline lavage could detect the presence of blood that could not be detected by simple paracentesis. Root et al. in 1965, and again in 1967, reported the clinical application of peritoneal lavage and experimental confirmation of its value [96,97]. The high degree of accuracy and low false-negative results achieved by these authors, using a single abdominal puncture site combined with a standard technique of lavage, has substantially improved the credibility of the peritoneal tap procedure. The test has become very reliable as a diagnostic tool, with application both in primary abdominal disorders and trauma. A variety of technical variations have been described for the lavage procedure. In addition, the experimental contributions of Olsen and others introduced the reliable quantitation of the lavage returns for volume of intraperitoneal blood, leukocytes, and other peritoneal substances [88].

Technique

The techniques used for the diagnostic peritoneal lavage have varied considerably over the last few years. The classic method for introducing lavage fluid was described by Root et al. [96]. The technique is based on the procedure for peritoneal dialysis and is performed under local anesthesia. An 18 French catheter of the type used for peritoneal dialysis is passed through a trocar after a midline incision; it is advanced 6 in. into the abdomen, and if blood or blood-tinged fluid is not immediately returned, 1000 cc of fluid is introduced slowly by gravity and allowed to return by gravity. The most commonly described site for the paracentesis is the infraumbilical midline area. This location is safe if the patient's bladder is empty and the patient has not had previous abdominal surgery. One can use a lateral site for paracentesis, either the lower quadrants or the point of maximum tenderness as recommended by Prout [94]. Injury to the epigastric vessels is the most frequent complication of a lateral lower-abdominal puncture site. Abdominal paracentesis in the upper quadrants may cause liver, gallbladder, or colon injury and should be performed with caution. In some reports, the catheter is introduced, using a very small laparotomy, with visualization and even palpation of the intraperitoneal contents beneath the incision site. Such a technique would reduce the likelihood of organ injury and may be applied in patients with previous surgery. Some authors have recommended culdocentesis as superior to abdominal tap for aspirating peritoneal fluid in traumatized females [17]. Although culdocentesis in a trauma setting is a reasonable procedure, it is not commonly used.

The fluids used for lavage are lactated Ringer's solution or saline. One thousand cubic centimeters of the solution is introduced slowly by gravity and allowed to return by placing the infusion bottle on the floor. The fluids should then return to the bottle. The acidity of the commercial lactated Ringer's solution may cause peritoneal irritation, especially if the patient has repeated examinations after the lavage fluid has been introduced. Baker has suggested adding 25 cc of a 7.5% sodium bicarbonate solution to prevent the development of confusing peritoneal signs [6]. After completion of the lavage and examination and analysis of the lavage fluid, it is occasionally beneficial to leave the catheter in the peritoneal cavity, especially if the results of the lavage are equivocally positive. Repeat aspiration of the catheter or repeat lavage can be performed after a period of observation.

Dialysis catheters, spinal needles, intracaths, and specially designed catheters have been used for paracentesis. The smaller 16-gauge catheters are packaged specifically for this purpose with a long needle and are convenient for paracentesis since all the necessary components are provided as a set. Central vein catheter sets are also readily available, but the catheter does not have multiple perforations. The intracath sets are more popular than dialysis catheters and are more familiar to house officers. The needle can be introduced percutaneously without making a skin incision and with little or no local anesthetic. A special Teflon needle with side holes and an internal needle obturator is used by Shaftan at the Kings County Hospital [102]. This type of catheter has the advantage of penetration of the abdomen with a small needle and is simple to use. A further development of this technique includes the use of a flexible guide wire (Fig. 3.37).

Indications for Paracentesis and Peritoneal Lavage

Peritoneal lavage is superior to clinical examination in its ability to detect intraabdominal-organ involvement in the patient subjected to blunt trauma. The reported indications for diagnostic peritoneal lavage vary considerably from one center to another. Perry and Strate, in 1972, used the criteria of unexplained hypotension, head injury with unconsciousness, severe chest injury, and multiple injuries if clinical findings did not very clearly suggest specific visceral injury [93]. They reported a 41.9% incidence of positive lavage in patients with unexplained hypotension, a 25.8% incidence of positive lavage in patients with chest injury, and a 12.9% positive lavage in patients with multiple injuries (Table 3.16). In 164 of the 252

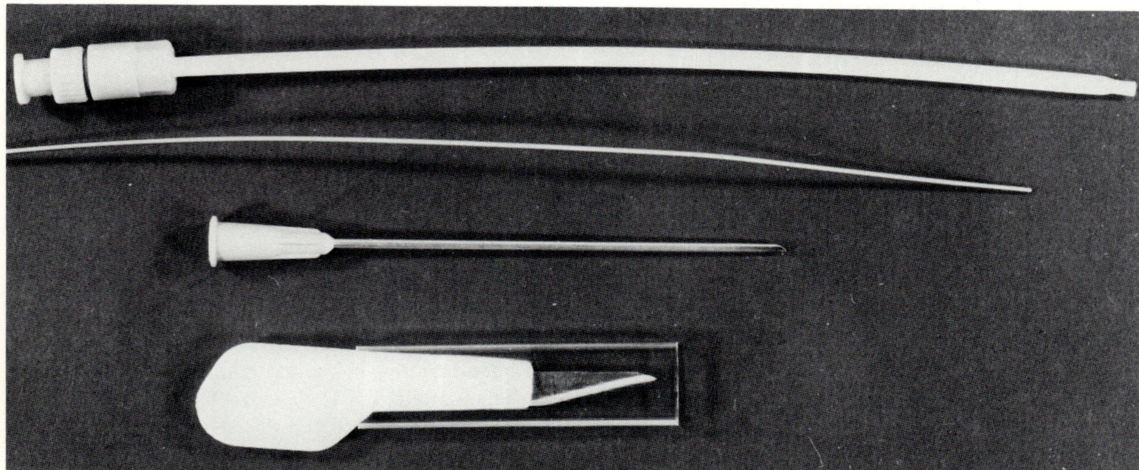

FIG. 3.37. The Lazarus-Nelson Peritoneal Lavage Kit contains a scalpel; blunt-nosed needle; flexible-tip wire; and a plastic, multiperforated, taper-tipped i.v. hub catheter. The kit is sterilely packaged for immediate use after abdominal skin preparation. The introduction of the multihole flexible catheter over the flexible wire introduced through the needle allows peritoneal lavage with minimal likelihood of bowel perforation or catheter occlusion.

TABLE 3.16. Indications for peritoneal lavage and results in patients with no specific symptoms or signs of abdominal injury

Indications	Total no. of patients	True positive	True negative	False positive	False negative
Arterial hypotension	29	13	16	0	0
Head injury with unconsciousness	42	8	33	0	1
Chest injury	33	6	27	0	0
Multiple injury	28	4	24	0	0
Circumstances of accident	10	0	10	0	0
Pelvic fracture	4	0	3	0	1
Falling hemoglobin	1	0	1	0	0
Other	2	0	2	0	0
Total	149	31	116	0	2

Source: Perry JF, Strate RG (1972) Diagnostic peritoneal lavage in blunt abdominal trauma: Indications and results. Surgery 71: 898

patients with clinical signs indicating the need for laparotomy, the lavage was negative and laparotomy was not performed. Thal and Shires found that their indications for lavage were a negative paracentesis in a patient with blunt trauma, closed injury to the head due to a motor vehicle accident, and equivocal physical findings on abdominal examination in a patient with multiple injury [109].

Currently, some trauma centers favor the use of peritoneal lavage in all cases associated with blunt abdominal trauma regardless of the physical findings or associated injury. The use of paracentesis has been extended as a means of confirming the clinical impression of hemoperitoneum in major organ injury and to provide an index of the severity of injury. An immediate recovery of gross blood from a paracentesis indicates acute bleeding and potentially massive hemoperitoneum. A pink return is less alarming but of major significance in terms of the patient's subsequent management. The widening scope of indications for paracentesis and lavage results from the simplicity of the procedure and the enthusiastic adoption of the technique by surgical trainees and emergency medical personnel.

Trauma to various areas of the body may have associated but unexpected peritoneal-cavity involvement and thus may necessitate aggressive diagnostic measures. Thoracoabdominal injuries are an example and can be especially perplexing. Penetration of the abdomen through the chest or visceral injury associated with trauma to adjacent areas must be identified, particularly if there is hypotension or unexplained blood loss. Lower thoracic area injuries are of special interest because of the potential for intraabdominal injury, especially to the spleen or liver [79]. Trauma to the flank may produce renal or other retroperitoneal injuries, and blood may enter the peritoneal cavity through a torn posterior peritoneum or from associated intraperitoneal-organ involvement.

Pelvic fractures can also produce intraperitoneal blood loss or actual intraabdominal-organ injury. Thus, paracentesis or lavage procedure may be a guide in determining subsequent therapy. Massive blood loss and lower abdominal clinical manifestation may develop owing to retroperitoneal and genitourinary-tract involvement. This combination of circumstances can produce a clinical presentation that is very difficult to evaluate. A tangential penetrating injury to the abdominal wall or flank may be associated with local abdominal tenderness and moderate peritoneal reaction with confusing physical findings. Paracentesis and lavage can accurately establish whether penetration of the peritoneal cavity actually occurred. Establishing peritoneal-wall penetration is important in evaluating gunshot wounds but less important for stab wounds. This distinction has significance in terms of whether, or not abdominal exploration should be performed (see section on gunshot wounds, p. 22).

Only a few clinical studies of paracentesis and lavage in injuries other than blunt trauma exist. Thal and Baxter reported a series of patients with abdominal stab wounds evaluated by both wound exploration and lavage [108]. Peritoneal lavage was performed if local exploration was positive, that is, with either penetration of the peritoneal cavity or nonvisualization at the end of an opacified sinus tract. Of 123 patients, 69.9% were treated conservatively on the basis of a negative lavage; 2.4% resulted in false-positive and 4.9% resulted in false-negative findings. In this series the incidence of negative laparotomies was reduced from 29% to 7.9%. Aragon and Eiseman reported a series of 172 patients from the Denver General Hospital with abdominal stab wounds [3]. Peritoneal aspiration and lavage were carried out in those cases where doubt existed as to the presence and type of a major intraperitoneal injury. Lavage was used in 10 cases, and 5 of the 6 patients with positive aspirations had significant intraperitoneal injury at the time of operation. Of the 2 cases with negative aspirations, 1 had extensive intraperitoneal soiling from multiple visceral injury. McAlvanah and Shaftan reported a large series of patients with penetrating injuries of the abdomen [62]. They emphasize the value of using objective indications for abdominal exploration in both penetrating and blunt abdominal injury. Their report discussed the value of paracentesis and lavage in assessing the patient with penetrating injury. A positive "tap/lavage" was the primary indication for surgery in 43.7% of patients with penetrating abdominal trauma (Table 3.17). In their experience with 90 patients with blunt trauma requiring surgery, 73.3% of the cases had surgery based primarily on the "tap/lavage."

TABLE 3.17. Abdominal trauma: Operative indications

	Penetrating		Blunt	
Initial peritoneal signs	54	(17.8)[a]	9	(10)
Development of signs	58	(19.2)	6	(6.7)
Positive tap/lavage	132	(43.7)	66	(73.3)
Shock/bleeding	22	(7.3)	7	(7.7)
Bowel evisceration	15	(5.0)		
Ancillary	13	(4.3)	2	(2.2)
Routine	8	(2.7)		
Total	302		90	

[a] Figures in parentheses are percentages.

Source: McAlvanah MJ, Shaftan GW (1978) Selective conservatism in penetrating abdominal wounds: A continuing reappraisal. J Trauma 18: 206

Lavage is a very useful technique for evaluating the abdominal injury in children. History taking is often unrewarding, particularly in the very young and in the "battered-child" syndrome. Physical findings are unreliable in small infants, and lavage can give considerable help in judging the abdominal status of the injured child. Drew et al. reported the use of peritoneal lavage in a series of 230 children aged 10 years or younger. They emphasized the importance of the procedure in deciding whether to perform exploratory laparotomy. The accuracy was 99.1% in determining the presence or absence of significant abdominal injuries. All 11 with extraperitoneal injury had positive lavage because of associated intraperitoneal injury [23].

The increasing list of indications for the use of lavage is the result of the clinical need for help in determining the status of the visceral organs. The more experience gained with the procedure, the more frequently it will be used. Patients with multiple trauma and hypotension of undetermined etiology represent the most clear-cut and appropriate indications for the study. It must be understood that, if the situation permits, paracentesis and lavage should be performed *after* abdominal films have been obtained. The introduction of a needle into the peritoneal cavity may introduce air and fluid that will confuse the interpretation of the roentgenograms.

Interpretation of Results of Lavage

Paracentesis and lavage are more than 90% reliable in establishing the presence or absence of intraperitoneal bleeding and intraabdominal-organ injury. Root

TABLE 3.18. Results of peritoneal lavage in diagnosis of blunt abdominal trauma

		No. (%)
True negative		935 (63.8)
True negative with extra-peritoneal injury	22	
False negative		19 (1.3)
True positive		505 (34.5)
True positive with trivial injury	31	
False positive		6 (0.4)
		1465
True-negative lavage with extraperitoneal injury (22 patients)		
Ruptured duodenum		3
Ruptured extraperitoneal bladder		9
Ruptured kidney		8
Other		2
True-positive lavage not requiring laparotomy (31 patients[a])		
Nonbleeding liver laceration		19
Retroperitoneal, omental, or mesenteric hematoma		13
False-negative lavage (20 patients,[b] 1.3%)		
Ruptured diaphragm		4
Ruptured intraperitoneal bladder		5
Ruptured spleen		4
Nonbleeding liver laceration		5
Small-bowel perforation		3
Lacerated mesentery		1

[a] One patient had two lesions.
[b] Two patients had more than one injury.
Source: Engrav LH, Benjamin CI, Strate RG, Perry JF Jr (1975) Diagnostic peritoneal lavage in blunt abdominal trauma. J Trauma 15: 854

reports a 96% accuracy in 403 cases in 1970. Engrav reports accurate results in 98% of patients. In some centers the procedure is performed in the emergency room as part of the initial evaluation. With the information that is gained, the timing of operative intervention and need for additional diagnostic studies can be assessed. The high degree of accuracy aids in determining the subsequent events in the workup and management of the patient.

Olsen and Hildreth compared simple paracentesis to lavage by evaluating the four-quadrant paracentesis method peritoneal lavage in 87 patients with abdominal trauma [87]. Using the four-site paracentesis, they found a 79% false-negative rate, a 21% accuracy rate in detecting significant sources of hemoperitoneum, and a 30% accuracy rate in detecting significant injuries in patients with equivocal or unreliable physical findings. However, using peritoneal lavage alone, the figures are 0% for false-negative injuries, and a 100% accuracy rate in detecting significant injuries in patients with equivocal or unreliable physical findings. The results favor the lavage technique for diagnosis and further confirm the unreliability of paracentesis alone, even when using the "four-quadrant tap" technique.

Several shortcomings exist in the use of peritoneal lavage. Failure to obtain a positive lavage in the presence of retroperitoneal injury is an important and frequently mentioned problem. However, failure to diagnose retroperitoneal injury has been overemphasized, especially in view of the low incidence of such errors in several recent large series. In the Perry and Strate report of 401 patients with abdominal injuries, false-negative results in patients with retroperitoneal injury occurred in 6 patients [93]. Two patients or 0.5% of their total group had otherwise false-negative results. In the Engrav et al. report of 1465 cases, duodenal and pancreatic injuries resulted in positive lavage returns in most cases. Three patients with negative lavage following retroperitoneal trauma had duodenal injuries. Engrav et al. reported a total incidence of 1.3% false-negative results [26] (Table 3.18). This overall incidence of error is rather small, and although important, it should not deter one from the use of lavage.

The high degree of sensitivity of the lavage test may produce a positive return without sufficient abdominal injury to justify laparotomy. Positive lavage returns led to unnecessary laparotomy in 7 patients in the Olsen et al. series of 87 patients studied [88]. Gill et al. reported an 8% incidence of clinically insignificant findings and 3% negative findings at laparotomy for trauma in patients with positive lavage [38]. In the Engrav et al. series, there were 6 false-positive and 31 trivial injuries or 2.7% of all patients in the study (Table 3.18). The occurrence of false-positive results is the major fault of the test. However, one must consider the fact that without the test, there would be many more unjustified laparotomies. This is especially significant in view of the established inaccuracy of clinical evaluation alone.

A quantitative definition of a significant tap or lavage is needed to avoid a high percentage of positive lavage results with negative laparotomy finding. Thal and Shires used a criterion of 100,000 red blood cells per cubic millimeter as a quantitative value indicative of a positive lavage [109]. It would require 22 cc of blood in 1000 cc of saline to produce this result in the average patient (Table 3.19). Olsen et al. used a color criterion that is simple and quick. A bright-red lavage return that permits the observer to read news-

TABLE 3.19. Visual quantitative of peritoneal lavage fluid

Lavage result	Appearance of fluid in bottle	Appearance of aliquot of fluid in tubing	Amount of blood necessary to produce this appearance
+++++	>20 ml of blood passes spontaneously from catheter without lavage	+++++ . . .	++++ . . .
++++	Gross blood	Gross blood, opaque	>100 ml/liter
+++	Bright red	Bright red, opaque	>25 ml/liter
++	Bright red	Pink, clear	5–15 ml/liter
+	Pink	Clear	2 ml/liter
Trace	Pale pink	Clear	8 drops/liter
Negative	Clear	Clear	0

Source: Olsen WR, Redman HC, Hildreth DH (1972) Quantitative peritoneal lavage in blunt abdominal trauma. Arch Surg 104: 536

print through the intravenous tubing used for collection of the lavage returns is considered 2+ or weakly positive [88] (Table 3.19). A breakdown of the degree and extent of abdominal injury with visual opacification of drainage returns after lavage is described by Olsen et al. [88] (Table 3.20). An alternative technique for crudely assessing lavage return is described by Barnes and Dennis [7]. They recommend diluting lavage returns in a liter bottle by 9 to 1 and holding the liter bottle to the light. If the fingers of the examiner can be counted through the glass of the bottle, the test is negative or consistent with a count of less than 100,000 red blood cells per liter [7]. The hematocrit of lavage fluid is also of value in the quantitative lavage return. A hematocrit of 1% represents a red blood cell count of 100,000/cc. Fullen achieved a 93%

TABLE 3.20. Comparison of quantitative peritoneal lavage with incidence of significant intraabdominal injuries

Lavage results	No. of patients	Significant intraabdominal injuries	
Lavage not performed	2	2	(100%)
+++++	21	21	
++++	11	10	(98%)
+++	12	12	
++	15	7	
+	7	1	(32%)
Trace	3	0	
Negative	29	0	(0%)
Total	100	53	(53%)

Source: Olsen WR, Redman HC, Hildreth DH (1972) Quantitative peritoneal lavage in blunt abdominal trauma. Arch Surg 104: 536

accuracy in 125 cases using the lavage-fluid hematocrit test [32]. This technique has the advantage of speed of interpretation especially if a microscope or laboratory is not immediately available.

Obtaining grossly bloody fluid returns with simple abdominal paracentesis is an obvious indication that exploratory surgery must be performed. Although the presence of bile or fecal material in the peritoneal cavity may indicate that the lavage needle or trocar has entered the bowel wall, the return of fluid that appears to contain bowel content can reflect the presence of massively ruptured or lacerated viscera. The return in peritoneal lavage may contain large numbers of leukocytes and high levels of amylase and other enzymes; in such a situation, appropriate analysis of the peritoneal fluid should be carried out. Detailed discussion of the importance of other peritoneal-fluid tests is reviewed in the chapter on laboratory evaluation.

The criteria for gross and quantative evaluation of lavage fluid in the 1465 patients studied by Engrav et al. are given in Tables 3.21 and 3.22. The general scheme for the use of lavage in the management of patients subjected to blunt injury is given in Fig. 3.38.

RADIONUCLIDE SCANNING

Introduction

Radioisotopic techniques may facilitate the early diagnosis of trauma to several intraabdominal organs and structures. These techniques are minimally invasive, safe, rapid, inexpensive, and easy to perform. Radiation exposure is less than when conventional radiologic diagnostic studies are used to obtain similar information. Radioisotope imaging procedures are particularly

TABLE 3.21. Criteria for interpretation of peritoneal lavage

1. Dialysis catheter fills with blood	Indeterminate
2. Free aspiration of blood	Positive
3. Passage of lavage fluid through chest tube or Foley catheter	Positive
4. Grossly bloody lavage fluid	Positive
5. More than 100,000 RBC/mm³	Positive
6. More than 500 WBC/mm³	Positive
7. More than 200 Karoway units amylase/100 cc	Positive
8. 50,000–100,000 RBC/mm³	Indeterminate
9. 100–500 WBC/mm³	Indeterminate
10. 100–200 Karoway units amylase/100 cc	Indeterminate

Source: Engrav LH, Benjamin CI, Strate RG, Perry JF Jr (1975) Diagnostic peritoneal lavage in blunt abdominal trauma. J Trauma 15: 854

useful screening techniques, and they may provide both morphologic images and functional evaluation of the organ studied. Postoperatively these techniques may aid in the diagnosis of complications. The equipment needed for performing these procedures is available in most hospitals.

TABLE 3.22. Distribution of red cell counts, white cell counts, and amylase values

	Total	Significant intraperitoneal injury
Distribution of red cell counts		
Under 50,000	806	34 (4%)
50,000–100,000	37	22 (59%)
Over 100,000	60	51 (85%)
Distribution of white cell counts		
0–99	773	28 (4%)
100–500	70	36 (51%)
Over 500	46	38 (83%)
Distribution of amylase values		
0–50	718	63 (9%)
51–100	86	11 (13%)
101–200	10	4 (40%)
Over 200	15	15 (100%)

Source: Engrav LH, Benjamin CI, Strate RG, Perry JF Jr (1975) Diagnostic peritoneal lavage in blunt abdominal trauma. J Trauma 15: 854

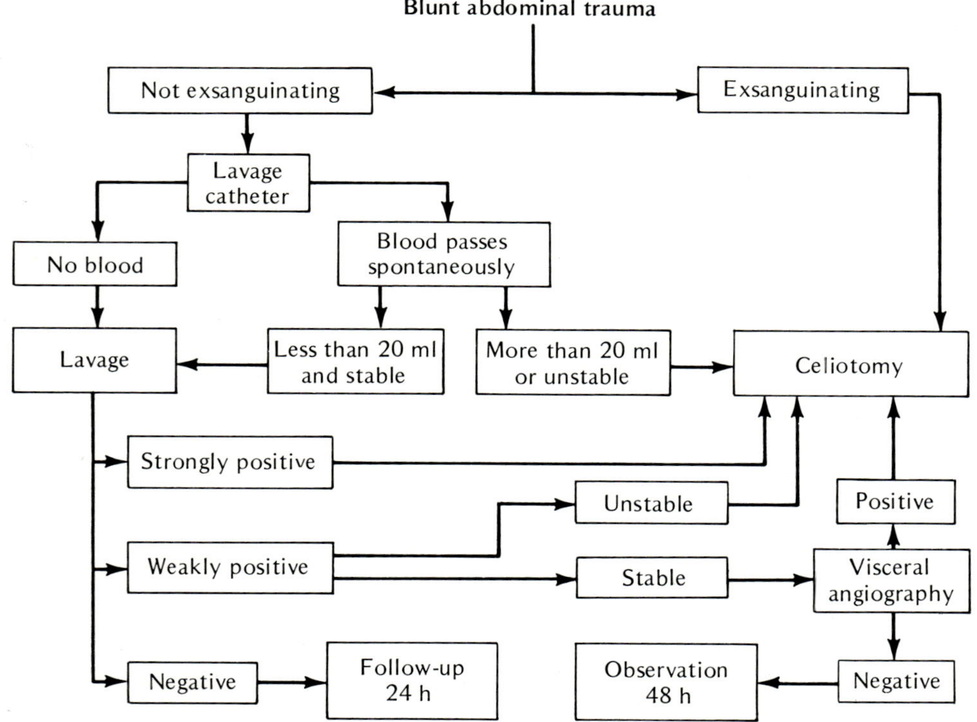

FIG. 3.38. Schematic diagram of selective management of patients with blunt abdominal trauma. From Olsen WR, Redman HC, Hildreth DH (1972) Quantitative peritoneal lavage in blunt abdominal trauma. Arch Surg 104: 536

History

Radioisotope scanning was first introduced in the 1950s to create a two-dimensional image of the thyroid gland. The development of commercial rectilinear scanners with photoscanning capabilities, coupled with the introduction of a number of organ- or system-specific radionuclides, made possible the static imaging of such organs as the liver, spleen, and kidney. Further refinements in radiopharmaceuticals afforded the physician the opportunity to study certain relatively slow physiologic processes (kidney, etc.) by the use of serial rectilinear scans or by coupling the output of appropriately placed probes to a chart recorder. The introduction of the gamma camera in the mid-1960s made it possible to visualize rapid changes in organ function by the use of appropriately timed serial images. Gamma cameras coupled with rapid-sequence photographic cameras permitted the performance of isotope angiograms (flow studies) using an intravenous injection of a bolus of a radiopharmaceutical. In recent years the interfacing of dedicated minicomputers to gamma cameras has significantly expanded the imaging and data-processing capabilities of radionuclide scanning equipment.

Technical Considerations

A radioisotope scan is a two-dimensional representation of the distribution of a radiopharmaceutical within an organ or organ system of interest. The radiopharmaceutical, which is usually administered intravenously, localizes within the organ or organ system of interest because of physiologic and structural considerations. Thus, the colloidal particles used to visualize the reticuloendothelial system of the liver localize within the hepatic Kupffer cells owing to the phagocytic activity of these cells. Radioiodinated rose bengal, as well as newer agents such as hepatic imino diacetic acid (HIDA), are excreted by the parenchymal cells of the liver into the bile and can be used to assess the integrity of the biliary tree. Autologous red blood cells may be tagged with a radioisotope and selectively sequestered within the spleen to delineate that organ without significant hepatic visualization. Certain radioactive chelates are preferentially concentrated, secreted, and excreted by the kidneys, providing a series of images that may be used to assess the renal vasculature, kidney parenchyma, and renal excretory system.

Ionic radiopertechnetate remains primarily in the vascular compartment during the first seconds following its injection and thus can be used to study the arterial tree. Radioactive agents chosen for in-vivo use have a relatively short physical and/or biologic half-life, minimizing radiation exposure to the patient. Maximum resolution and sensitivity with presently available equipment is achieved by choosing a radioactive tag that is primarily a gamma emitter (energy between 100 and 200 keV). The most commonly used radionuclide with these characteristics is technetium 99m which can be tagged to a variety of substances, is a pure gamma-ray emitter, has a 140-keV energy and a 6-h half-life. Technetium 99m is available in most hospitals as the product of a molybdenum-technetium generator system and is available on a 24-h basis for emergency procedures. The whole-body radiation exposure sustained by a patient undergoing a technetium 99m scan is equal to or less than that of a PA and lateral chest roentgenogram.

Radionuclide imaging, though lacking the resolution of available radiologic procedures, can yield much useful information about the morphology and function of various intraabdominal organs.

Spleen

The spleen is the intraabdominal organ most commonly found to be injured following blunt injury. Penetrating wounds of the spleen are less frequent but may result in varying degrees of injury ranging from simple laceration following knife wounds to complete rupture following gunshot wounds.

The diagnosis of splenic injury can be difficult despite the availability of plain film, radiologic examination, paracentesis and lavage, and careful clinical assessment. The clinical findings in patients with blunt injury are well known to be unreliable in a significant proportion of patients (see section on blunt trauma, p. 24). Contrast arteriography and laparoscopy have been utilized to examine the spleen for injury, but both procedures are invasive and not without risk. Most traumatologists prefer the isotope splenic scan for the initial screening of these patients (Figs. 3.39–3.44).

Method

Scans of the spleen are usually performed using a dose of 1–4 mCi of technetium 99m sulfur colloid which is concentrated in both hepatic and splenic tissue. Careful positioning of the patient and multiple views usually separate splenic uptake from hepatic uptake and clearly delineate the spleen. Either the gamma camera or rectilinear scanner may be used to image the patient, although the greater mobility and flexibility of the gamma camera in obtaining multiple and oblique views are of distinct advantage in imaging the spleen. In studies where the liver overlies the spleen and the two organs cannot be separately visualized,

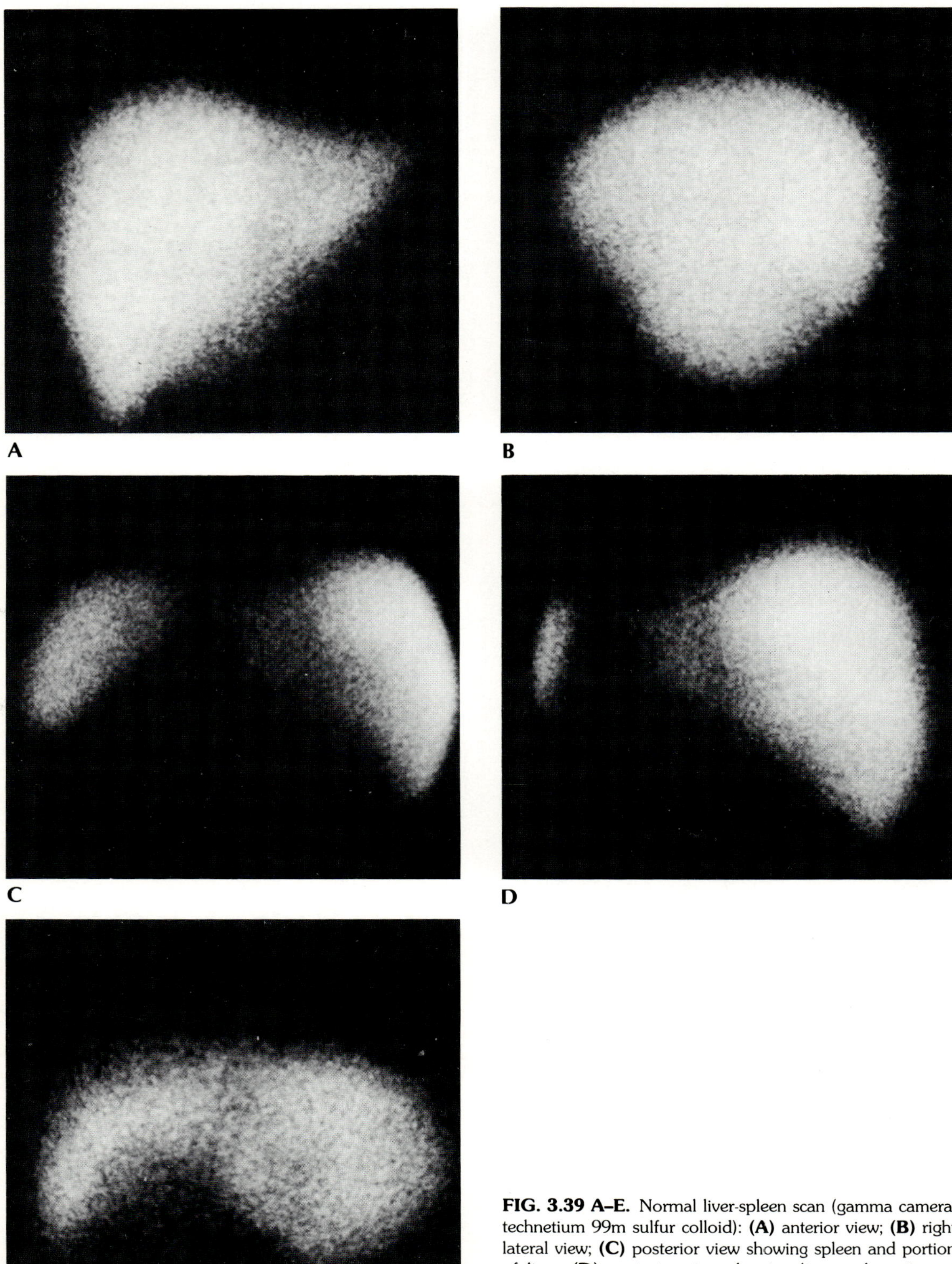

FIG. 3.39 A–E. Normal liver-spleen scan (gamma camera, technetium 99m sulfur colloid): **(A)** anterior view; **(B)** right lateral view; **(C)** posterior view showing spleen and portion of liver; **(D)** posterior view showing liver and portion of spleen; **(E)** left lateral view, larger organ is spleen.

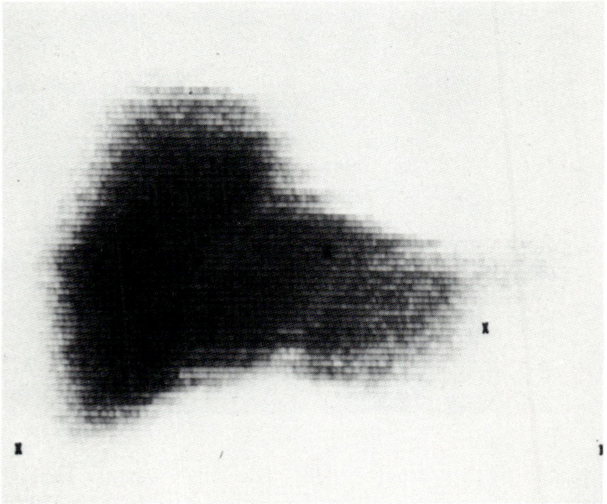

A

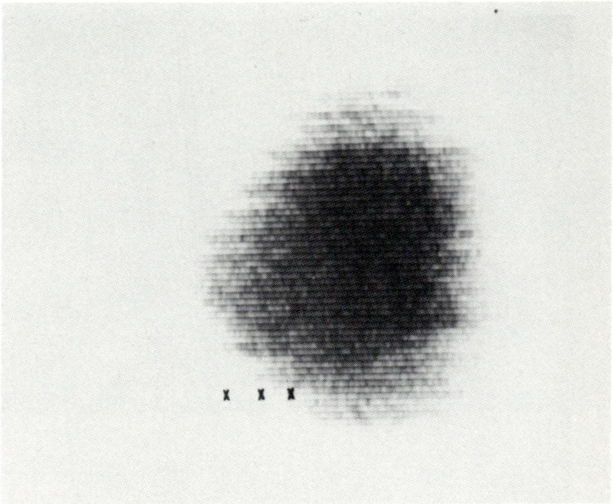

B

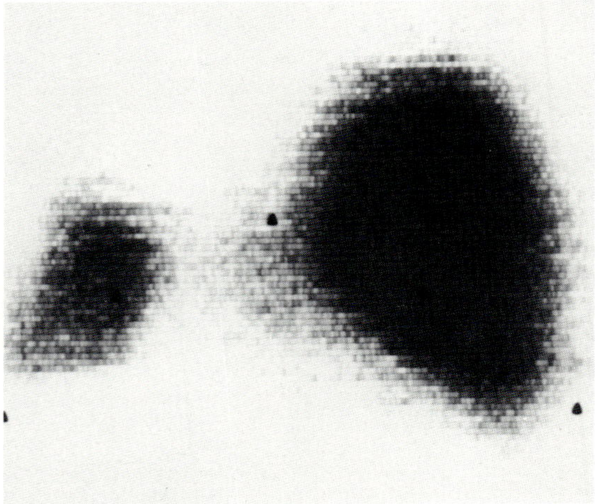

C

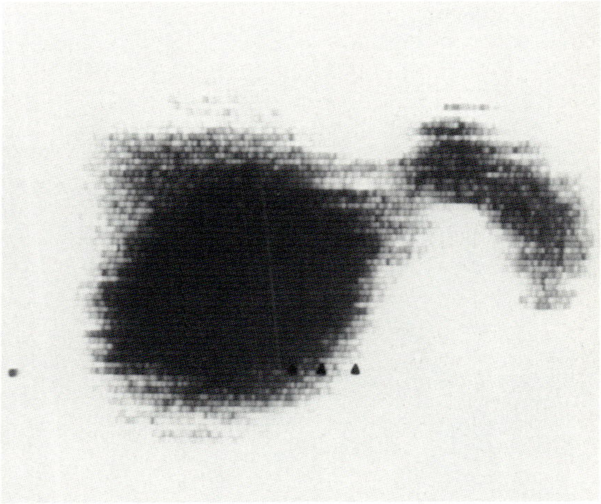

D

FIG. 3.40 A–D. Normal liver-spleen scan (rectilinear scanner, technetium 99m sulfur colloid): **(A)** anterior view, markers represent outline of costal margin; **(B)** right lateral view; **(C)** posterior view, liver is larger organ; **(D)** left lateral view, liver is larger and darker organ.

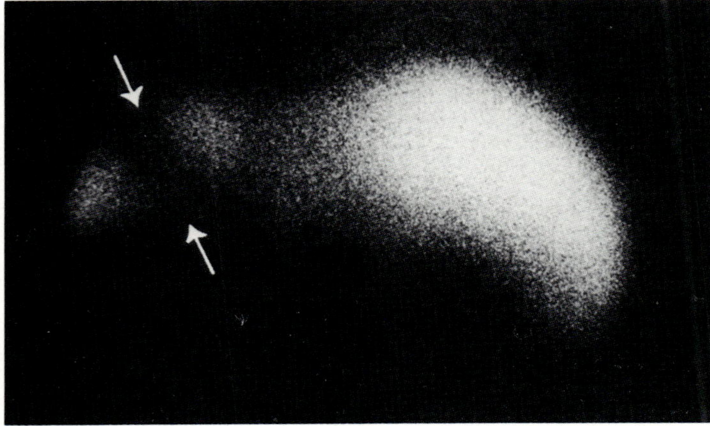

FIG. 3.41. This 60-year-old man fell down stairs 2 weeks prior to coming to the emergency room for evaluation of severe persistent (LUQ) pain. Posterior view of spleen (gamma camera, technetium 99m sulfur colloid) clearly shows intrasplenic defect *(arrows)*.

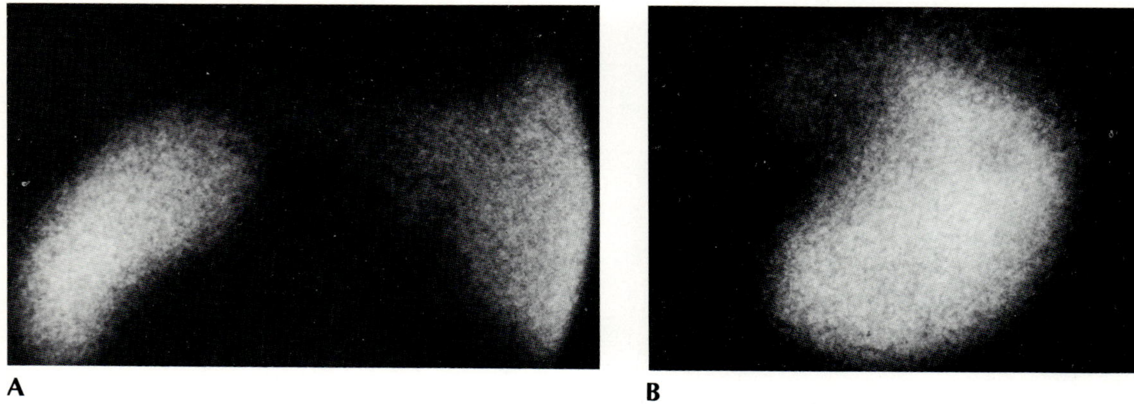

FIG. 3.42 A and B. This 25-year-old man sustained a gunshot wound through the left axilla. The bullet was not located on plain-film studies, but the patient complained of LUQ pain. Spleen scan (gamma camera, technetium 99m sulfur colloid): **(A)** posterior view appears normal; **(B)** left lateral view shows tunnel wound of spleen.

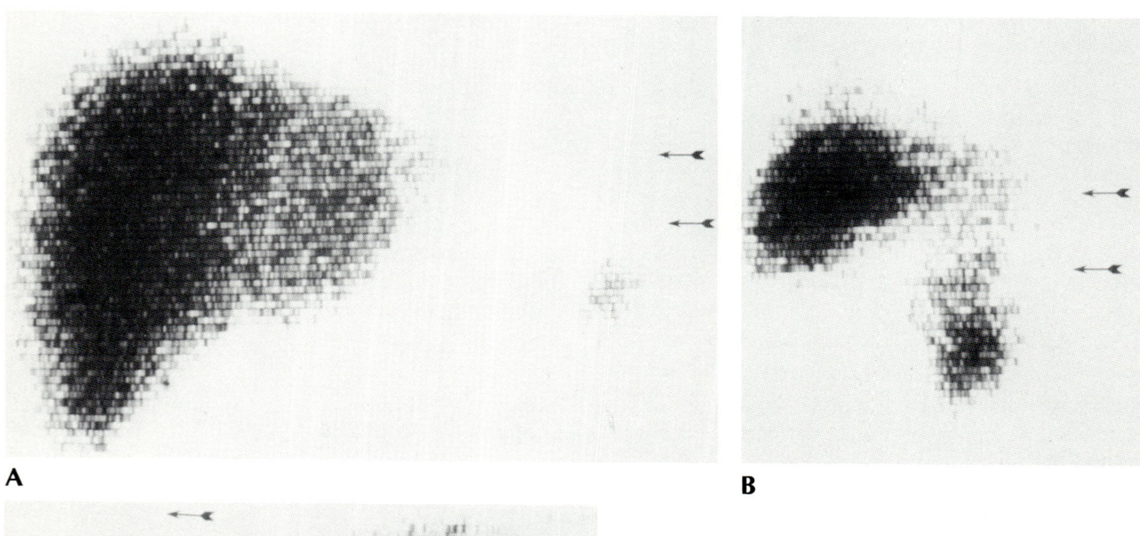

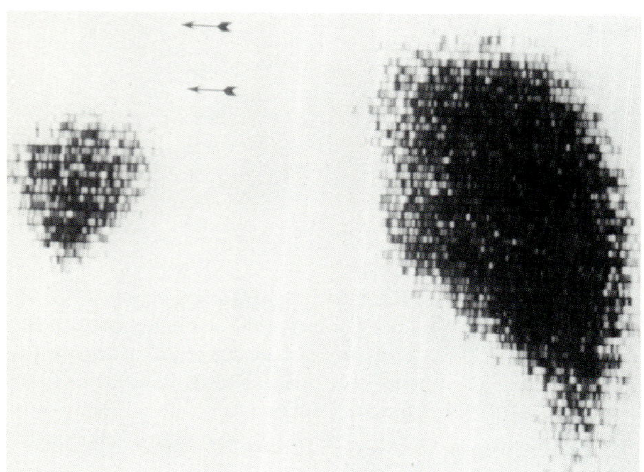

FIG. 3.43 A–C. This 17-year-old boy sustained multiple trauma in an altercation. Patient was admitted complaining of severe LUQ pain. Liver-spleen scan (rectilinear scanner, technetium 99m sulfur colloid): Anterior, left lateral, and posterior views all demonstrate decreased uptake in superior one-half of spleen *(arrows)*. **(A)** Anterior view; **(B)** left lateral view; **(C)** posterior view.

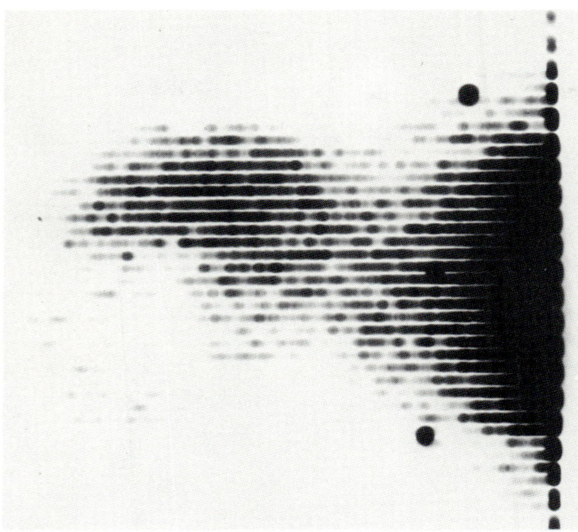

A

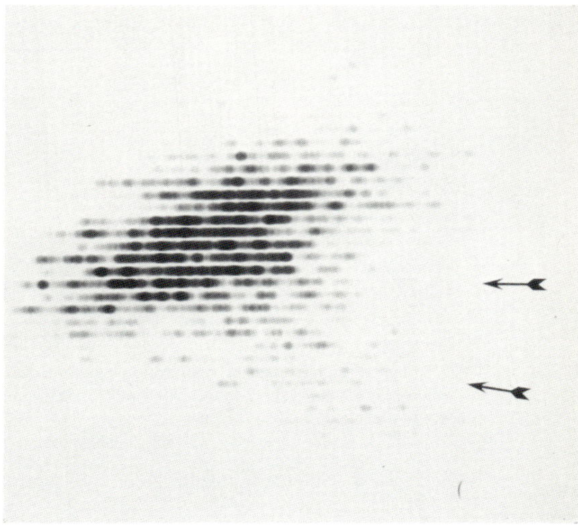

B

FIG. 3.44 A and B. This 21-year-old man fell two stories from an open window 4 days before scan was obtained. Patient presented no signs or symptoms of intraabdominal trauma. Spleen scan (rectilinear scanner, technetium 99m sulfur colloid): **(A)** posterior view showing an area of decreased uptake in the inferolateral portion of the spleen; **(B)** left lateral view demonstrating that this area of decreased uptake *(arrows)* lies posteriorly. The scan impression of a subcapsular splenic hematoma was confirmed at surgery.

autologous red blood cells which have been denatured either by chemical or heat treatment may be tagged with technetium 99m or chromium 51 to image the spleen with little hepatic interference. Since chromium 51 has a much higher energy than technetium 99m and thus can be used in the presence of technetium 99m, red blood cells tagged with chromium 51 may image the spleen immediately following an unsuccessful attempt with technetium 99m sulfur colloid. With either agent, splenic abnormalities due to trauma appear as areas of decreased uptake in the splenic parenchyma or as irregularities of the splenic border. A minimum of three splenic projections should be obtained including anterior, posterior, and left lateral views. When feasible, oblique views and views obtained with the collimator tilted caudad may be of considerable value. A complete series of scans for splenic evaluation can be obtained in 30 min or less at an isotope cost (for technetium 99m sulfur colloid) of $3–$4 [28,55,60,80].

Results

The results of splenic scanning have been correlated with those of arteriography and/or operation in several clinical series, as well as in an animal model.

In dogs subjected to minor (1- to 2-cm diameter) subcapsular hematomas at laparotomy, splenic scanning did not reveal any focal defects in the immediate postoperative period. By the fifteenth postinjury day, scanning indicated a slight increase in splenic size and uptake of isotope (technetium 99m sulfur colloid). Neither of these findings can be considered diagnostic of splenic injury. Larger (5- to 7-cm diameter) subcapsular hematomas regularly showed focal defects on early splenic scanning. However, by the ninth day the scans reverted to normal. This study suggests that positive splenic scintiscanning reveals only injuries of clinical significance. There are significant differences between the canine and human spleen; smooth-muscle tissue in the dog's spleen allows the spleen to contract, counteracting slow bleeding. This may prevent extrapolation of the results to the human.

Several series of scans in patients with suspected splenic injuries have been reported, indicating an excellent correlation between operative and contrast angiographic findings and nuclear medicine techniques. Review of several series indicates that the false-positive incidence of splenic scans is 7.2% and the false-negative incidence is 1.5% [37] (Tables 3.23, 3.24). The number of false-positive interpretations may be minimized by performing scans in multiple projections, including oblique views.

Repeat splenic scans may be used to assess completeness of surgical removal of the splenic tissue following splenectomy or to confirm the stability of a splenic injury when the patient is treated expectantly. The presence of splenosis may be detected by scans performed at a time remote from splenic rupture.

TABLE 3.23. Liver injury in abdominal trauma

Hospital	Patients	Negative	False negative	Positive	False positive
St. Mary's	119	100	0	19	2[a]
Winchester	19	16	0	3	0
Royal Prince Alfred	8[b]	3	0	5	0
Hospital for Sick Children	16	15	0	1	0
Total	162	134	0 (0%)	28	2 (7%)

[a] Normal laparotomy.

[b] Four cases excluded as scan done postoperatively.

Source: Gilday DL, Alderson PO (1974) Scintigraphic evaluation of liver and spleen injury. Semin Nucl Med 4(4): 357–370

TABLE 3.24. Splenic injury in abdominal trauma

Hospital	Patients	Negative	False negative	Positive	False positive
St. Mary's	119	91	0	28	4[a]
Winchester	19	14	0	5	0
Mass. General–Cardinal Cushing	32	19	1	11	0
Albert Einstein–Bronx Municipal Hospital	16	3	1[b]	13[c]	1
Upstate Medical Center	—	—	—	5	0
Hospital for Sick Children	16	9	0	7[d]	0
Total	202	136	2 (1.5%)	69	5 (7.2%)

[a] Laparotomy normal.

[b] Questionable minor injury by angiography.

[c] Two patients had negative angiograms, but the scintigraphic defects subsequently returned to normal. Contusion was the accepted diagnosis.

[d] Four patients had abnormal scans return to normal and were not operated upon.

Source: Gilday DL, Alderson PO (1974) Scintigraphic evaluation of liver and spleen injury. Semin Nucl Med 4(4): 357–370

Liver

Direct trauma, such as bullet, stab, or blunt wounds to the right upper abdominal quadrant, will often involve the liver. Radionuclide visualization of the liver or the hepatic excretory system is not necessary in cases where obvious trauma to the hepatic or biliary system has occurred. When no definite clinical or laboratory evidence of hepatic injury is present following abdominal trauma, the static liver scan can provide evidence of the benign nature of the injury. A positive liver scan may give the initial indication that hepatic trauma, unsuspected on clinical grounds, has occurred [55]. Though the wound itself may not be visualized, the resultant hematoma occurring in the highly vascular liver tissue will cause a scan defect which provides evidence of the injury (Figs. 3.39, 3.40, 3.45–3.47). Trauma may involve the extrahepatic biliary system, leaving the hepatic parenchyma intact. The biliary system may be visualized by administration of a radiopharmaceutical that is excreted into bile by parenchymal cells. Biliary-system imaging is not attempted without some suspicion that the integrity of the biliary ducts has been compromised, because of the time-consuming nature of the procedure.

Because of the considerable regenerative capability of the liver, rapid healing may occur following repair or resolution of hepatic trauma and/or resection of devitalized tissue. Follow-up liver scans may be helpful in documenting this healing. Repeat excretory studies may likewise confirm the adequacy and functional status of repairs to the biliary ducts.

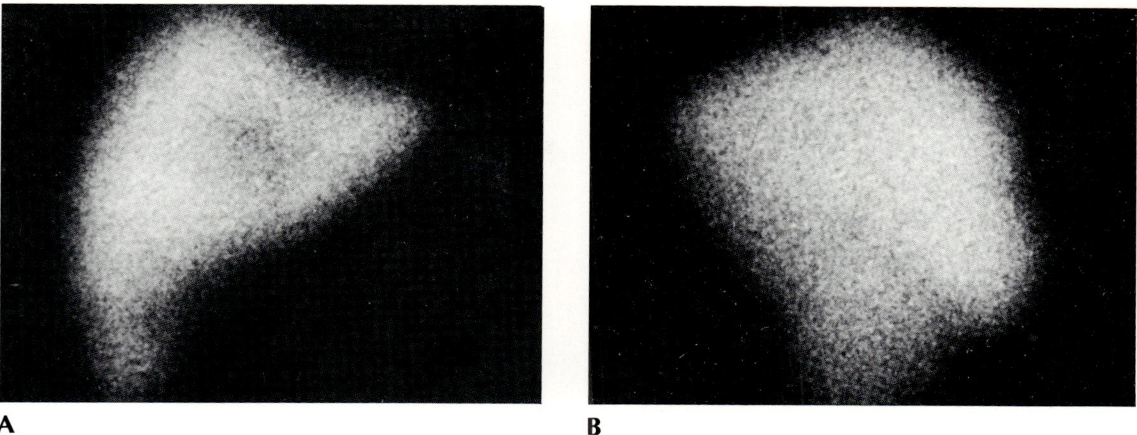

FIG. 3.45 A and B. This 67-year-old woman sustained a gunshot wound to the RUQ of the abdomen. Liver scan (gamma camera, technetium 99m sulfur colloid): **(A)** anterior view shows circular area of decreased uptake representing a tunnel wound to the liver; **(B)** right lateral view shows no abnormality. Bullet was removed from liver at operation.

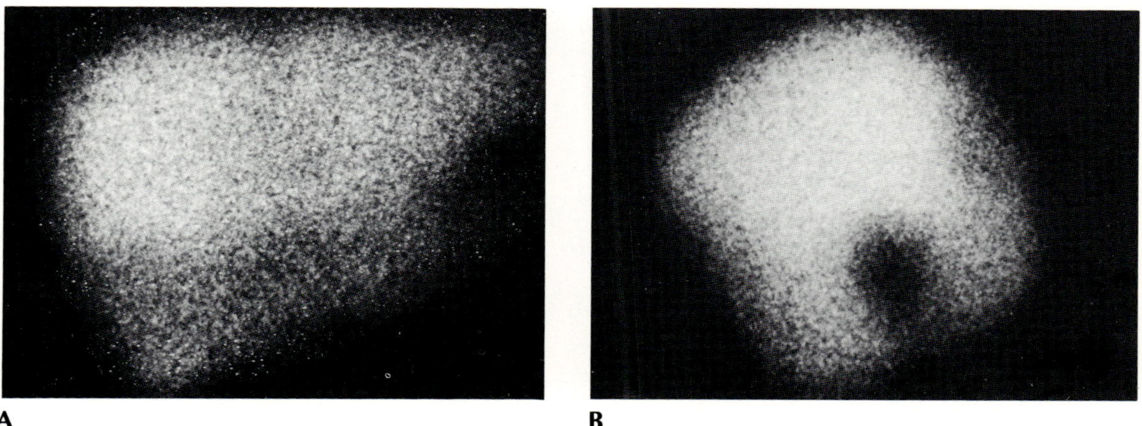

FIG. 3.46 A and B. This 24-year-old man sustained a gunshot wound to the abdomen. Liver scan (gamma camera, technetium 99m sulfur colloid): **(A)** anterior view showing decreased uptake along inferior one-third of the liver; **(B)** right lateral view demonstrating spheroid area of decreased uptake in inferior portion of the liver. Tunnel wound of liver was found at laparotomy.

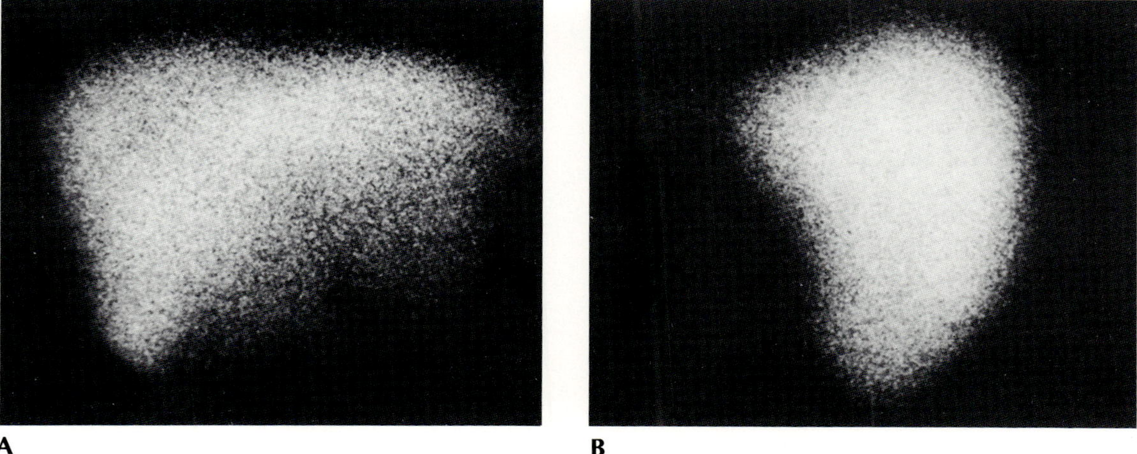

FIG. 3.47 A and B. This 47-year-old man sustained a stab wound to the RUQ of his abdomen several days before scan was performed. Liver scan (gamma camera, technetium 99m sulfur colloid): **(A)** anterior view shows area of decreased uptake in the superior portion of the right lobe of the liver; **(B)** right lateral view appears normal. Hepatic laceration was confirmed at laparotomy.

Methods

Static liver scans to delineate the hepatic parenchyma are performed following the administration of 1–4 mCi of technetium 99m sulfur colloid. The colloid particles are selectively phagocytized by the reticuloendothelial or Kupffer cells of the liver and remain fixed in the cells for several hours before undergoing degradation. The spleen may also be visualized by this injection. Other radiopharmaceuticals may be used, but from the point of view of cost and availability, technetium 99m sulfur colloid is the radionuclide of choice. Either the rectilinear scanner or the gamma camera will produce satisfactory liver images. The entire procedure including anterior, right and left lateral, and posterior views can be completed within 30 min following administration of the radionuclide. Abnormalities appear as cold areas on the scan. Radiopharmaceutical cost for the static liver scan is about $3–$4 per dose.

Visualization of the biliary ducts, gallbladder, and excretory system has been accomplished in the past using radioiodinated (I 131) rose bengal, which is excreted by the parenchymal cells of the liver into the bile ducts and gallbladder. Unfortunately, the significant radiation exposure resulting from the use of this compound has limited the dose that could be used. In addition, the high-energy (364 keV) gamma radiation of I 131 is poorly imaged by the thin crystal of the gamma camera. A new group of technetium pharmaceuticals has become available; these compounds are in the imino diacetic acid family and include HIDA, BIDA, and PIPIDA. They are rapidly removed from the blood by the liver and promptly appear in the bile. Because of the rapidity of their excretion, they are best imaged with the gamma camera, obtaining serial images every 15–30 min. Since these radiopharmaceuticals are tagged with technetium 99m, a relatively high dose can be administered with minimal radiation exposure and high detection efficiency.

Radiopharmaceuticals that extravasate from the biliary system can be readily identified as an area of increased activity in an aberrant location within the abdomen. Likewise, areas of ductal stenosis or occlusion can be demonstrated. When there is a possibility that hepatic parenchymal injury and bile-duct injury coexist, use of this new class of pharmaceuticals will given an image of intrahepatic architecture in the early phases of the study and an opportunity to evaluate the biliary system later in the examination.

Liver-Lung Scans

Liver-lung scans are useful in detecting the presence of an abnormal space between the inferior border of right-lung activity and the superior border of hepatic activity. Normally, no separation between these two organs exists on the anterior, right lateral, posterior, or oblique views. Because of the compressibility of these organs, the liver and lung scans obtained independently of each other may appear to be normal, despite a collection of fluid, blood, or pus between the two organs. Though it is relatively unusual for a bullet or penetrating missile to cause intrathoracic or abdominal trauma without affecting the lung or liver directly, this does occasionally occur. The combined liver-lung scan is of greater utility in detecting the presence of a subphrenic abscess, which is not an uncommon result of thoracoabdominal trauma. Following treatment of a subphrenic abscess, the healing of the lesion can be evaluated by sequential liver-lung scans (Figs. 3.48–3.51).

Because of anatomic considerations, liver-lung scans are much more useful in evaluating right-sided thoracoabdominal trauma than left-sided trauma. Though the spleen is usually juxtaposed below the left lung, this anatomic configuration is not so constant as the relationship between the liver and the right lung. As previously noted, the spleen is a relatively mobile organ when compared to the liver and may be located somewhat below the diaphragm. Thus lung-spleen scans are of considerable clinical value when they demonstrate the absence of a separation between the inferior border of left-lung activity and the superior border of splenic activity, confirming the absence of fluid collection between the two organs. Such scans are of little value when the combined lung-spleen scan

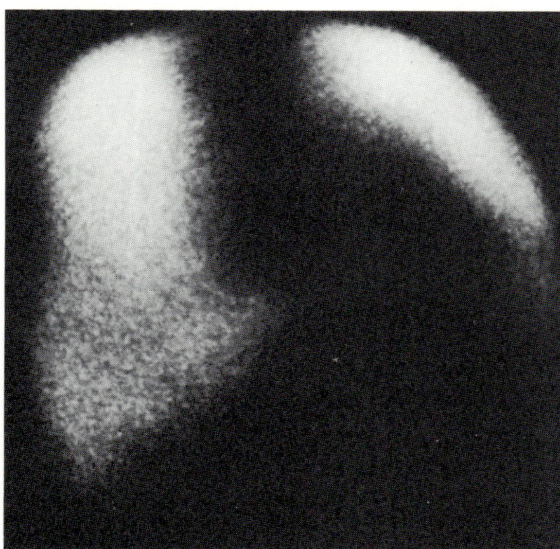

FIG. 3.48. Normal liver-lung scan, anterior view; gamma camera, technetium 99m sulfur colloid (liver), technetium 99m, macroaggregated albumin (lung). Note that inferior border of pulmonary (right lung) activity is contiguous with superior border of hepatic activity.

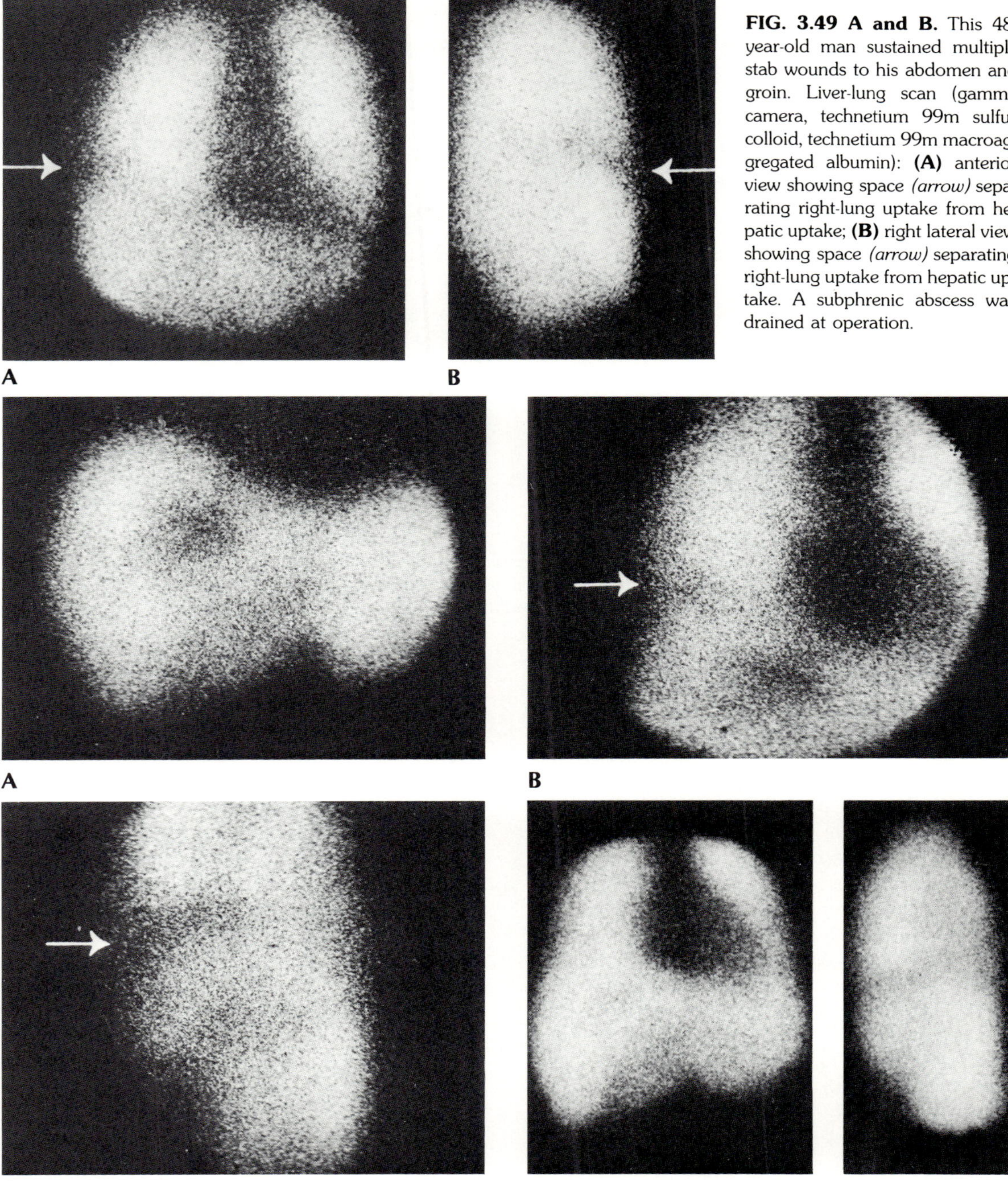

FIG. 3.49 A and B. This 48-year-old man sustained multiple stab wounds to his abdomen and groin. Liver-lung scan (gamma camera, technetium 99m sulfur colloid, technetium 99m macroaggregated albumin): **(A)** anterior view showing space *(arrow)* separating right-lung uptake from hepatic uptake; **(B)** right lateral view showing space *(arrow)* separating right-lung uptake from hepatic uptake. A subphrenic abscess was drained at operation.

FIG. 3.50 A–E. This 29-year-old woman sustained multiple thoracoabdominal gunshot wounds. Liver and liver-lung scans (gamma camera, technetium 99m sulfur colloid, technetium 99m macroaggregated albumin): **(A)** anterior liver scan demonstrating an area of decreased uptake representing a tunnel wound of the liver; **(B)** anterior liver-lung scan demonstrating a suspicious area of decreased uptake *(arrow)* separating right-lung uptake from liver; **(C)** right lateral liver-lung scan demonstrating a definite space *(arrow)* separating right-lung uptake from liver uptake—the abnormality is located posteriorly, and the hepatic wound is also seen; **(D)** anterior liver-lung scan obtained 3 weeks following initial study showing significant interval resolution of the intrahepatic defect and almost complete resolution of the space separating the right lung from the liver; **(E)** right lateral liver-lung scan obtained 3 weeks following initial study showing significant interval healing of the intrahepatic defect as well as almost complete resolution of the space separating the right lung from the liver. Both the intrahepatic tunnel wound and the subphrenic lesion were confirmed at laparotomy performed after the initial studies. The patient was treated with surgical drainage and antibiotics.

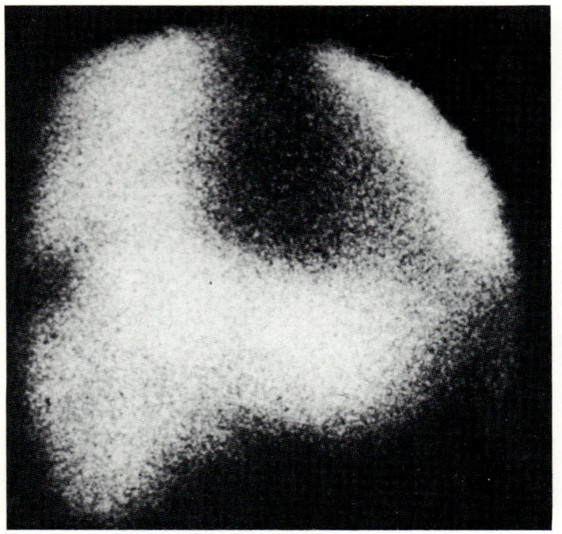

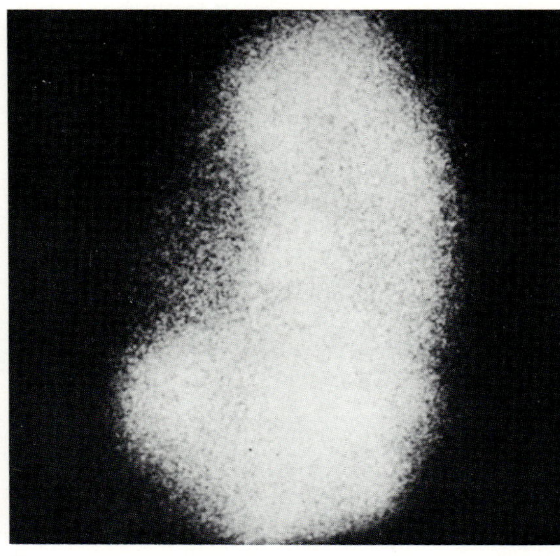

A B

FIG. 3.51 A and B. This 30-year-old man sustained a gunshot wound of the lower thorax. The patient developed a fever and drainage of bile. Liver-lung scan (gamma camera, technetium 99m sulfur colloid, technetium 99m macroaggregated albumin): **(A)** anterior view showing discrete area of decreased uptake separating lung from liver; **(B)** right lateral liver view appears normal.

shows a space between the margins of the two organs, since this finding may be demonstrated when no abnormality exists. For these reasons the lung-spleen scan is considerably less useful than the liver-lung scan.

Liver-lung scans are performed by administering two radiopharmaceuticals, one to visualize the liver and one to visualize the lung. In order to visualize both organs on the same image it is desirable to choose two radiopharmaceuticals that are tagged with radionuclides of the same or similar energies. Currently, radiopharmaceuticals tagged with technetium 99m are routinely used to visualize both organs. Technetium 99m sulfur colloid is used as described above to visualize the liver, and macroaggregated human serum albumin tagged with technetium 99m (Tc 99mMAA), is used to obtain the lung scan. In order to obtain comparatively equal activities in both organs so that they may be satisfactorily visualized on a single exposure, approximately equal doses of technetium 99m sulfur colloid and technetium 99m macroaggregated human serum albumin are administered.

It is important that the radiopharmaceutical for lung visualization be injected when the patient is in a supine position to ensure even distribution of the Tc 99mMAA throughout the lungs. Imaging may be done in either a supine, sitting, or standing position; the latter two positions may cause some ptosis of the intraabdominal organs, falsely indicating the presence of a space between the lung and the liver. It is prudent to obtain a liver scan in multiple views prior to injecting the radiopharmaceutical to visualize the lung, since frequently the liver scan alone will reveal an unsuspected lesion and obviate the need for the combined study. When the liver-lung scan is performed, the patient is positioned so that the dome of the liver is centered under the detector of the gamma camera or in the field of view of the rectilinear scanner, and multiple views are obtained. As a minimum these views should include the anterior, right lateral, and posterior views. When a lung-spleen scan is indicated, the same technical considerations apply and the radiopharmaceuticals are identical to those used to obtain a liver-lung scan, since technetium 99m sulfur colloid will also visualize the spleen.

Kidney

The kidney is less commonly involved in abdominal trauma then either the liver or spleen. However, because it is a paired organ with compensatory capabilities, significant trauma to a single kidney or excretory system may not be evident initially. Fractures, lacerations, and hematomas may appear as areas of decreased uptake on static kidney scans, whereas dynamic studies may be helpful in elucidating trauma to the renal vascular system or excretory system [9].

The radioisotope renogram was introduced in the 1950s as a nonimaging method to study kidney function. The accumulation and excretion of radioiodinated hippuran were plotted against time (for 30 min) to give evidence of renal arterial stenosis, kidney malfunction, and/or pelvic or ureteral obstruction. Because of its lack of specificity, the radioisotope renogram is not commonly used today. Static renal scans using mercury compounds were used in the 1960s to determine the presence of structural lesions within the kidneys. The introduction of technetium 99m–labeled DTPA (diethylene triamine pentaacetate) as well as other technetium 99m–labeled agents that are specific for kidney scanning has allowed the nuclear medicine physician to obtain visualization of the renal arteries, renal parenchyma, and excretory system with a single injection. These technetium-labeled radiopharmaceuticals are selectively localized in the kidney and then secreted and excreted into the urine.

Renal scans are currently obtained by using one of the technetium-labeled radiopharmaceuticals in a dose of 10–15 mCi injected as a bolus into a vein in the anticubital fossa. The patient, who may be in either a supine or a sitting position, is positioned in front of a gamma-camera detector for a posterior view of the renal area. It is important that the patient be well hydrated. Serial 2- to 6-s images are obtained during the first 30–45 s after injection to visualize the renal vasculature. A static image is secured between 30 and 90 min following administration of radiopharmaceutical to delineate renal structure, location, and configuration. Since the technetium 99m–labeled pharmaceutical is excreted into the urine, interval images of the kidneys, ureters, and bladder may be obtained to determine sites of extravasation or ureteral obstruction and to ascertain the adequacy of renal function.

Arteries

Isotope angiography permits the visualization of the major branches of the arterial tree following the intravenous administration of a bolus of radioactive material [98]. After the patient is properly positioned under the gamma camera, technetium 99m (as the pertechnetate or tagged to albumin or DTPA) is administered as a bolus by the Oldendorf technique and the gamma camera activated. Images obtained every 1–2 s following administration of the radioactive material will delineate the major arteries in the field of view of the detector. Excellent visualization of the truncal arteries (including the aorta, and iliac and femoral arteries) as well as the arteries of the extremities (to the level of the ankle or the level of the wrist) can be accomplished by this technique. The renal arteries may also be visualized (see p. 187). Sites of arterial transection appear as an abrupt cut-off in the column of radioactive material. True and false aneurysms appear as saccular collections of radioactive material that often increase in activity with time. Extrinsic pressure on an artery (as from a hematoma) may also be successfully demonstrated by this technique. The demonstration of an intact artery precludes the need for conventional angiography for confirmation of arterial integrity.

During the past decade the advances in nuclear imaging techniques have facilitated the use of this modality for the evaluation of intraabdominal trauma.

Radionuclide methods of evaluating the patient subjected to abdominal trauma are especially valuable because they are associated with no morbidity or mortality and require minimal handling of the patient once he is in the nuclear medicine facility. Since radioisotope techniques are based on physiological considerations, they often give information that is at best difficult and sometimes impossible to obtain by other noninvasive techniques. Radioisotope imaging techniques have frequently obviated the need for more complex and invasive radiologic procedures and exploratory surgery. Where an abnormality has been demonstrated by radioisotope techniques, the preoperative knowledge gained has simplified subsequent examinations of varying types.

PERITONEOSCOPY

The use of peritoneoscopy in the diagnosis of abdominal injuries is a new concept. There is a very limited experience with its value in trauma management primarily because laparoscopy has not been a standard diagnostic tool for the general surgeon. As the quality of instrumentation has improved, gynecologists have used the laparoscope as both a diagnostic and therapeutic aid. Endoscopic surgical procedures are of increasing importance and consequently laparoscopy should be viewed as a technique of growing value.

Indications

Despite the established contribution of careful physical examination, peritoneal lavage and radiologic examination, laboratory data, and scanning techniques, there is still a small percentage of patients with abdominal trauma who have "trivial" injuries. This group of patients will often have the physical findings and peritoneal lavage and tap findings that justify exploratory laparotomy. Kazarian et al. reported a negative laparotomy rate of 10.5% for a large group of stab-wound patients [51]. Engrav et al. reported an unnecessary laparotomy rate of 7.1% in patients with blunt abdominal trauma selected for surgery utilizing paracentesis with lavage [26]. Of 40 unnecessary laparotomies, 31 were performed in patients with trivial injuries. This unnecessary surgery can be avoided only if a fairly accurate, direct assessment of the injury can be made visually. Laparoscopy can be viewed as an extension of the paracentesis-lavage procedure in that a limited but direct set of conclusions can be drawn based on the direct inspection of portions of abdominal cavity. The firm conclusions that can be made from laparoscopy include the presence or absence of anterior and lateral abdominal-wall penetration, the presence and extent of injury to the anterior lateral and superior surface of the liver, the existence of injury to the anterior surface of the stomach, and the presence and extent of intraperitoneal blood and other fluids. The laparoscopic evaluation of the retroperitoneum, pelvic structures, and spleen is more limited. A significant assessment of bowel injury cannot be made with the laparoscope by current techniques.

A number of variables relevant to the clinical application of peritoneoscopy in trauma need assessment: whether all or only some patients suffering abdominal trauma should have laparoscopy, whether blunt or penetrating injury or both are most appropriate for laparoscopy, and whether laparoscopy should be highly selective and used only after lavage and very careful clinical and radiologic examination. Experience with the laparoscopic examination of 20 patients suffering trauma of all types was reported by the Morrisania Hospital group in 1976 [14].

The patients with abdominal stab wounds admitted to Morrisania Hospital were selectively explored based upon the clinical criteria advocated by Shaftan. The attitude of the authors is to perform exploratory operations for all patients with abdominal gunshot wounds, unless the injury is obviously tangential to the abdominal wall. The decision to explore the abdomen in patients with blunt trauma has been based on the physical and radiologic findings, laboratory data, and quantitative analysis of aliquots of aspirated peritoneal fluid obtained using paracentesis with lavage [14].

A group of 20 patients with abdominal trauma had peritoneoscopy performed at the Morrisania City Hospital during a 15-month interval. Laparoscopy was performed as a preliminary diagnostic procedure before exploratory celiotomy. The principal objective was to avoid unnecessary laparotomy in patients with a trivial visceral injury that would not require definitive surgical correction. All patients were examined by members of the resident surgical staff and one of the authors. The need for exploratory celiotomy was based upon the interpretation of findings in one or more of the following categories: general physical and abdominal examinations, radiologic studies, laboratory data, and peritoneal tap and lavage. None of the patients had signs of cardiovascular instability.

Technique

All patients were prepared and draped for exploratory celiotomy. General endotracheal anesthesia was administered, although local anesthesia can be utilized in cooperative patients. A 1.5-cm incision was made through the skin and subcutaneous tissue in either the supraumbilical or infraumbilical position. A stab incision in the linea alba was made to facilitate intraperitoneal insertion of a spring-loaded pneumoperitoneum needle and subsequent passage of the trocar and valve sleeve. The Verres needle provides a point to pierce the peritoneum as the spring sleeve is retracted. Release of the spring sleeve upon entry into the peritoneal cavity advances the blunt needle point to prevent bowel perforation.

Nitrous oxide was administered through the needle to effect gaseous distension of the peritoneal cavity. Observation and abdominal percussion monitored the degree of pneumoperitoneum. More recently, carbon dioxide pneumoperitoneum given through the Semm insufflator permitted flow control and pressure monitoring of the administered gas.

The trocar and cannula with valve (outer diameter, 11 mm) were then inserted into the peritoneal cavity at an angle directed toward the true pelvis. After removal of the trocar, the cannula was directed toward the region of interest, and the sheathed Hopkins forward-oblique telescope (outer diameter, 5.8 mm) was inserted. Fiberoptic light transmission was generated by an ACMI-FCB 1000 light source. If needed, a palpation probe was inserted into the peritoneal cavity through a separate, conveniently localized, abdominal site to facilitate intraabdominal exposure by gentle depression or pulsion of either the organ of interest or adjacent viscus. The recent availability of a flexible-tipped fiberoptic peritoneoscope has broadened the diagnostic potential of laparoscopy for the diagnosis of hepatobiliary and splenic injuries. Moreover, the ability to visualize anterior and lateral parietal peritoneal penetration has been facilitated.

ILLUSTRATIVE CASE REPORTS

D.J., a 26-year-old man, was hospitalized 2 h after he was stabbed in the right side of the neck and in the right seventh intercostal space at the anterior axillary line. The blood pressure was 140/80 mmHg, pulse 80 per min, respirations 24 per min, and temperature 99°F. The neck injury penetrated the platysma muscle but there was no hematoma, bleeding, or wound crepitation. The abdominal examination disclosed right-upper-quadrant (RUQ) rigidity and tenderness. Bowel sounds were decreased. Aspiration through the nasogastric tube and the rectal examination were unremarkable. Laboratory values included a hematocrit of 46%, and white blood cell (WBC) count of 7000/mm³. Urinalysis revealed 45 WBC/hpf, and the red blood cells were too numerous to count. The plain abdominal roentgenograms and the intravenous pyelogram were normal. Abdominal paracentesis and lavage disclosed bloody fluid with a hematocrit of 1%.

Peritoneoscopy disclosed a nonbleeding 2-cm laceration in the dome of the right hepatic lobe and bloody peritoneal fluid. The remainder of the intraabdominal examination was normal. Exploratory laparotomy was not performed. There was no deep structural injury found at neck exploration. The patient's hospital course was unremarkable, and he was discharged on the fifth hospital day.

P.M., a 4-year old boy, was struck by a car. There was no loss of consciousness, and he was alert on hospital admission; however, he complained of abdominal pain. The vital signs were blood pressure 110/70 mmHg, pulse 120 per min, respirations 24 per min, temperature 101.4°F. The important physical findings were upper-abdominal rigidity and tenderness more pronounced on the right side. Bowel sounds were hypoactive. Serial laboratory values showed a fall in the hematocrit from 37% to 32% associated with hydration; serum amylase 106 dye units; urinalysis 100 RBC/hpf. Plain abdominal roentgenograms were normal. An intravenous urogram showed delayed function of the right kidney. Paracentesis with lavage disclosed bloody fluid with more than 10,000 RBC/mm³.

Peritoneoscopy revealed a 3-cm laceration of the right hepatic lobe and a torn falciform ligament. Dilute bloody fluid was observed in the peritoneal cavity, but there was no active bleeding. The patient's RUQ abdominal findings were normal 2 days later. The repeat excretory urogram 6 days later was normal.

B.B., an inebriated 45-year-old man with a history of psychotic illness, was hospitalized after a self-inflicted stab wound of the left side of the epigastrium (Fig. 3.52). The vital signs were normal. Abdominal physical examination revealed diffuse epigastric tenderness without rigidity. The laboratory values and plain-film studies were normal.

Peritoneoscopy disclosed a small hemoperitoneum. There was a nonbleeding penetrating wound through the lateral segment of the left hepatic lobe. Examination of the left infrahepatic area revealed omentum. Exploratory laparotomy was not performed. The pa-

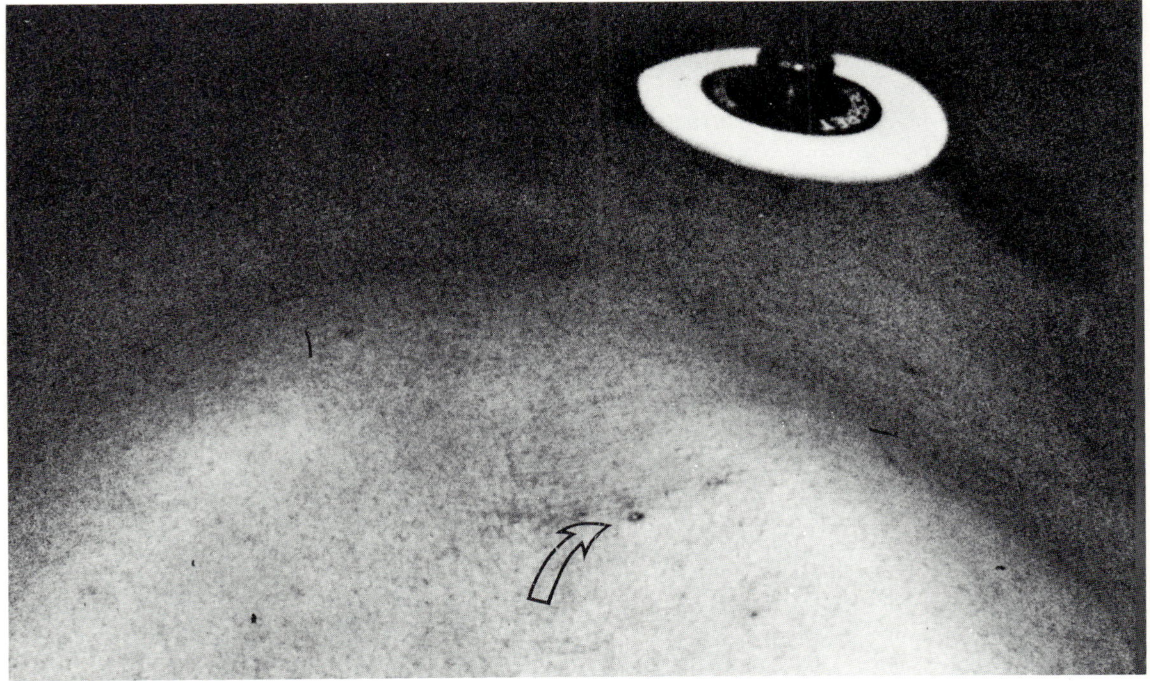

FIG. 3.52. The patient depicted sustained a self-inflicted "pig sticker" wound of the epigastrium 2 cm to the left of the midline. The patient fashioned a pointed weapon from a thick, stiff wire. Laparoscopy revealed a puncture wound through the left lobe of the liver into the supergastric retroperitoneum. Despite the presence of direct tenderness by physical examination, surgical exploration was not required.

tient was discharged to a mental institution 3 days later.

Twenty patients with abdominal trauma judged to require exploratory laparotomy had peritoneoscopy as a preliminary diagnostic procedure. The group was composed of 14 males and 6 females ranging in age from 4 to 67 years.

The types of abdominal injury in the 20 patients included 11 stab wounds, 3 gunshot wounds, 5 blunt trauma, and 1 shotgun injury (Table 3.25).

An exploratory laparotomy was avoided in 12 of 20 patients (60%) because of the peritoneoscope findings (Table 3.26). In three patients with abdominal stab wounds, exploratory laparotomy was avoided because peritoneal-cavity penetration had not occurred. Four patients in the group of twelve had peritoneal-cavity penetration; however, no visceral injury was observed. Five patients in this group did not have exploratory laparotomy although visceral injury was observed at peritoneoscopy. Two of these patients had hepatic lacerations confined to the right lobe. A third patient had a stab wound through the lateral segment of the left hepatic lobe and a nonexpanding hematoma in the gastrohepatic omentum. The fourth individual had a 3.0-cm subcapsular hematoma of the right hepatic lobe due to blunt trauma. The fifth patient was found to have a 3-cm laceration of the right hepatic lobe and a lacerated falciform ligament. None of the hepatic injuries were drained, and the average hospitalized period for the group with visceral injury was 3.4 days.

Exploratory laparotomy was performed subsequent to peritoneoscopy in eight patients (40%) (Table 3.27). In seven of the eight individuals, the injuries observed at peritoneoscopy were repaired during laparotomy. The eighth patient had normal peritoneoscopy findings 24 h after blunt trauma to the scrotum that clinically resulted in fever and right-lower-quadrant abdominal rigidity. The appendix was not detected during the peritoneoscopy. A normal retroceal appendix was removed at laparotomy.

The hospitalization period for the 12 patients who avoided exploratory laparotomy because of the peritoneoscopic findings averaged 4.5 days. The minimum hospitalization time for the exploratory celiotomy group was 7 days.

There were no complications in the group of patients who had peritoneoscopy only, nor were there complications attributable to peritoneoscopy in those individuals who also had exploratory laparotomy.

Heselson [46], Tostivint et al. [111], and Gazzaniga et al. [35] have published reports on the use of peritoneoscopy in trauma (Table 3.28). In their experience, peritoneoscopy was found to be a most valuable diagnostic technique in trauma. Gazzaniga et al. reported

TABLE 3.25. Types of injuries

Types	No. of cases
Stab wound	11
Gunshot wound	3
Blunt trauma	5
Shotgun	1
Total	20

Source: Carnevale N, Baron N, Delany HM (1977) Peritoneoscopy as an aid in the diagnosis of abdominal trauma. A preliminary report. J Trauma 17: 634–641

TABLE 3.26. Exploratory celiotomy not performed after laparoscopy

Reason	No. of cases
A. No peritoneal-cavity penetration	3
B. Peritoneal-cavity penetration: no visceral injury	4
C. Visceral injury seen: judged to be minor	5
Total	12

Source: Carnevale N, Baron N, Delany HM (1977) Peritoneoscopy as an aid in the diagnosis of abdominal trauma. A preliminary report. J Trauma 17: 634–641

TABLE 3.27. Exploratory celiotomy performed after laparoscopy

Findings	No. of cases
A. Negative exploratory celiotomy	1
B. Positive exploratory celiotomy	7
Total	8

Source: Carnevale N, Baron N, Delany HM (1977) Peritoneoscopy as an aid in the diagnosis of abdominal trauma. A preliminary report. J Trauma 17: 634–641

TABLE 3.28. Peritoneoscopy (personal series): 18 percent cases analyzed[a]

Type	No.	Laparotomy	No laparotomy
Blunt	16	11	5
Stab	2	2	0
Total	18	13	5

[a] One case showed negative sinogram followed by positive peritoneoscopy 24 h later.

Source: Heselson J (1970) Peritoneoscopy in abdominal trauma. S Afr J Surg 8: 1

37 patients from the University of California at Irvine: 22 of their 37 patients required laparotomy, and 15 patients were spared laparotomy based on the laparoscopic findings. Gazzaniga et al.'s experience was similar to the authors' in terms of indications, except that their group approached all penetrating injuries with laparoscopy. In the authors' series the patients with penetrating injury were selected for laparoscopy if they had the standard clinical indications for laparotomy. The patients with blunt injury had surgery if the tap/lavage was positive.

The limited nature of this examination has to be emphasized in order to avoid the inappropriate use of the procedure. The authors' experience led to the conclusion that laparoscopy is indicated as an adjunctive diagnostic technique to clinical examination and peritoneal tap and lavage. It is not an alternative procedure and should not be used for primary diagnosis. Gazzaniga et al. and the authors were able to avoid false-negative examinations by exploration of all patients when there was doubt about the severity of injury based on the peritoneoscopy. It is clear that peritoneoscopy has its greatest value in the assessment of limited but potentially significant upper-abdominal injuries. It is of most help in evaluating liver injuries, tangential abdominal stab wounds, gunshot wounds to determine penetration, and to confirm the extent of blunt injury in patients with borderline positive peritoneal lavage results. The potential of peritoneoscopy is enhanced with the use of flexible peritoneoscopy with simultaneous manipulation of the visceral structures. A more extensive experience with the technique is needed.

EXPLORATORY LAPAROTOMY

The first principle in the exploratory surgical procedure for abdominal injury is thorough and systematic evaluation. The complete examination of the abdominal contents is vital for proper care in abdominal trauma, regardless of the nature of the abdominal wound. The failure to identify all intraabdominal-organ injuries is a tragedy with ominous consequences. The postoperative complications of persistent fever, abdominal tenderness, or ileus cannot be properly evaluated if there is doubt whether a satisfactory repair of all injured organs was performed at the time of surgery.

A step-by-step approach to abdominal exploration should be standard procedure for the responsible surgeon regardless of the extent of injuries or the difficulties inherent in the situation. Life-threatening hemorrhage must be dealt with as soon as the origin and nature of such hemorrhage has been identified. However, multiplicity of injury is quite common, and thorough examination of all intraabdominal structures should follow the control of hemorrhage. A missed injury cannot be excused.

The Incision

The midline incision is most suitable for emergency abdominal exploration (Fig. 3.53). This incision can be performed quickly and allows access to all areas of the abdomen. The length of the incision is based on the individual circumstances. An ample abdominal exploratory incision is important for a prompt and complete evaluation. Exploration with an inadequate incision should not be attempted. Extension of the incision into the right or left chest may become necessary, depending on whether access to the retrohepatic vena cava or the dome of the liver is required. A separate thoracic incision on the left or right side is an alternative approach, but may be more cumbersome.

Access to the thoracic vena cava and retrohepatic vena cava has been described through a sternal split-

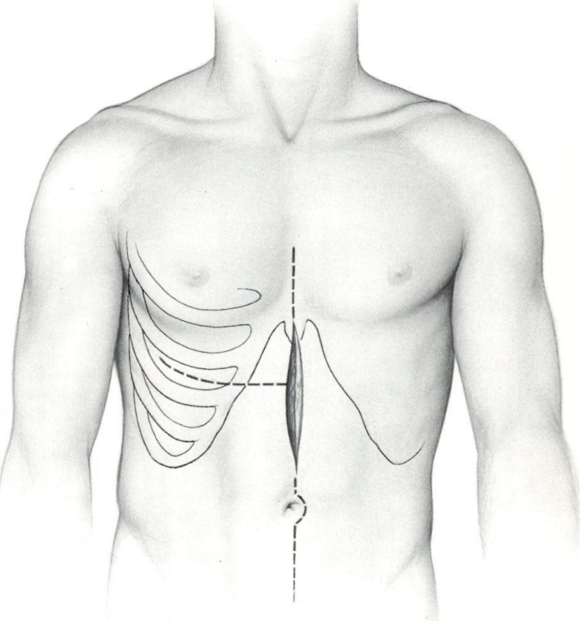

FIG. 3.53. *Abdominal incision.* The ideal incision for exploratory laparotomy for abdominal trauma is the midline incision. This incision can be extended upward into the mediastinum through a sternal split or downward to the pubis. In multiple abdominal injuries, an incision extending from the xyphoid to well below the umbilicus is ideal for thorough exploration. An extension into the right chest at the 7th or 8th intercostal space allows access to the retrohepatic vena cava.

ting incision as an extension of the midline abdominal incision [71]. On occasion, paramedian or rectus muscle splitting incisions are indicated if the patient has had a previous midline incision or multiple operative procedures have been performed in the past. Although a transverse incision can be used for laparotomy and exploration, it is not the optimal incision to use. If the circumstances necessitate the use of a transverse incision, it must be ample in length to allow evaluation of all areas. The selection of an incision should not be dictated by the location of the penetrating injury or the area of maximum abdominal tenderness. Even if the surgeon is fairly confident that he is dealing with a lacerated spleen or liver, a transverse incision in the upper or lower abdomen can lead to difficulty if the possibility of injury to another organ exists. The limitation of the midline incision, in terms of increased postoperative pain, is accepted in exchange for the flexibility that this incision offers.

Controlling Hemorrhage

The first basic technical step is to deal with acute intraabdominal hemorrhage. If bleeding is from the spleen or liver or other supracolonic structures, immediate control should be gained using the appropriate measures. If the bleeding is from the bowel wall, bowel mesentery, or the retroperitoneal region, immediate evisceration should be performed, if possible. This ma-

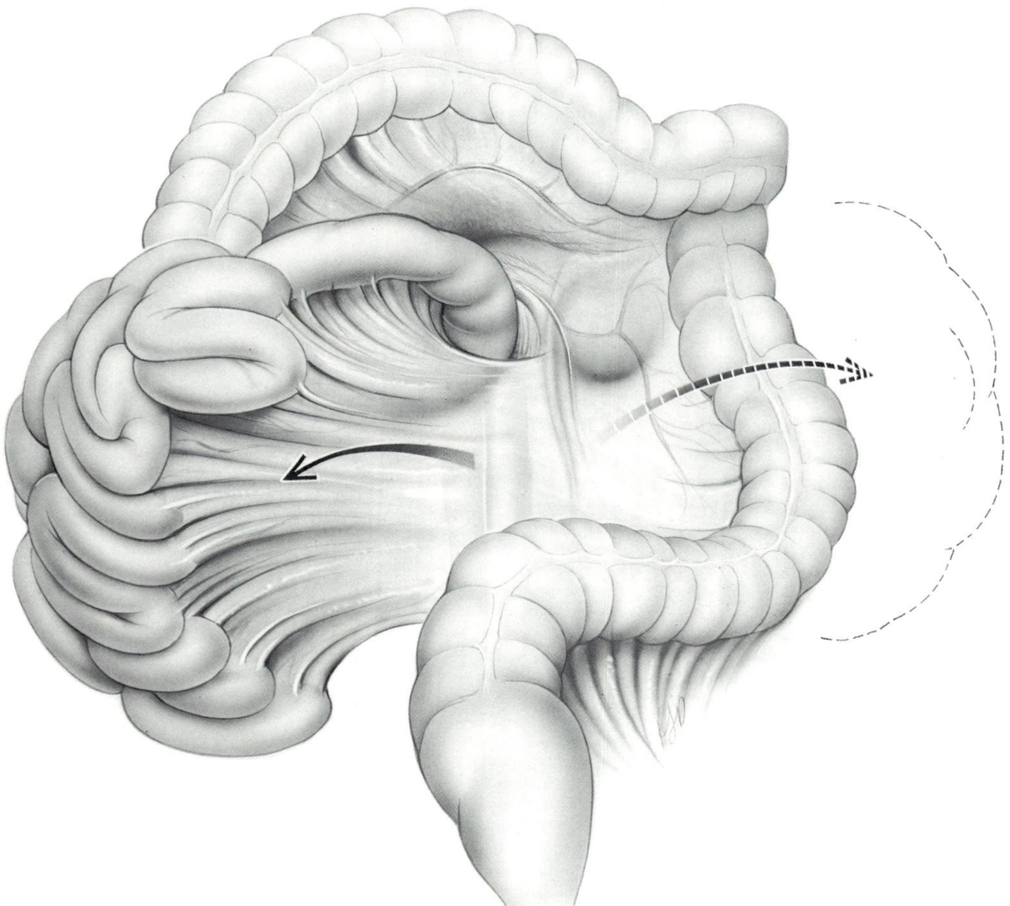

FIG. 3.54. *Evisceration.* Evisceration of the small bowel permits visualization of the mesentery of the left colon when the bowel is swept to the right and allows visualization of the mesentery of the right colon when the small bowel is swept to the left. Inspection of the small-bowel mesentery can be accomplished with this maneuver. Control of bleeding from the mesentery can be easily obtained by manual compression. In view of the anatomical location of the aorta and the left ureter, some impression of the extent of retroperitoneal-organ injury is evident immediately upon evisceration. In the illustration showing the small bowel on the right side, the tip of the left kidney, the mesentery of the small bowel, the left colon, and sigmoid are readily seen.

neuver offers an opportunity for rapid control of the bowel mesentery by hand-squeeze or compression of the retroperitoneum by pressure. Evisceration also offers a good view of the retroperitoneal space to evaluate the location and size of a retroperitoneal hematoma (Fig. 3.54). It is difficult to deal with bleeding, or leaking viscera or mesentery if the bowel mesentery is in its normal position. The use of dry lap pads pressed about the area of active bleeding can be an alternative to immediate evisceration. If adhesions are present, an attempt must be made to gain in-situ control of hemorrhage until the surgeon has sufficient time to divide the adhesions.

Once immediate control of life-threatening bleeding from visceral or vascular injuries has been accomplished, the second step should be the identification of any source of contamination of the peritoneal cavity. Obviously, contamination from colonic or multiple lower-small-bowel injuries carries greater danger than a gastric or upper-small-bowel injury. Spillage from injuries producing fecal contamination should be immediately controlled. Definitive repair of the bowel or exteriorization is not necessary immediately, but the leakage of contaminating fluid should be prevented.

Inspection of Abdominal Organs

Careful exploration of the abdominal organs should then be carried out beginning with the esophagus and continuing to the stomach, liver, spleen, retrogastric spaces, duodenum, small bowel, and colon. Several maneuvers should be considered as a standard part of complete intraoperative evaluation. The duodenum, the head of the pancreas, the hepatoduodenal ligament, and vena cava must be carefully inspected. In order to accomplish thorough demonstration of these structures, the Kocher maneuver may be required. This procedure is justified for every case with injuries near the areas described (Fig. 3.55). Inspection of the duodenum in its posterior and retroperitoneal course is then completed by medial displacement of the jejunum at the ligament of Treitz and direct visualization of the posterior surface of the third and fourth portions of the duodenum beneath the superior mesenteric vessels (Fig. 3.56). It is important to be familiar with this "blind" retroperitoneal area and to examine it thoroughly. Injuries to this area may not result in significant findings; therefore, any retroperitoneal hemorrhage or bile-staining must be investigated [59].

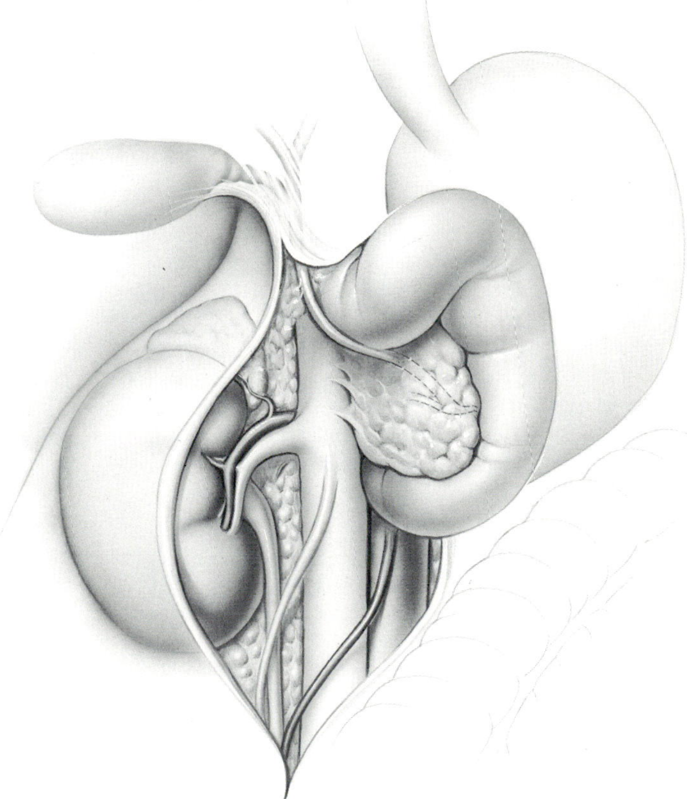

FIG. 3.55. *Kocher maneuver.* Mobilization of the second portion of the duodenum and the head of the pancreas using the Kocher maneuver provides access to several important intraabdominal organs. This maneuver is valuable in the management of patients with retroperitoneal hematomas or pancreatic, renal, and vena caval injuries. The number of structures that can be visualized and palpated with this maneuver include head of pancreas, duodenum, vena cava, right renal artery and vein, right kidney, the common duct, and portal vein. The Kocher maneuver often requires mobilization of the hepatocolic attachments with displacement of the hepatic flexure.

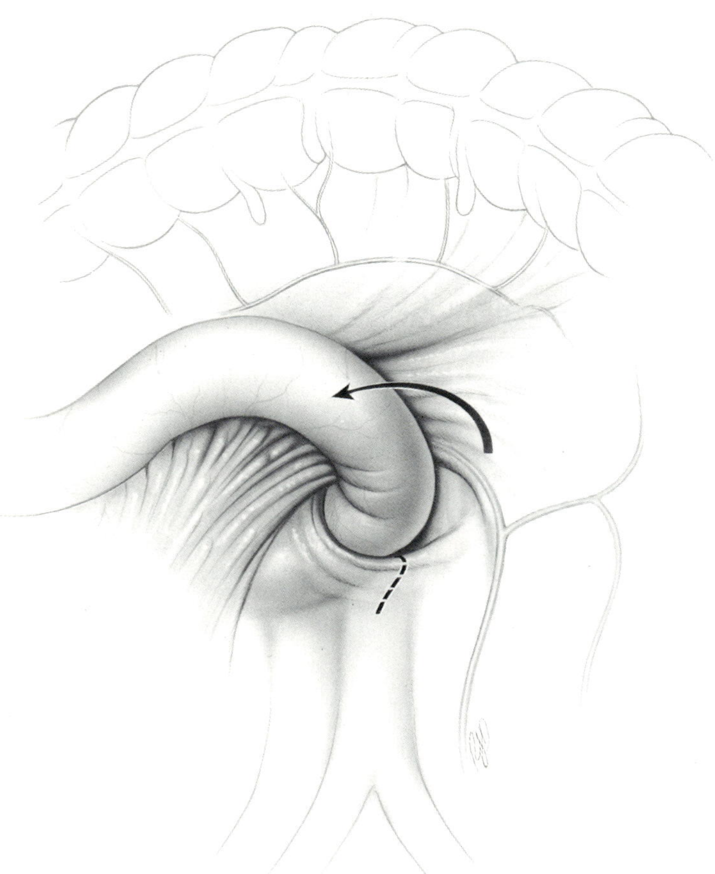

FIG. 3.56. *Visualization of retroperitoneal duodenum.* Mobilization of the duodenojejunal junction and retroperitoneal dissection of the duodenum gives opportunity to visualize and palpate the entire duodenum. It is important to visualize this area in patients who have retroperitoneal hematomas. Combined with a Kocher maneuver, this procedure allows examination of the posterior and inferior surface of the third and fourth portion of the duodenum.

Running the Bowel

The small bowel should be inspected in its full length, with examination of all surfaces. This procedure is performed by folding the bowel from side to side (Fig. 3.57). The cecum and right side of the colon should be mobilized if there is the slightest evidence or suspicion of injury to this area. Small-bowel and colonic injuries are usually accompanied by a serosal or mesenteric hematoma. When such a finding is present, careful inspection of the bowel-wall surfaces must be carried out to look for lacerations or perforations (Fig. 3.58). A foul odor or bubbles issuing from the area is an obvious signal that a large-bowel injury has occurred. Injuries to the bowel mesentery can be particularly troublesome. If blind ligation of mesenteric tissue is performed, hematomas can develop and intact mesenteric vessels may be inadvertently compromised. Care should be taken to secure the single or multiple mesenteric vessels injured. After repair of the mesentery there should be close attention to the result in terms of bowel viability. Dissection in the mesenteric fat may be necessary to identify the mesenteric vessels. Palpation by hand is a good technique for identifying the major vessel bundles.

If the hepatic flexure of the colon is not readily visualized, it can be mobilized with relative ease. The transverse colon and sigmoid are readily accessible. However, redundancy, abundant omentum, and mesenteric fat can obscure colonic injuries unless great care is taken with the inspection process.

The Spleen, Pancreas, and Retroperitoneum

Although mobilization of the splenic flexure is not a routine part of exploration for trauma, it should be considered if it is necessary to visualize the colon in this area or if a specific injury to structures in the left upper quadrant is suspected. Unexplained continuing bleeding from the upper abdomen is likely to come from the spleen. Injury and laceration of the spleen

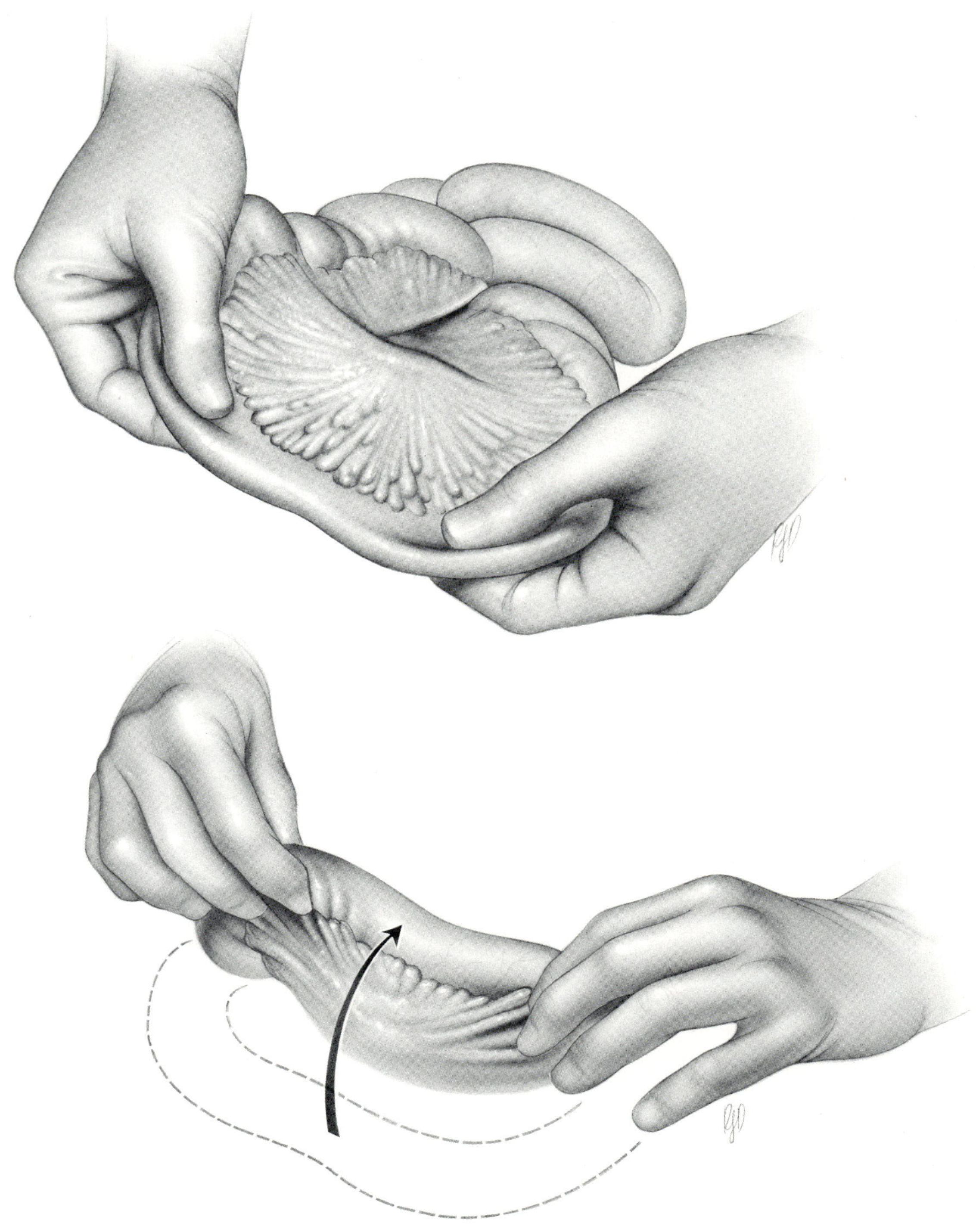

FIG. 3.57. *Running the bowel.* Proper examination of the full length of the small bowel is achieved by flipping the intestine back and forth. This procedure must be carried out thoroughly, beginning at the ligament of Treitz and continuing to the ileocecal junction.

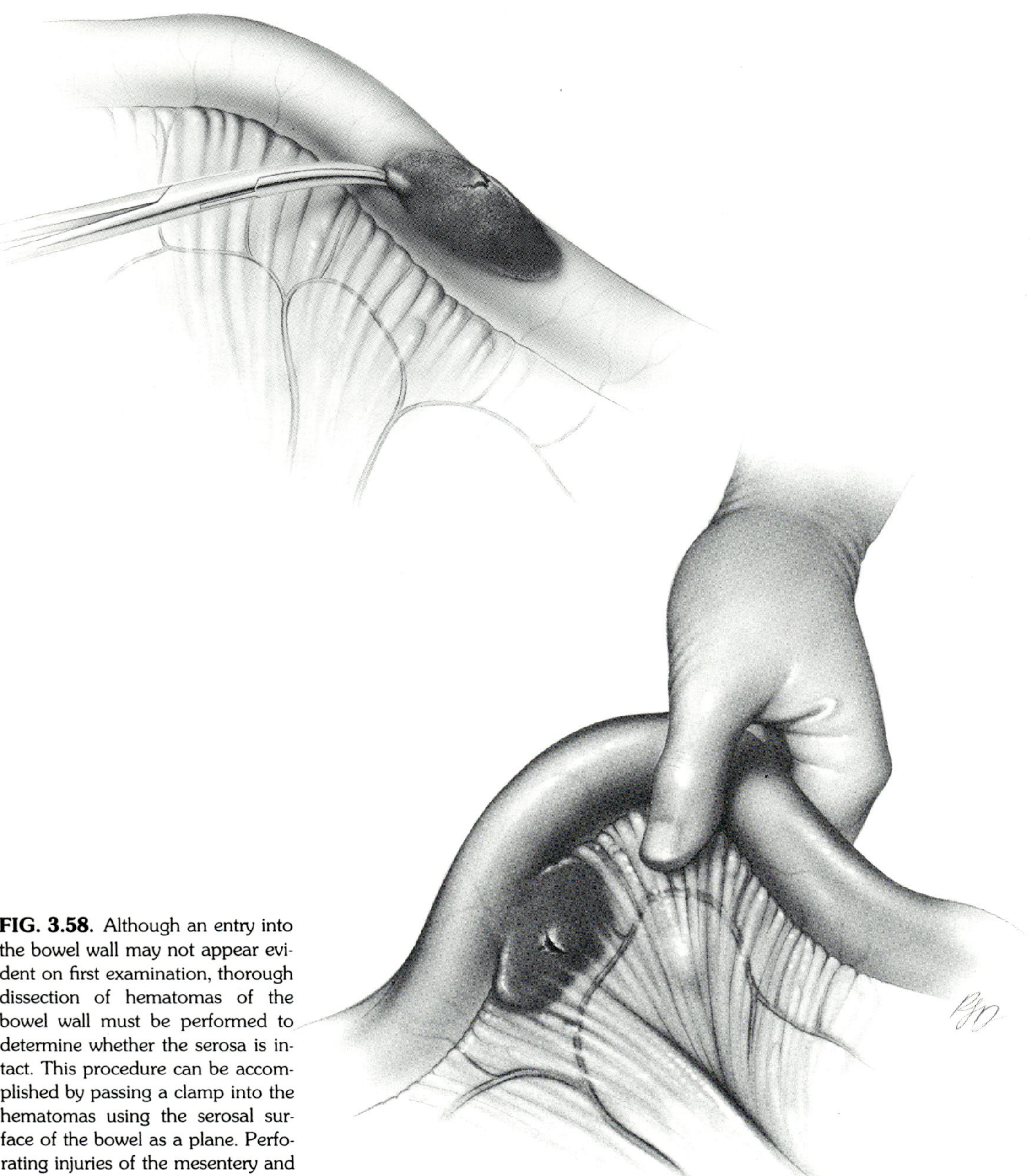

FIG. 3.58. Although an entry into the bowel wall may not appear evident on first examination, thorough dissection of hematomas of the bowel wall must be performed to determine whether the serosa is intact. This procedure can be accomplished by passing a clamp into the hematomas using the serosal surface of the bowel as a plane. Perforating injuries of the mesentery and bowel may be manifest as varied-sized hematomas.

can sometimes be identified by palpation alone. However, visualization of the anterior and lateral surface of the spleen should be attempted. Mobilization of the spleen routinely is contraindicated. However, the risks associated with spleen mobilization are justified when there is suspicion that there is significant injury to the body of the spleen, splenic pedicle, or tail of the pancreas.

The retroperitoneal space should be opened and explored to identify the kidneys, ureter, pancreas, vena cava, and aorta, if retroperitoneal hemorrhage or bile staining is present (Fig. 3.59). The anterior surface of the vena cava should be visualized to rule out the presence of a controlled injury to the vena cava. Abdominal stab wounds or gunshot wounds can completely or partially transect the ureter. If doubt exists

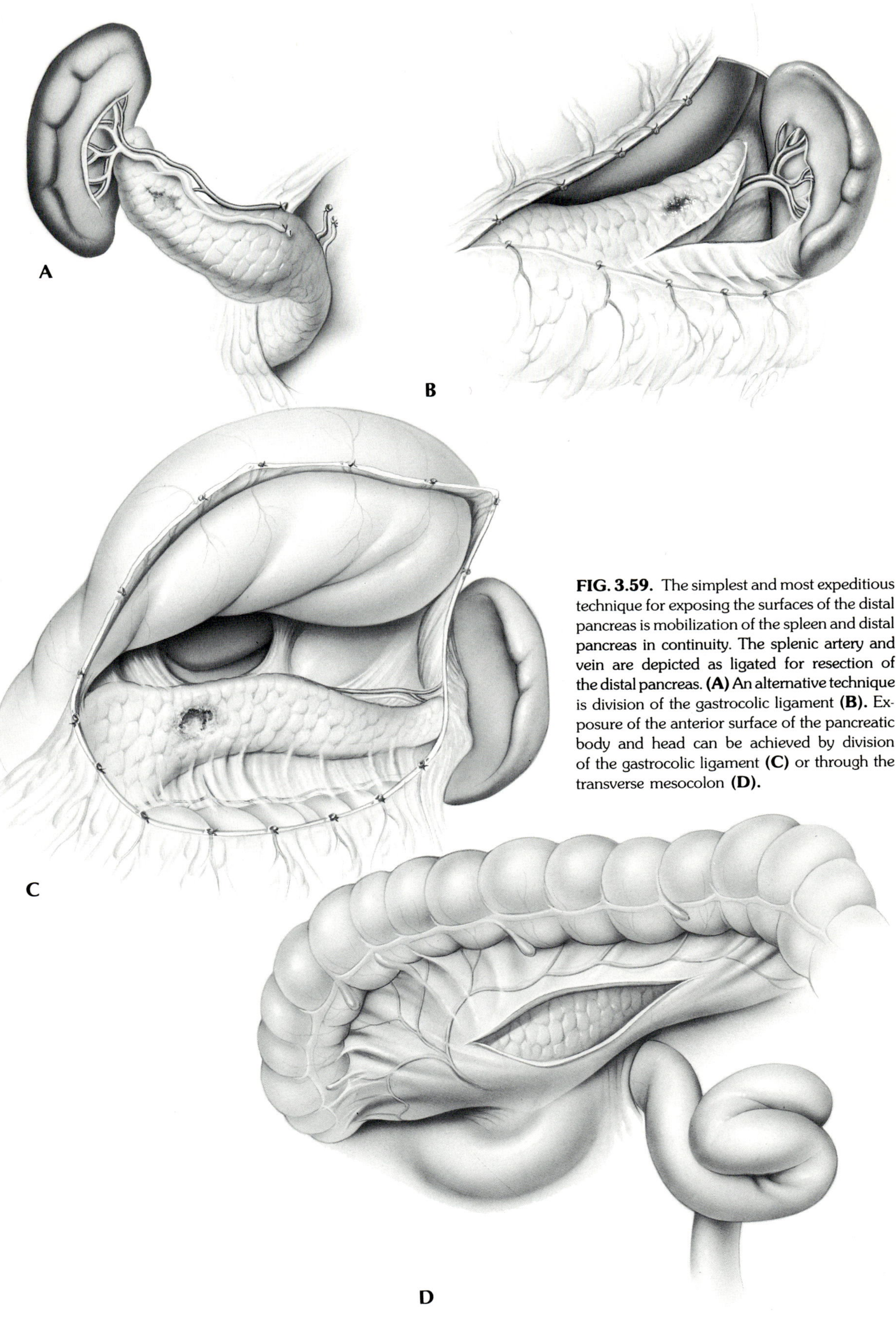

FIG. 3.59. The simplest and most expeditious technique for exposing the surfaces of the distal pancreas is mobilization of the spleen and distal pancreas in continuity. The splenic artery and vein are depicted as ligated for resection of the distal pancreas. **(A)** An alternative technique is division of the gastrocolic ligament **(B).** Exposure of the anterior surface of the pancreatic body and head can be achieved by division of the gastrocolic ligament **(C)** or through the transverse mesocolon **(D).**

concerning ureteral injury, 10% indigo carmine should be injected intravenously and the dye will appear at an ureteral injury site. The historic distaste for performing retroperitoneal-space exploration is based on the fear of exsanguinating hemorrhage from retroperitoneal vascular structures. The well-trained surgeons of today have sufficient skill and familiarity with the anatomy of the retroperitoneal vasculature to deal decisively with major injuries outside the pelvis. A large, bulging retroperitoneal hematoma often connotes a vena cava injury; and once identified, the defect can be controlled by pressure applied against the spine above and below the injury site. The retroperitoneal hematoma in the pelvis is different and should be dealt with cautiously. Most pelvic hematomas do not require exploration. If the hematoma is very large and rapidly expanding, suggesting major vascular injury, exploration is indicated to control either venous or arterial injury in this area. When multiple pelvic fractures are present, retroperitoneal pelvic bleeding may be extensive and uncontrollable. When this situation is encountered, extraordinary measures may be necessary. It must be emphasized, however, that an attempt should be made to identify the course of the iliac arteries and veins. A good general rule is to explore pelvic hematomas above the pelvic brim and to leave intact the hematomas below. If continued bleeding occurs, angiography for identification of the bleeding site and endovascular occlusion may be necessary.

For penetrating injury it is worthwhile to attempt exploring the injury tract for its full length in order to assess the traumatized structure. Although the procedure is simple for victims of a knife wound, it is difficult in patients who have suffered gunshot wounds. If a thorough, systematic exploration of the important abdominal structures has been accomplished, retrieval of a bullet or exact delineation of the course of the bullet or knife is not necessary. It is generally considered appropriate to find an even number of bowel-wall entry and exit wounds when exploring penetrating injuries. However, tangential and single-entry wounds frequently occur to confuse the surgeon.

REFERENCES

1. Adams JT, Libertino JA, Schwartz SI (1968) Significance of an elevated serum amylase. Surgery 63: 877–884
2. Ahmad W, Polk HC (1976) Blunt abdominal trauma: A prospective study with selective peritoneal lavage. Arch Surg 111: 489–492
3. Aragon GE, Eiseman B (1976) Abdominal stab wounds; Evaluation of sinography. J Trauma 16: 792
4. Bach RD, Frey CF (1971) Diagnosis and treatment of pancreatic trauma. Am J Surg 121: 20
5. Baker RJ, Dippel WF, Freeark FJ, Strohl EL (1963) The surgical significance of trauma to the pancreas. Arch Surg 86: 1038
6. Baker R (1976) Discussion of paper by Ahmad; Blunt abdominal trauma: A prospective study with selective peritoneal lavage. Arch Surg 11: 489–492
7. Barnes JP, Dennis DS (1975) Quick method of estimating red cell count in peritoneal lavage. Tex Med 71(5): 62–64
8. Benjamin CI, Engrav LH, Perry JF (1976) Delayed rupture or delayed diagnosis of rupture of the spleen. Surg Gynecol Obstet 142: 171–172
9. Berger BC (1974) Radionuclide studies after urinary tract injury. Semin Nucl Med 4(4): 371–393
10. Berman JK, Habegger ED, Fields DC, Kilner WL (1958) Blood studies as an aid in differential diagnosis of abdominal trauma. JAMA 165(12): 1537–1541
11. Calman C, Hersey FB, Skaggs JO, Spencer A (1958) Serum lactic dehydrogenase in the diagnosis of the acute surgical abdomen. Surgery 44: 43
12. Canizaro PD, Fitts CJ, Sawyer RB (1964) Diagnostic abdominal paracentesis—A proposed adjunctive measure. US Army Surg Research Unit Annual Report. June
13. Cantor MO (1970) Abdominal Trauma. Charles C Thomas, Springfield, Illinois
14. Carnevale N, Baron N, Delany HM (1977) Peritoneoscopy as an aid in the diagnosis of abdominal trauma. A preliminary report. J Trauma 17: 634–641
15. Cimmino CV (1964) Ruptured spleen: Some refinements in its roentgenologic diagnosis. Radiology 82: 57–62
16. Cimmino CV, Southworth LE (1978) Further refinements in the plain radiologic diagnosis of splenic rupture: The air enema. Radiology 127: 649–653
17. Clark JM (1969) Culdocentesis in evaluation of blunt abdominal trauma. Surg Gynecol Obstet 129: 809
18. Clark OH, Lim RC, Margarettey W (1975) Spontaneous delayed splenic rupture—Case report of a five year interval between trauma and diagnosis. J Trauma 15: 245
19. Cleveland HC, Reinschmidt JD, Waddel WR (1963) Traumatic pancreatitis: An increasing problem. Surg Clin North Am 43(2): 402
20. Delany HM, Moss CM, Carnevale N (1976) The use of enzyme analysis of peritoneal blood in the clinical assessment of abdominal organ injury. Surg Gynecol Obstet 142: 161–167
21. DeMuth WE (1966) Bullet velocity and design as determinants of wounding capability: An experimental study. J Trauma 6(2): 222–232
22. Drapanas T, McDonald J (1967) Peritoneal tap in abdominal trauma. Surgery 50: 742–746
23. Drew R, Perry JF Jr, Fisher RP (1977) The expediency of peritoneal lavage for blunt trauma in children. Surg Gynecol Obstet 145(6): 885–888
24. Elman R, Arneson N, Graham EA (1929) Value of blood amylase estimations in the diagnosis of pancreatic disease. Arch Surg 19: 943–967
25. Elkin M, Cohen G (1962) Diagnostic value of psoas shadow. Clin Radiol 13: 210–217

26. Engrav LH, Benjamin CI, Strate RG, Perry JF Jr (1975) Diagnostic peritoneal lavage in blunt abdominal trauma. J Trauma 15: 854
27. Epstein LJ, Lempke RE (1968) Rupture of the right hemidiaphragm due to blunt trauma. J Trauma 8: 19–28
28. Evans GW, Curtin G, McCarthy HF, Kieran JH (1972) Scintiography in traumatic lesions of liver and spleen. JAMA 222(6): 665–667
29. Fiss TW, Cigtay OS, Miele AJ, Twigg HL (1975) Perforated viscus presenting with gas in the soft tissues. (Subcutaneous emphysema.) Am J Roentgenol Radium Ther Nucl Med 125(1): 226–233
30. Fitzgerald JB, Crawford ES, DeBakey ME (1960) Surgical consideration of non-penetrating abdominal injuries. An analysis of 200 cases. Am J Surg 100: 22
31. Frimann-Dahl J (1973) The acute abdomen. In: Margulis AR, Burhenne HJ (eds) Alimentary Tract Roentgenology, Vol. I. C. V. Mosby Company, St. Louis, pp 172–227
32. Fullen WD (1973) Discussion of paper by Thal and Shires: Peritoneal lavage in blunt abdominal trauma. Am J Surg 125: 64–68
33. Gambill EE, Mason HF (1963) One hour value for urinary amylase in 96 patients with pancreatitis. JAMA 186: 24
34. Garvey JW, Delany HM (1974) Giant cyst of the spleen. J Trauma 14: 974
35. Gazzaniga AB, Stanton WW, Bartlett RH (1976) Laparoscopy in the diagnosis of blunt and penetrating injuries to the abdomen. Am J Surg 131(3): 315–323
36. Giacobine JW, Siler VE (1960) Evaluation of diagnostic abdominal paracentesis with experimental and clinical studies. Surg Gynecol Obstet 110: 676
37. Gilday DL, Alderson PO (1974) Scintigraphic evaluation of liver and spleen injury. Semin Nucl Med 4(4): 357–370
38. Gill W, Champion HR, Long WB, Jamaris J, Cowley RA (1975) Abdominal lavage in blunt trauma. Br J Surg 62: 121
39. Godley DR, Smith TK (1977) Some medicolegal aspects of gunshot wounds. J Trauma 17: 866–871
40. Goldberg BB (ed) (1977) Abdominal Gray Scale Ultrasonography. John Wiley & Sons, New York.
41. Gould JR, Thorworth WT (1963) Retroperitoneal rupture of duodenum due to blunt, nonpenetrating abdominal trauma. Radiology 80: 743–747
42. Griffen WO, Belin RP, Ernst CB, Sachatello CR, Daugherty ME, Mulcahy JJ, Chuang VA, Maull KI (1978) Intravenous pyelography in abdominal trauma. J Trauma 18(6): 387–392
43. Griswold RA, Collier HS (1961) Collective review: Blunt abdominal trauma. Surg Gynecol Obstet (Int Abstr Surg 112: 309–329 April 1961)
44. Hassani N (1976) Ultrasonography of the Abdomen. Springer-Verlag, New York
45. Health, Education and Welfare Report: Child abuse and neglect: The problem and its management, Vol. I. U.S. Department of Health, Education and Welfare, Children's Bureau, National Center on Child Abuse and Neglect, 1976.
46. Heselson J (1970) Peritoneoscopy in abdominal trauma. S Afr J Surg 8: 1
47. Hobson RW, Conant C, Mahoney WD, Baugh JH (1972) Serum creatine phosphokinase. Am J Surg 125: 625
48. Howell HW, Bartizal JF, Freeark RJ (1976) Blunt trauma involving the colon and rectum. J Trauma 16: 624
49. Howell JF, Burrus GR, Jordan GL Jr (1968) Surgical management of pancreatic injuries. J Trauma 1: 32–40
50. Jacobson G, Carter R (1951) Small intestinal rupture due to nonpenetrating abdominal injury: Roentgenological study. Am J Roentgenol 66: 52–64
51. Kazarian KK, DiSpaltro FL, McKinnon WMP, Mersheimer WL (1971) Stabwounds of the abdomen: An analysis of 500 patients. Arch Surg 102: 465–468
52. Koenigsberg M, Blaufox D, Freeman LM (1974) Traumatic injuries of the renal vasculature and parenchyma. Semin Nucl Med 4(2): 117–132
53. Krausz M, Manny J, Durst AL (1976) A simplified method for abdominal lavage in patients with blunt trauma. Surg Gynecol Obstet 142: 741–742
54. Lawson NS, Waters MD, Amato JJ, Billy LJ (1971) Serum enzymes in experimental ballistic injury to extremities. Arch Surg 103: 741
55. Little JM, McRae J, Smitananda N, Morris, JG (1967) Radioisotope scanning of liver and spleen in upper abdominal trauma. Surg Gynecol Obstet 125(4): 725–729
56. Love L (1975) Radiology of abdominal trauma. JAMA 231(13): 1377–1380
57. Love L, Greenfield GB, Braun TW, Moncada R, Freeark RJ, Baker RJ (1968) Angiography of splenic trauma. Radiology 91: 96–102
58. Lowenfels AB (1966) Kehr's sign—A neglected aid in ruptures of the spleen. N Engl J Med 274(18): 1019
59. Lucas CE, Ledgerwood AM (1975) Factors influencing outcome after blunt duodenal injury. J Trauma 15: 839–846
60. Lutzker L, Koenigsberg M, Meng C, Freeman LM (1974) The role of radionuclide imaging in spleen trauma. Radiology 110: 419–425
61. Matsumoto T, Wyte SR, Moseley RV, Newhauser GM, Henry JN, Aaby G (1969) Surgical research in the communication zone. Arch Surg 99: 537
62. McAlvanah MJ, Shaftan GW (1978) Selective conservatism in penetrating abdominal wounds: A continuing reappraisal. J Trauma 18:206
63. McCort JJ (1973) Abdominal trauma. In: Margulis AR, Burhenne HJ (eds) Alimentary Tract Roentgenology, Vol I. C. V. Mosby Company, St. Louis, pp 228–270
64. McCort JJ (1964) Radiographic examination in blunt abdominal trauma. Radiol Clin North Am 2: 121–143
65. McCort JJ (1966) Radiographic Examination in Blunt Abdominal Trauma. W. B. Saunders Company, Philadelphia
66. McCort JJ (1962) Rupture or laceration of the liver by nonpenetrating trauma. Radiology 78: 49–57
67. McDonald EJ, Korobkin M, Jacobs RP, Minagi H (1976) The role of emergency excretory urography in evaluation of blunt abdominal trauma. Am J Roentgenol 126: 739–742

68. Meschan I (1975) An Atlas of Anatomy Basic to Radiology. W. B. Saunders Company, Philadelphia
69. Meyers MA (1976) Dynamic Radiology of the Abdomen: Normal and Pathologic Anatomy. Springer-Verlag, New York
70. Meyers MA (1974) Radiographic features of spread and localization of extraperitoneal gas and their relationship to its sources: An anatomical approach. Radiology 111: 17–27
71. Miller DR (1972) Median sternotomy extension of abdominal incision for hepatic lobectomy. Ann Surg 175: 193
72. Miller DW Jr, Kelley DL (1972) Splenic trauma in children. Arch Surg 105: 561–563
73. Miller RE (1973) The technical approach to the acute abdomen. Semin Roentgenol 8: 267–279
74. Mokrohisky J (1958) Pseudopneumoperitoneum. Am J Roentgenol 79: 293–300
75. Moretz WH, Erickson WG (1954) Peritoneal tap as an aid in the diagnosis of acute abdominal disease. Am J Surg 20: 363–377
76. Moss CM, Caron N, Bernstein L, Delany HM (1977) The origin of elevated alkaline phosphatase activity in small intestinal injury. J Surg Res 23: 172–176
77. Mullen JT (1974) Editorial: The magnitude of the problem of trauma. J Trauma 14(12): 1070–1072
78. Murr P, Moore EE, Dunn EL (1979) Stabbed stuffed stomach syndrome. N Engl J Med 300(11): 625
79. Nance CF, Cohn I Jr (1969) Surgical judgment in the management of the stabwounds of the abdomen: A retrospective and prospective analysis based on a study of 600 stabbed patients. Ann Surg 170(4): 569–580
80. Nebesar RA, Rabinov KR, Potsaid MS (1974) Radionuclide imaging of the spleen in suspected splenic injury. Radiology 110: 609–614
81. Neuhof H, Cohen I (1926) Abdominal puncture in the diagnostics of acute intraperitoneal disease. Ann Surg 83: 454–462
82. Nevins MA, Saran M, Bright M, Lyon LD (1973) Pitfalls in interpreting serum creatine phosphokinase activity. JAMA 224: 1382
83. Nickell WK, Albritten FF (1957) Serum transaminase content related to tissue injury. Surgery 42: 240
84. Olsen WR (1974) Delayed rupture of the spleen as an index of diagnostic accuracy. Surg Gynecol Obstet 138: 82
85. Olsen WR (1973) The serum amylase in blunt abdominal trauma. J Trauma 13(3): 200–204
86. Olsen WR, Folley TZ (1977) A second look at delayed splenic rupture. Arch Surg 112: 422–425
87. Olsen WR, Hildreth DH (1971) Abdominal paracentesis and peritoneal lavage in blunt abdominal trauma. J Trauma 11: 824
88. Olsen WR, Redman HC, Hildreth DH (1972) Quantitative peritoneal lavage in blunt abdominal trauma. Arch Surg 104: 536
89. Oppenheim WL (1977) The "battered alcoholic syndrome." J Trauma 17: 850–856
90. Osborn DJ, Glickman MG, Graja V, Ramsby G (1973) The role of angiography in abdominal nonrenal trauma. Radiol Clin North Am 11: 579–592
91. Pacey J, Forward AD, Preto AJ (1971) Peritoneal tap and lavage in patients with blunt abdominal trauma: Their contribution to surgical decisions. Can Med Assoc J 105: 365
92. Perry JF (1965) A five year survey of 152 acute abdominal injuries. J Trauma 5: 53–61
93. Perry JF, Strate RG (1972) Diagnostic peritoneal lavage in blunt abdominal trauma. Indications and results. Surgery 71: 898
94. Prout WG (1968) An evaluation of diagnostic paracentesis in the acute abdomen. Br J Surg 55: 853
95. Richter MW, Lytton B, Myerson D, Gruja V (1973) Radiology of genitourinary trauma. Radiol Clin North Am 11: 593–631
96. Root HD, Hauser CW, McKinley CR, LaFare JW, Mendiola RP (1965) Diagnostic peritoneal lavage. Surgery 57: 633
97. Root HD, Keizer P, Perry JJ (1967) Peritoneal trauma, experimental and clinical studies. Surgery 62: 679
98. Rosenthal L (1974) Intravenous radionuclide angiography in the diagnosis of trauma. Semin Nucl Med 4(4): 395–409
99. Rudolph LA, Schaefer JA, Dutton RE, Lyons R II (1957) Serum glutamic oxalectic transminase in experimental tissue injury. J Lab Clin Med 49: 31
100. Rutkow IM (1978) Rupture of the spleen in infectious mononucleosis. Arch Surg 113: 718
101. Sanders RC (ed) (1975) Symposium on B-scan ultrasound. Radiol Clin North Am 13(3): 417–434
102. Shaftan GW (1975) Penetrating wounds of the abdomen. Resident and Staff Physician 102: 1–10
103. Shaftan GW (1960) Indications for operation in abdominal trauma. Am J Surg 99: 657–664
104. Solomon H (1906) Die Diagnostische Funktion des Bauches. Berl Klin Wochenschr 43: 45–46
105. Sperling L, Rigler LG (1937) Traumatic retroperitoneal rupture of duodenum. Radiology 29: 521–524
106. Strauch GO (1973) Major abdominal trauma in 1971. A study of Connecticut by the Connecticut Society of American Board Surgeons and the Yale Trauma Program. Am J Surg 125: 413–418
107. Terry JH, Self MM, Howard JM (1956) Injuries of the spleen. A report of 102 patients. Surgery 40: 615–619
108. Thal ER, Baxter CR (1976) Evaluation of peritoneal lavage in abdominal stab wounds. Abstract. American Association for Surgery of Trauma. Colorado Springs, September
109. Thal ER, Shires GT (1973) Peritoneal lavage in blunt abdominal trauma. Am J Surg 125: 64–68
110. Ting YM, Renter SR (1973) Hollow viscus injury in blunt abdominal trauma. Am J Roentgenol 119: 408–413
111. Tostivint R, Rosenberg A, Chauveinc L, et al. (1971) Plaidoyer pour la Laprascopie das les Traumatismes Abdominaux Fermes. J Chir (Paris) 102: 77
112. White PH, Benfield JR (1972) Amylase in the management of pancreatic trauma. Arch Surg 105: 158–163
113. Williams RD, Zollinger RM (1959) Diagnostic and prognostic factors in abdominal trauma. Am J Surg 97: 575–581

114. Wilson H, Sherman R (1961) Civilian penetrating wounds of the abdomen. Factors in mortality and differences from military wounds in 494 cases. Ann Surg 153: 639–649
115. Wolf BS, Khilnani MT (1973) Plain film diagnosis of gastrointestinal lesions. In: Margulis AR, Burhenne HI (eds) Alimentary Tract Roentgenology. C. V. Mosby Company, St. Louis, pp 137–171
116. Yeh HC, Wolf BS (1977) Ultrasonography in ascites. Radiology 124: 783–790

4

Specific Organ or Supporting-Structure Injury

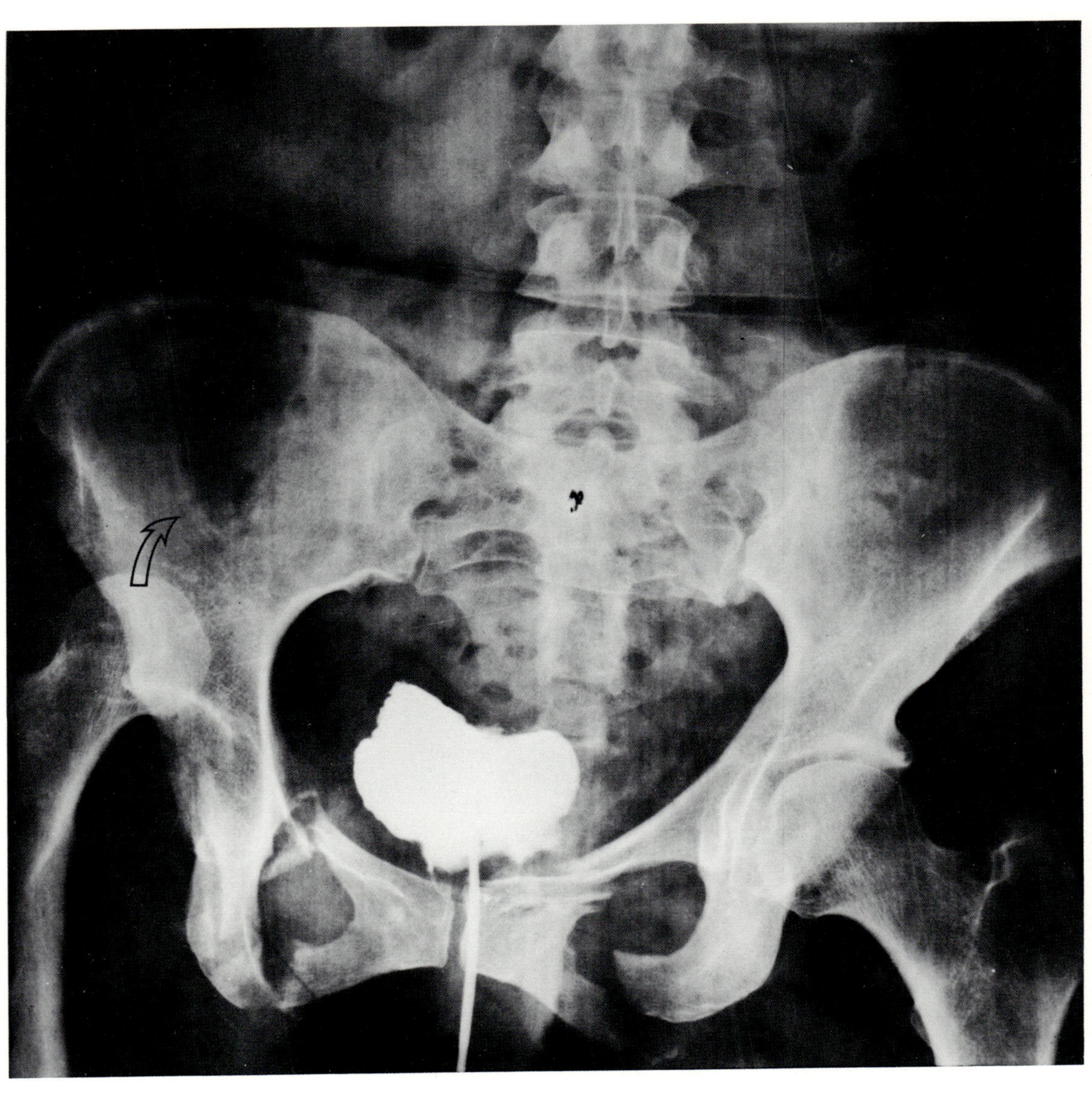

DIAPHRAGM

General Aspects of Injury

Injury to the diaphragm occurs as a result of both penetrating and blunt trauma. BeKassy et al. reported 19 cases of ruptured diaphragm from Leeds; 14 of the patients had a history of trauma, and 4 of these were bullet wounds. The other 5 patients had "spontaneous" rupture of the diaphragm secondary to severe exertion [13,52,95]. Seat belts have also been implicated in diaphragmatic injury. Bergquist et al. reported 6 patients who suffered diaphragmatic tear out of 435 cases of blunt trauma; 4 of the patients wore seat belts. They describe a specific injury combination consisting of diaphragmatic injury, costal fractures, and pelvic or vertebral fracture [16].

Injury to the diaphragm following blunt trauma was first mentioned in the world literature by Ambrose Paré in 1580. The first report in the American literature was by Dowditch in 1853, and the first repair was reported by Walker in 1899 [60]. This injury was a medical rarity prior to the introduction of the automobile. In the United States today, vehicular accidents account for 75% of diaphragmatic injuries due to blunt trauma, with the remaining 25% due to sport and industrial accidents [67]. Injury to the diaphragm rarely occurs as an isolated entity, and its presence may be obscured by findings related to other organ-system injury. Diaphragmatic tear due to blunt trauma is present in 4.5% of patients hospitalized with multiple injuries. It should always be suspected in cases of fracture of the lower thoracic and upper lumbar spine, particularly when these fractures are due to acute flexion [47]. The common association of diaphragmatic rupture with fractures of the pelvic or lumbar spine has been described in the review of the literature by Carlson and associates [26]. In 95% of cases, the left hemidiaphragm is injured probably because the liver acts as a protective buttress for the right diaphragmatic leaflet [66]. Injury to both leaves of the diaphragm is a medical rarity, but when it occurs it is usually fatal. A series of 27 patients with blunt injury to the diaphragm was reported by McCune et al. [111] (Tables 4.1–4.4).

Unfortunately, diaphragmatic lesions are often overlooked at the initial examination, and the average delay between injury and diagnosis ranges from 3.5–4.5 years [47,67,108]. Evidence of diaphragmatic rupture or laceration may develop long after the injury and present as latent incarceration of the bowel. According to Carter and Brewer [27] and Hill [67], 90%

TABLE 4.1. Etiology of rupture of diaphragm

Causes	Rupture left diaphragm	Rupture right diaphragm
Automobile accidents	18	6
Ditch cave-in	1	
Fall from a height	1	
Thrown from tractor	1	
Totals	21	6

Source: McCune RP, Roda CP, Eckert C (1976) Rupture of the diaphragm caused by blunt trauma. J Trauma 16(7): 531–537

TABLE 4.2. Age and sex incidence as related to site of rupture of diaphragm

Age (years)	Rupture left diaphragm		Rupture right diaphragm	
	Male	Female	Male	Female
1–9	1			
10–19	4	1	1	
20–29	3	2	1	
30–39	2		1	
40–49	1		2	
50–59	5			1
60–69	1			
Over 70	1			
Totals	18	3	5	1

Source: McCune RP, Roda CP, Eckert C (1976) Rupture of the diaphragm caused by blunt trauma. J Trauma 16(7): 531–537

TABLE 4.3. Rupture of diaphragm—Associated injuries

	Early		Late	
	L	R	L	R
Rib fractures	6	4	3	1
Pelvic fractures	5	1	1	
Other skeletal fractures	8	3		3
Pneumohemothorax	1	1		1
Ruptured spleen	7			
Laceration of liver	1	4		
Intracranial injury	6	2		
Ruptured urinary bladder	2	1	1	
Necrosis of stomach			1	
Paraplegia	1			

Source: McCune RP, Roda CP, Eckert C (1976) Rupture of the diaphragm caused by blunt trauma. J Trauma 16(7): 531–537

TABLE 4.4. Symptoms of rupture of diaphragm

	Early	Late
Chest pain	8	2
Difficulty in breathing	6	3
Abdominal pain	3	4
Shoulder pain	3	1
Pelvic pain	4	
Pain in extremities	3	
Nausea & vomiting	1	1
Back pain	2	
Hemoptysis	1	
Gas & belching		3
Heartburn		2

Source: McCune RP, Roda CP, Eckert C (1976) Rupture of the diaphragm caused by blunt trauma. J Trauma 16(7): 531–537

of strangulated diaphragmatic hernias are traumatic in origin. In a recent report of delayed presentation of traumatic diaphragmatic hernia by Hegarty et al. [66] in South Africa, 25 cases are described occurring 5 months or more after injury. Only 3 of the 25 patients suffered blunt injury. The majority of the patients had stab wounds. In 1 patient the hernia was found on the right side. The diagnosis was usually made on chest or abdominal radiologic examination. In 10 cases, a barium enema confirmed the diagnosis. It was emphasized that physical examination is of limited value in establishing the diagnosis (Tables 4.5, 4.6). Jarrett and Bernhardt [73] reported on a series of 6 patients with traumatic right-sided diaphragmatic rupture. In this series, 5 patients had visceral injury. It was suggested that the true incidence of right-sided diaphragmatic rupture is greater than is generally appreciated. One additional significant aspect of diaphragmatic injury was pointed out by Hill [67], who showed that paralysis of one hemidiaphragm resulted in a 25% decrease in respiratory function.

TABLE 4.5. Delayed diaphragm rupture—Symptomatology

Symptoms	No.
No symptoms	3
Chronic dyspepsia	5
Acute symptoms	
Intestinal obstruction	8
Upper abdominal or chest symptoms	9
Total	25

Source: Hegarty MM, Bryer JV, Angorn IB, Baker LW (1978) Delayed presentation of traumatic diaphragmatic hernia. Ann Surg 188(2): 229–233

TABLE 4.6. Delayed diaphragm rupture—Herniated viscera

Viscera	No.	Gangrene
Colon	18	2
Stomach	10	2
Small bowel	4	1
Spleen	2	—

Source: Hegarty MM, Bryer JV, Angorn IB, Baker LW (1978) Delayed presentation of traumatic diaphragmatic hernia. Ann Surg 188(2): 229–233

Radiologic Features

Fluoroscopic evaluation of the patient may reveal decreased or absent function on the side of the injury. Plain-film radiologic findings include (a) a high diaphragmatic leaflet; (b) an archlike shadow resembling an abnormally high hemidiaphragm, which may represent either the diaphragm or portions of herniated viscera through the rent in the diaphragm; (c) gas bubbles, homogeneous densities, or abnormal markings extending above the anticipated level of the normal hemidiaphragm; (d) shift of heart and mediastinal structures away from the side of the injury; and (e) discoid or platelike atelectasis at the lung base on the side of the injury [47] (Fig. 4.1).

One radiologic feature that may be confusing and require an additional diagnostic workup is the presence of a soft-tissue homogeneous density at the lung base silhouetting with the diaphragm (Fig. 4.2). Without the findings of gas bubbles or the presence of an air-fluid level within the density, it may be impossible to determine the exact etiology of the mass. Contrast evaluation, using barium in either the upper or lower gastrointestinal tract, may clarify the problem (see Fig. 4.1). However, a solid viscus or portions of the omentum may herniate through a rent in the diaphragm without herniation of hollow viscera. Angiographic demonstration of visceral vessels or an organogram above the level of the diaphragm may be helpful in making the diagnosis. However, it must be remembered that this soft-tissue mass may have pre-dated the trauma and be unrelated to it. Additional differential possibilities must include subdiaphragmatic, diaphragmatic, pleural, and parenchymal nontraumatic lesions.

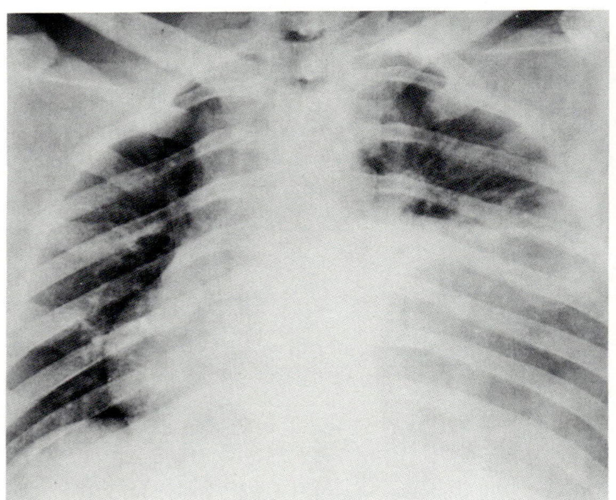

A

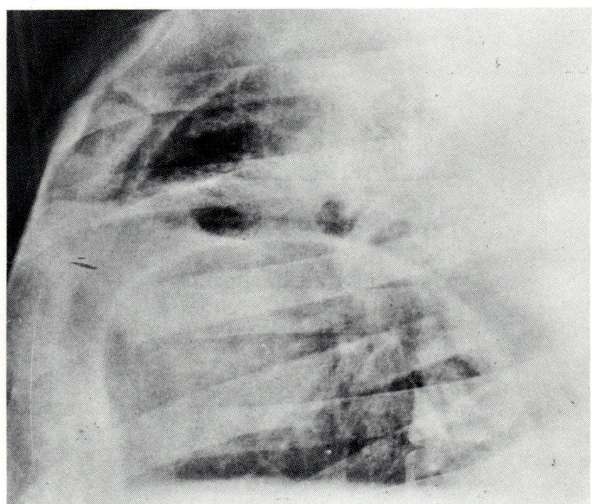

B

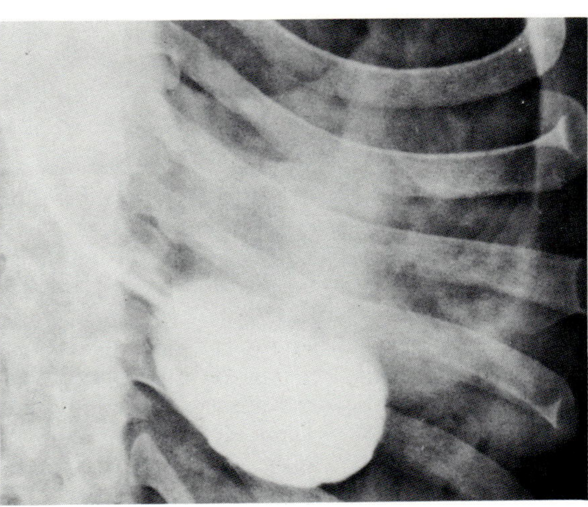

C

FIG. 4.1A–C. This young male patient was a victim of blunt abdominal trauma. The **(A)** frontal projection of his admission chest examination revealed elevation of the left hemidiaphragm with a large lucent collection beneath it, platelike atelectasis at the left lung base, and rightward shift of mediastinal structures. The **(B)** lateral projection confirmed these findings. A **(C)** contrast evaluation of the upper GI tract demonstrated contrast entering the lucent collection at the base of the left lung. Just lateral to the confined contrast collection was an area of mottled density, suggestive of the splenic flexure of the colon. At exploration, a rent in the left diaphragm was discovered through which there was herniation of a volvulated stomach and colon.

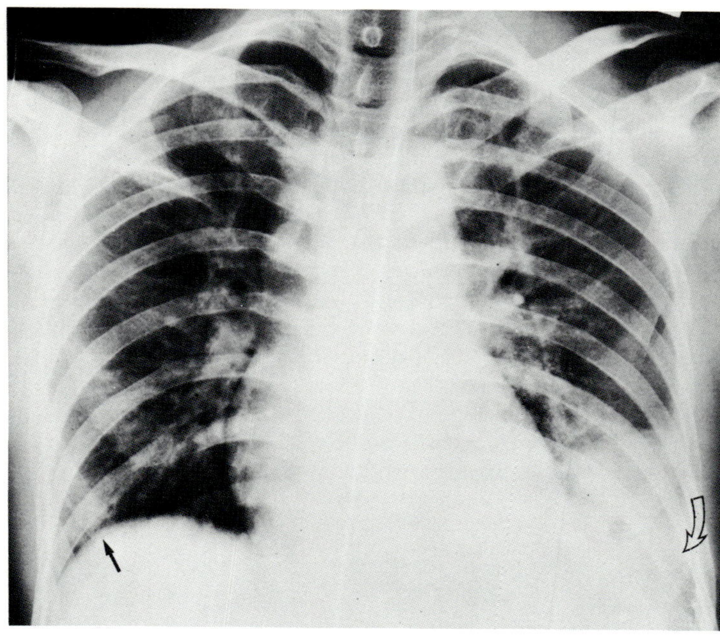

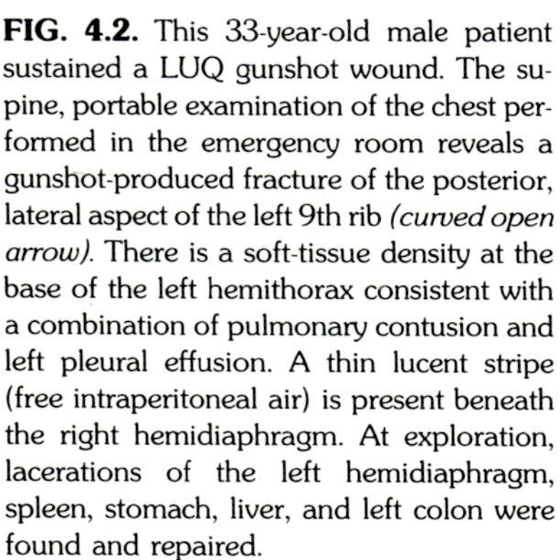

FIG. 4.2. This 33-year-old male patient sustained a LUQ gunshot wound. The supine, portable examination of the chest performed in the emergency room reveals a gunshot-produced fracture of the posterior, lateral aspect of the left 9th rib *(curved open arrow)*. There is a soft-tissue density at the base of the left hemithorax consistent with a combination of pulmonary contusion and left pleural effusion. A thin lucent stripe (free intraperitoneal air) is present beneath the right hemidiaphragm. At exploration, lacerations of the left hemidiaphragm, spleen, stomach, liver, and left colon were found and repaired.

SPLEEN

General Aspects of Injury

Unlike the medical history of diaphragmatic lacerations, blunt injury to the spleen was well known before the common use of the automobile. The ancient Chinese used a sharp blow over the region of the spleen as a method of assassination. While this method of assassination did not uniformly accomplish results, it was a satisfactory assault technique since 75% to 95% of patients with splenic rupture die without appropriate surgical intervention [60,127]. The etiology of splenic injury can be varied. Whereas blunt trauma is the most frequent cause of splenic injury, penetrating trauma to the spleen is still significant in the civilian population. The injuries reported in a 1975 review by Steele and Lim [171] lists the causes of splenic injury in a series of 247 cases (Table 4.7).

The first reported case of splenic rupture in the world medical literature was presented by Celsus in the fifteenth century, and the first splenectomy following splenic laceration was performed by Zaccarelli in 1549 [60]. Prior to the beginning of the twentieth century, the operative mortality for this condition was well over 50%. In 1900, Bessel-Hagen reported a 46% operative mortality. In 1941, in the reported series of Rousselot and Illeyn, the mortality had decreased to 29%. By 1956, the operative mortality reported by Terry et al. had dropped to approximately 17%.

TABLE 4.7. Causes of splenic rupture (247 cases)

Cause		No.
Blunt trauma		183
Motor vehicle accidents	87	
Motor vehicle vs pedestrian	29	
Falls	29	
Assaults	35	
Other	3	
Penetrating trauma		58
Gunshot wounds	29	
Stab wounds	29	
Iatrogenic injuries		6

Source: Steele M, Lim RC (1975) Advances in management of splenic injuries. Am J Surg 130: 159–169

In that same year, Bollinger and Fowler reported an operative mortality of 4.8% [60] (Table 4.8). Currently, the overall mortality for traumatic splenic rupture is in the range of 10% to 15%. This mortality rate is largely attributable to the associated injuries and complications (Table 4.9).

Steele reported 118 injuries to other structures or organs in 58 penetrating injuries to the spleen, and 291 associated abdominal injuries in 183 splenic ruptures caused by blunt trauma (Table 4.10) (Fig. 4.3). With splenic laceration as the only injury, the mortality is in the range of 5% [171].

TABLE 4.8. Mortality rates after traumatic rupture of spleen

Author	Year	No. of cases	Total mortality (%)	Operative mortality (%)
Bessel-Hagen	1900	37	46	46
Lotsch	1908	138	38	38
Michelsson	1913	298	—	33.2
Buxton	1922	37	46	46
Robitshck	1923	124	21.7	—
Connors	1928	25	40	40
McIndoe	1932	46	37	27
Wright and Prigot	1939	30	43	27
Rousselot and Illyne	1941	17	29	29
Roetting et al.	1943	22	32	7
Byrne	1950	101	17	17
Mayo Clinic	1950	22	18	14
Larghero and Guiria	1951	18	6	6
Terry et al.	1956	102	24	17
Bollinger and Fowler	1956	24	16.6	4.8
Miller and Lewlyn	1972	56	0	0
Steele and Lim	1975	298	13	—

Source: Griswold RA, Collier HS (1961) Collective review: Blunt abdominal trauma. Surg Gynecol Obstet 112: 309–329

TABLE 4.9. Associated injuries in 58 patients with penetrating injuries[a]

Associated injury	No.
Diaphragm	25
Chest	19
Stomach	17
Liver	16
Kidney	9
Pancreas	8
Colon	8
Small bowel	7
Major vascular structures	7
Other	2
Total	118

[a] 41 of the patients (71%) had 118 associated injuries.
Source: Steele M, Lim RC (1975) Advances in management of splenic injuries. Am J Surg 130: 159–169

TABLE 4.10. Associated injuries in 183 patients with blunt splenic rupture[a]

Associated injury	No.	
Abdominal		67
Liver	35	
Kidney	10	
Colon	8	
Pancreas	7	
Small bowel	6	
Stomach	1	
Extraabdominal		224
Long bones	72	
Ribs	45	
Head	37	
Chest	31	
Pelvis	25	
Major vascular structures	5	
Diaphragm	2	
Other	7	

[a] 116 of the patients (63%) had 291 associated injuries.
Source: Steele M, Lim RC (1975) Advances in management of splenic injuries. Am J Surg 130: 159–169

The literature varies as to whether the spleen or kidney is the most frequently injured organ in patients who sustain blunt abdominal trauma. Those series that evaluate only the frequency of intraperitoneal-organ injury all agree that the spleen is the most frequently injured viscus. Although all ages are susceptible to this condition, the peak incidence is in the second or third decade. Seventy-six percent of splenic injuries occur in patients between the ages of 3 and 40, with a male/female predominance of 3 to 1 [60,173].

The automobile is the etiologic factor in 50% to 84% of cases of blunt splenic injury [60,192]. As a result, there is a high frequency of associated organ injury with splenic rupture: 27% to 50% of patients

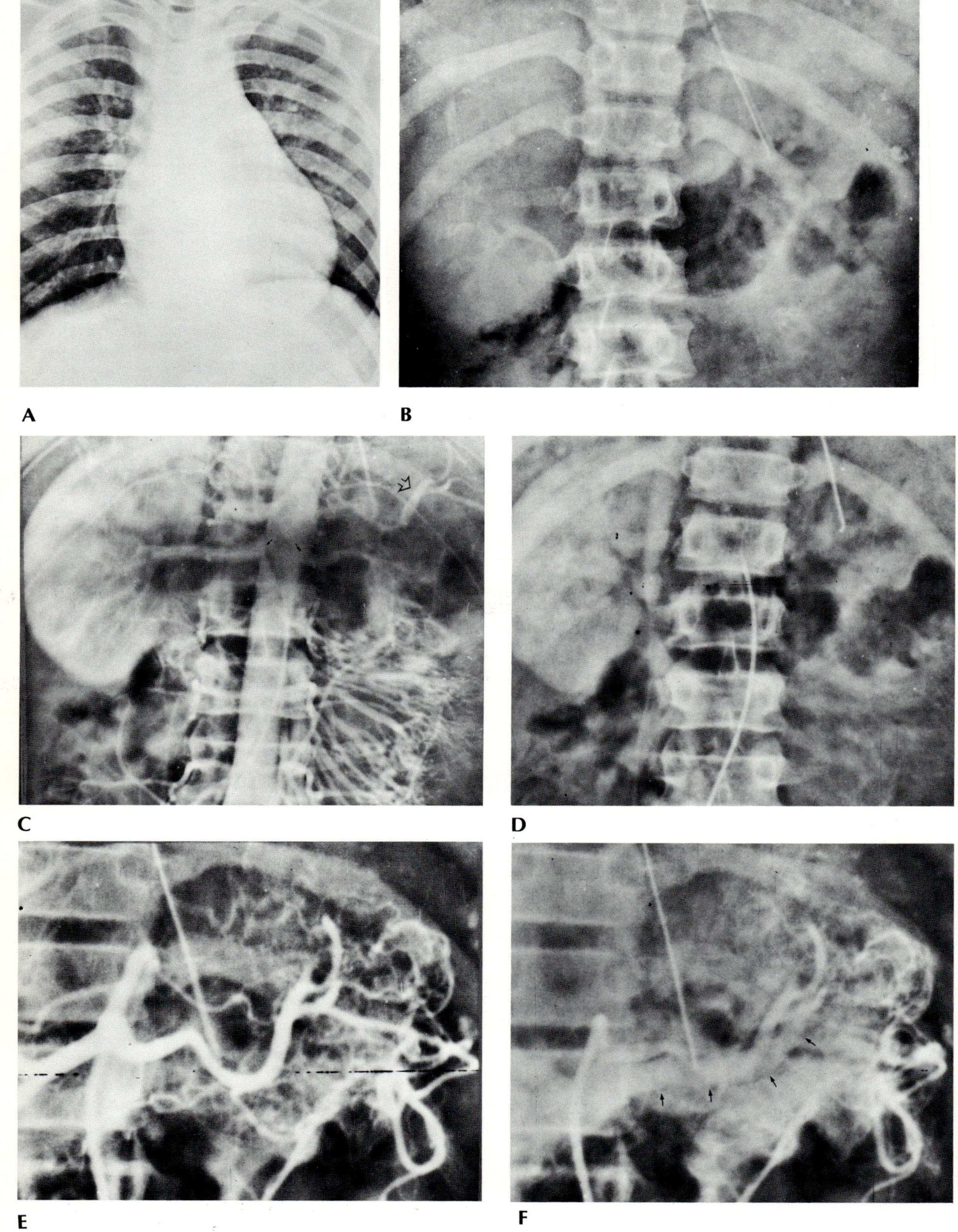
A
B
C
D
E
F

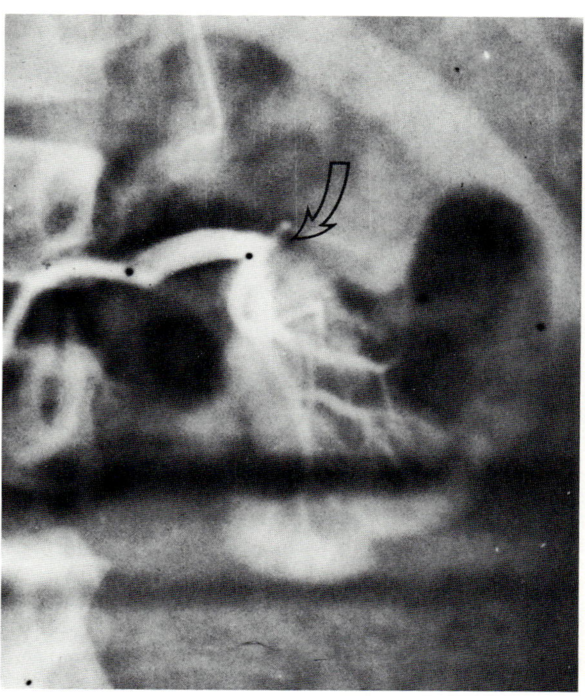

G

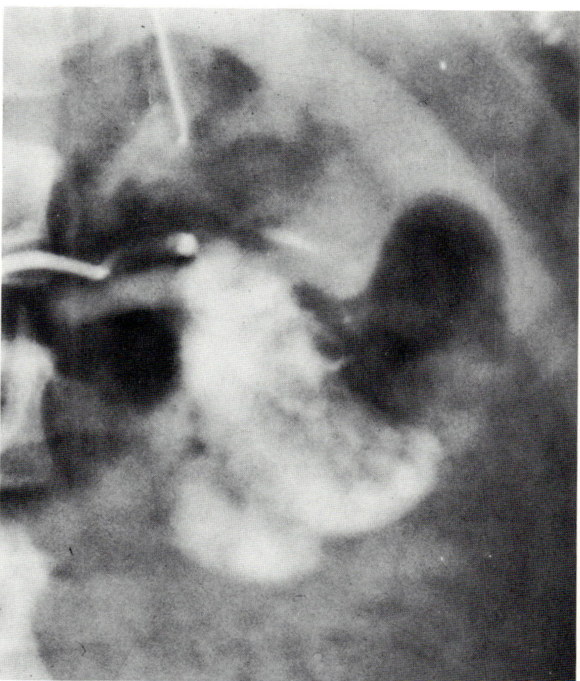

H

FIG. 4.3A–H. This 12-year-old male, while "hitching a ride" on the outside of a city bus, was crushed between the bus and a passing truck. No rib fractures were present on the **(A)** admission chest examination. The left hemidiaphragm was elevated by a LUQ mass containing several small calcifications. An emergency **(B)** IVP confirmed the presence of a LUQ mass depressing the splenic flexure of the colon and containing several calcifications. Gastric dilatation and prominent rugal folds were also revealed. The right kidney appeared normal but there was "nonvisualization" of the left. The **(C)** arterial phase of a flush aortogram showed that both renal arteries *(small solid arrows)* were present but failed to reveal the distal end of the left renal artery. Abnormalities of the splenic artery *(open arrow)* and spleen were also suspected. The **(D)** venous phase of this examination showed a good nephrogram on the right but a poor to absent nephrogram on the left. The **(E)** early arterial phase of a selective celiac axis injection revealed upward dislocation and narrowing of the midsplenic artery, abrupt termination of many intrasplenic branches, and a generally chaotic intrasplenic arterial pattern. A **(F)** later arterial phase of this same injection revealed early splenic vein filling *(small solid arrows)*. The **(G)** arterial phase of a selective left renal artery injection showed amputation of the dorsal branch *(open arrow)* of this vessel. The **(H)** venous phase of this injection revealed the absence of an upper-pole nephrogram and a linear lucent defect through the lower pole.

At exploration, lacerations of the spleen and left kidney were found, resulting in splenectomy and left nephrectomy. The spleen weighed 142 g and had several deep lacerations. There were areas of infarction and multiple calcified nodules consistent with tuberculosis or histoplasmosis. The left kidney weighed 146 g and was completely divided into two parts with a deep laceration through its lower pole.

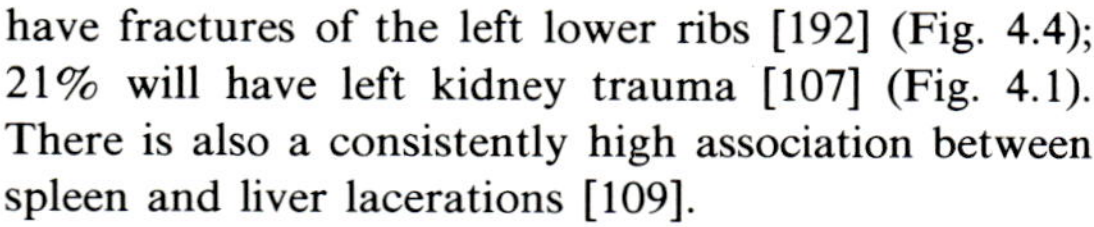

have fractures of the left lower ribs [192] (Fig. 4.4); 21% will have left kidney trauma [107] (Fig. 4.1). There is also a consistently high association between spleen and liver lacerations [109].

The force producing splenic lacerations need not be excessive. This is particularly true when the spleen is abnormally enlarged by disease. Under these conditions, minimal trauma can result in significant injury. The conditions which are most frequently associated with increased splenic susceptibility are malaria, infectious mononucleosis, congestive splenomegaly, sarcoidosis, and Gaucher's disease [109].

Types of Splenic Injury

Splenic trauma can be separated into three broad categories: contusion or parenchymal injury with an intact capsule, parenchymal injury with a small capsular tear allowing oozing of blood from the spleen, and splenic laceration or rupture with massive intraperitoneal bleeding [57,60,92,107–109,127,154,173,179].

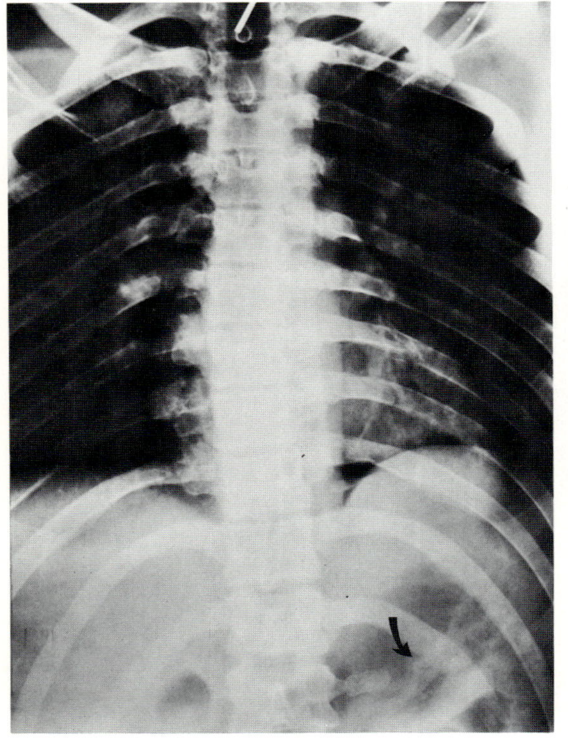

A

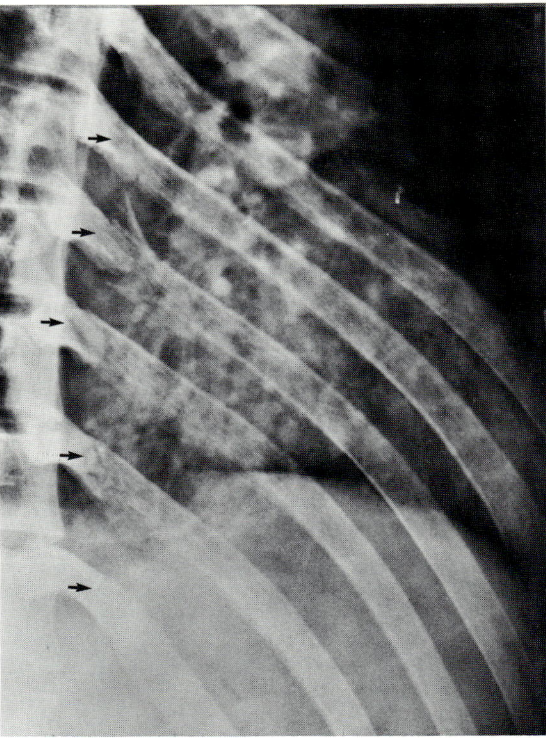

B

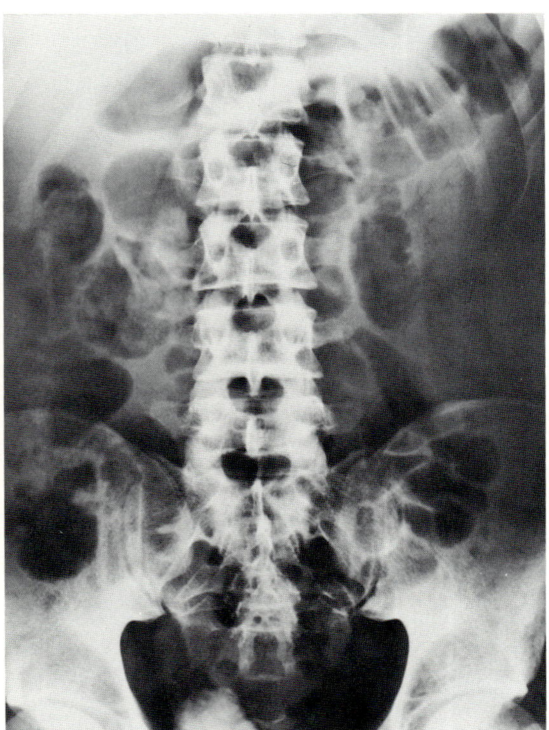

C

FIG. 4.4A–C. This 20-year-old male sustained thoracic and upper abdominal injury in an automobile accident, requiring abdominal exploration and splenectomy. Examination of the **(A)** chest and **(B)** left ribs reveal multiple left rib fractures *(straight arrows)* with gastric dilation and mucosal fold prominence *(curved arrow)*. The **(C)** abdominal examination failed to reveal any evidence of mass, free fluid, or free air.

D and E This 55-year-old male sustained blunt abdominal trauma requiring abdominal exploration and splenectomy. Evaluation of **(D)** the left ribs failed to reveal any fractures but did disclose blunting of the left costophrenic angle consistent with an effusion and atelectasis at the lung base. The examination of the **(E)** abdomen in AP supine projection reveals subtle fractures of the medial left 9th and 10th ribs *(straight arrows)*, a soft-tissue LUQ mass, and gastric dilation with mucosal fold prominence.

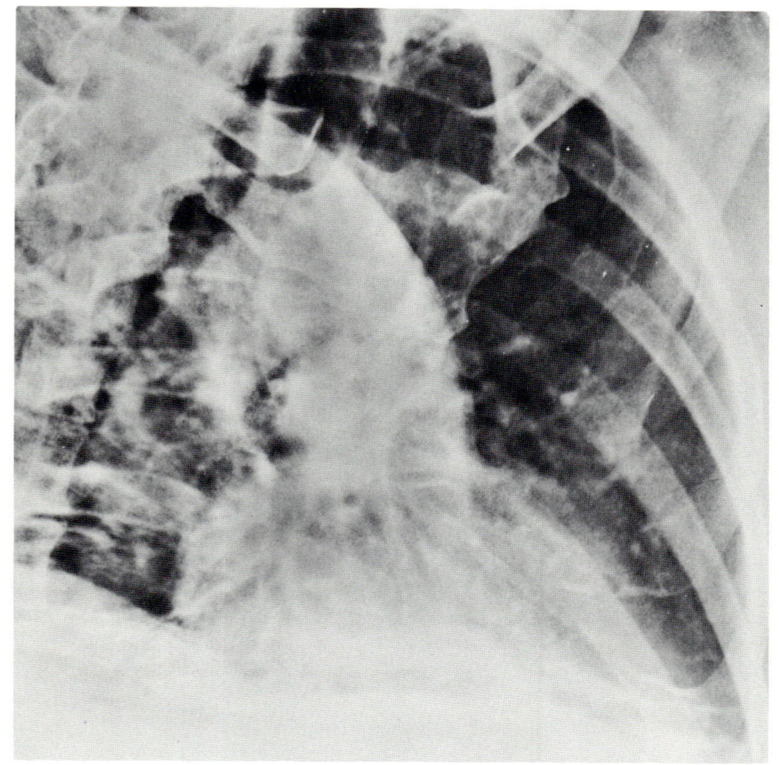

D

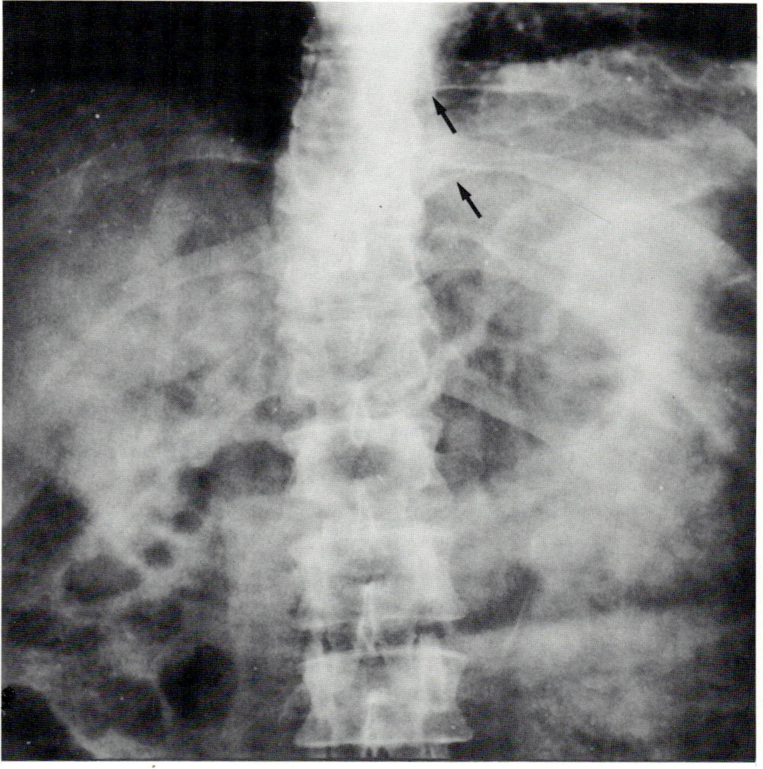

E

Splenic Contusion with an Intact Capsule

In this setting, there has been minor or significant parenchymal injury with bleeding into the splenic pulp, but the bleeding is confined by the intact splenic capsule. If the bleeding is diffuse with massive involvement of the splenic parenchyma, there may be a generalized enlargement of the spleen with resultant displacement of surrounding viscera. However, as long as the capsule is intact, or as long as there is no other source of free intraperitoneal bleeding, the splenic outline remains sharp and distinct. Because of the mass effect of the enlarging spleen, the left hemidiaphragm may be elevated and show decreased motion; the stomach may be shifted to the right with downward displacement of the cardia; the left kidney may show displacement (usually downward) either by the enlarging mass of the spleen or by the accumulation of a retroperitoneal hematoma (the signs of a retroperitoneal hematoma, obliteration of the renal and psoas outline, should strongly suggest the possibility of an associated renal injury) (see Fig. 4.3); and there may be depression and medial displacement of the splenic flexure. If the bleeding is less diffuse and more localized but still confined by the intact capsule, there may be localized changes in the splenic contour at sites of blood and fluid accumulation. These localized bulges can also result in displacement of contiguous viscera.

Capsular Tear with Oozing

The injury has resulted in parenchymal as well as capsular tears. This combination of lesions allows blood to escape out of the splenic capsule and may result in localized obscuration of portions of the splenic outline contiguous to the hematoma. Since the hematoma is relatively confined, little if any evidence of free intraperitoneal fluid is present (see Fig. 4.7).

Splenic Laceration or Disruption with Hemorrhage

With massive injury of the spleen and of its capsule, blood is released into the peritoneal cavity, producing the signs of free intraperitoneal accumulation of fluid. In addition, there is significant disruption and obscuration of the splenic outline (see Fig. 3.34). While none of the plain-film findings just described is diagnostic by itself, a certain constellation of findings should alert the radiologist and clinician that further diagnostic procedures are needed to rule out the possibility of significant splenic injury (Fig. 4.5). These signs include alteration of splenic size, contour, and definition; the presence of lower left rib fractures; pleural reaction and/or effusion at the left base (this may be seen in approximately one-third of cases); the presence of free intraperitoneal fluid (detection of small amounts of free fluid is more significant for early diagnosis and treatment than is the identification of massive amounts of fluid); severe gastric dilatation; prominent mucosal folds along the greater curvature aspect of the stomach; anterior, medial, and downward displacement of the stomach with or without indentation by an expanding left upper quadrant mass; obliteration of the left psoas and renal silhouettes; elevation of the left hemidiaphragm with decreased motion; spasm of the descending colon just below the splenic flexure; widening of the lower thoracic paravertebral soft tissues due to upward extension of the retroperitoneal hematoma; and depression and medial displacement of the splenic flexure. None of these plain-film radiologic features is pathognomonic in itself. It is the presence of these findings in the appropriate clinical setting that should suggest a significant abnormality and lead to additional procedures for a definitive diagnosis. A more detailed evaluation of certain of these plain-film findings may demonstrate the degree of diagnostic difficulty that their interpretation presents.

Plain-Film Findings

Alteration of Splenic Size, Position, and Contour

Frequently in medical practice, one pathologic entity may be superimposed on another. Thus, splenic enlargement demonstrated on a roentgenogram may be secondary to a known or unknown abnormality unrelated to the patient's trauma. In addition, the position of the spleen in the left upper quadrant is quite variable in normal patients. Its superior border is usually indistinct or not visualized. The visualized margin may demonstrate abnormal bulges and angulations secondary to fetal lobulation. Wyman states that the spleen is not visualized on abdominal roentgenograms in approximately 42% of patients, regardless of the underlying condition necessitating radiologic studies [207].

Gastric Dilatation

Severe dilatation of the stomach is a frequent finding in splenic trauma (see Fig. 4.4). Its significance and exact cause are unknown. Gastric dilation accompanying splenic injury is of debatable significance since it may be observed in inflammatory disease and other disorders. In fact, it may simply be the result of aerophagia secondary to anxiety or stress.

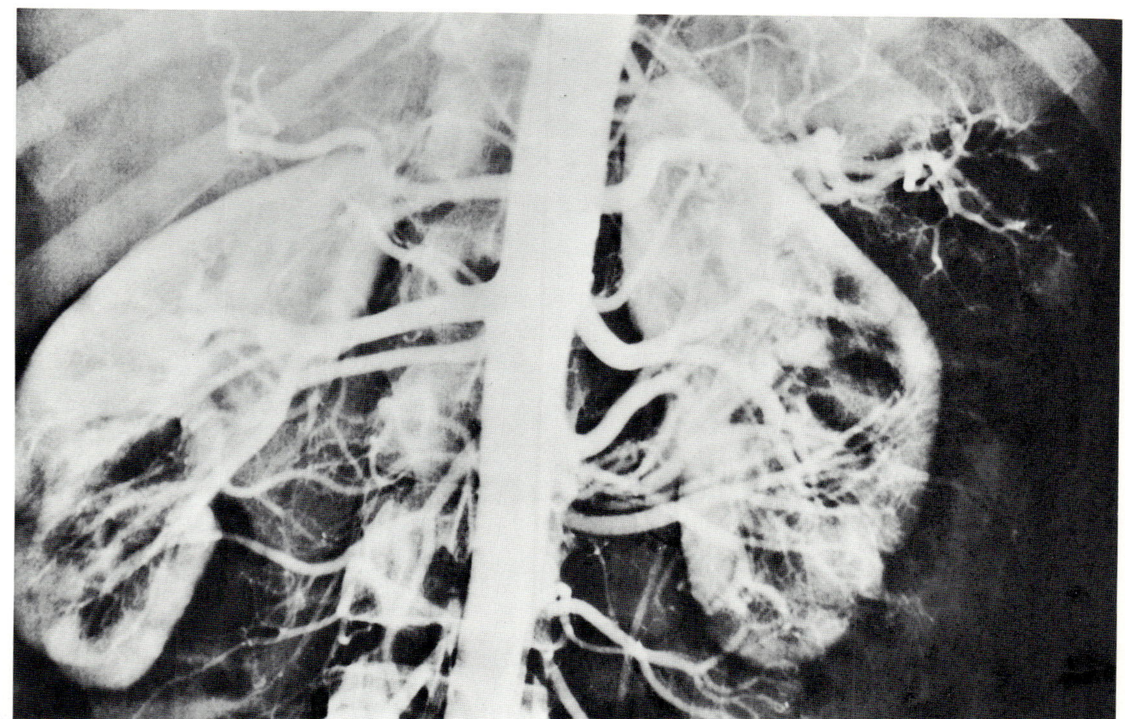

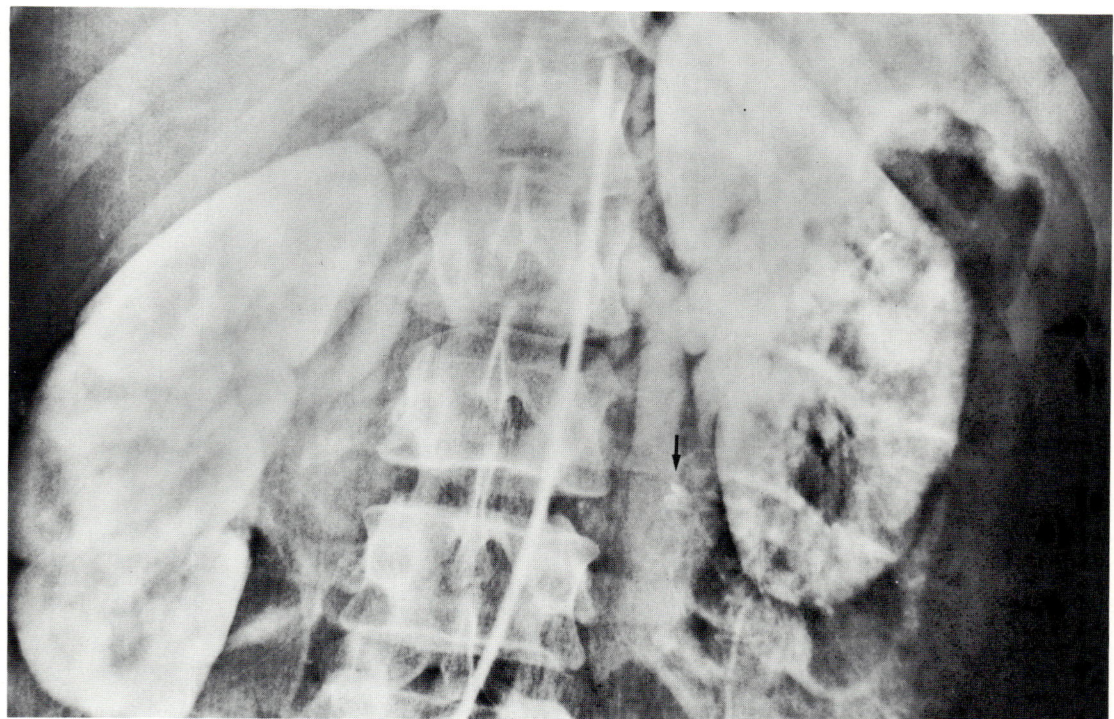

FIG. 4.5A–E. This 24-year-old female was stabbed in the left flank. The admission abdominal examination suggested questionable enlargement of the spleen with prominent gastric folds. A splenic scan revealed decreased uptake in the lower pole of the spleen. The **(A)** arterial phase of a flush aortogram suggested a normal spleen. This was confirmed on the **(B)** venous phase of this examination. However, this phase revealed evidence of contrast extravasation *(solid arrow)* just below the left transverse process of L3. *(Continues)*

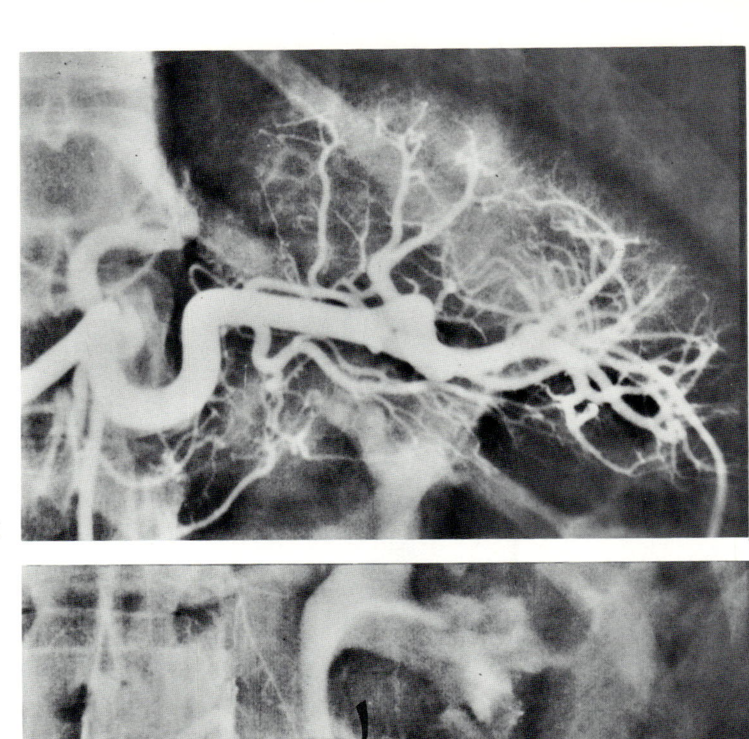
C

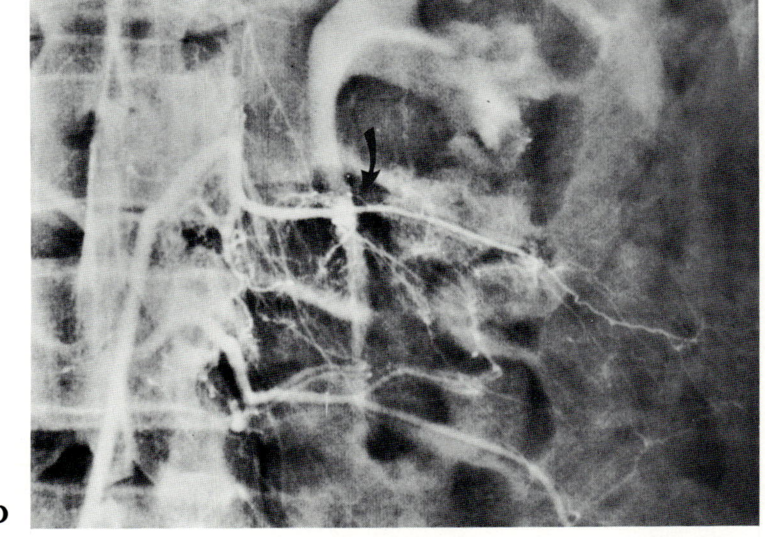
D

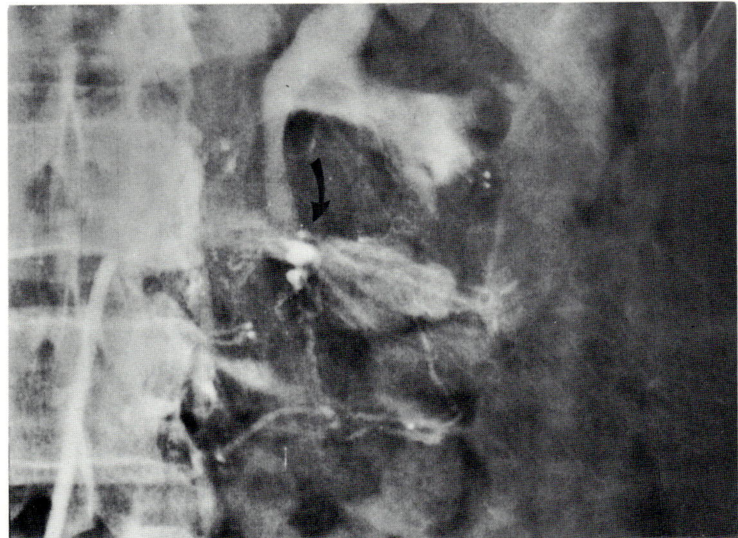
E

FIG. 4.5 ***(Continued).*** Selective catheterization of the **(C)** celiac axis confirmed the lack of splenic injury. Selective catheterization of the left third lumbar artery revealed contrast extravasation *(curved arrow)* on **(D)** the arterial and **(E)** venous phases.

Serration of the Greater Curvature of the Stomach

This finding (see Figs. 4.3 and 4.4A) is believed to be due to the dissection of blood at the site of splenic trauma through the splenogastric ligament with subsequent infiltration of the wall of the greater curvature of the stomach and accumulation of fluid along the greater curvature. Unfortunately, it has been noted by a number of observers, including Williams and Zollinger [199], that serration of the greater curvature of the gas-filled stomach is more frequently present when the spleen is undamaged than when it is ruptured (see Fig. 4.5).

Sonographic Evaluation

Ultrasonic scanning of the abdomen with particular attention to the left upper quadrant may identify not only the presence of intraperitoneal fluid but also the effects of trauma on the spleen. According to Carlsen [161], small subcapsular hematomas may be difficult to diagnose by ultrasound, but large subcapsular hematomas are clearly visualized by ultrasonic gray-scale imaging as echo-free areas separated from the remainder of the spleen by an acoustic interface. Cystic collections within the spleen may indicate the presence of an unorganized hematoma. However, with organization of the hematoma, the level of return echoes increases and makes a definitive diagnosis difficult. Carlsen suggests combined ultrasonic and radioisotope examination to rule out acute trauma to the spleen.

Contrast Evaluation

When clinical and laboratory findings suggest significant splenic abnormalities, contrast studies may be of benefit in confirming the diagnosis (Fig. 4.6). Bancrof and others [208] have suggested the use of barium examination of the stomach with the patient in the Trendelenburg position in order to delineate an impression of an enlarged spleen on the fundus of the stomach or displacement of the stomach by a splenic mass (Fig. 4.7).

Angiographic evaluation of the patient with splenic trauma gives the most information about vascular and parenchymal abnormalities produced by the injury [3,57,84,93,107–110,135,145]. The signs of significant splenic trauma, arranged in order of decreasing reliability are as follows:

1. Extravasation of contrast material. The most reliable sign of splenic injury is the visualization of frank contrast extravasation from the confines of the vascular channels of the spleen. This extravasation may take the form of an amorphous collection of contrast within the splenic capsule or extending into

A

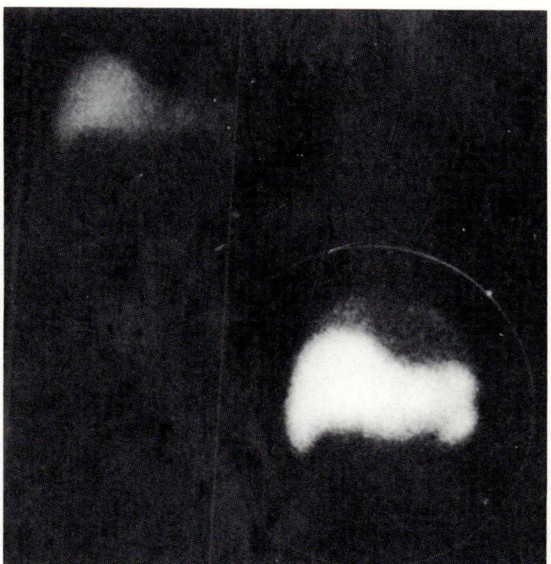

B

FIG. 4.6A–D. This 54-year-old female was admitted to the hospital with chest and abdominal injury following an automobile accident. Evaluation of **(A)** the right ribs revealed multiple fractures *(small arrows)*. *A* **(B)** liver-spleen radionuclide scan demonstrated a linear defect in the lower pole of the spleen consistent with a laceration. The **(C)** arterial and **(D)** venous phases of a selective celiac axis injection revealed a normal spleen. *(Continues)*

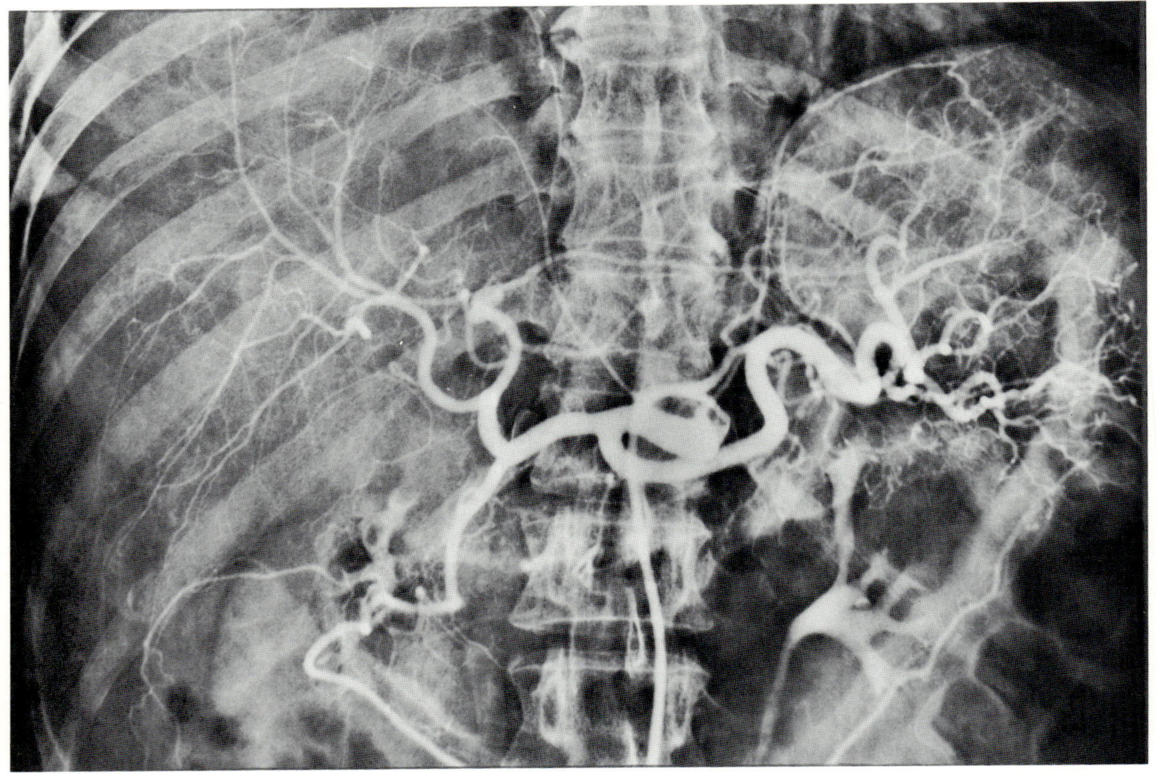

C

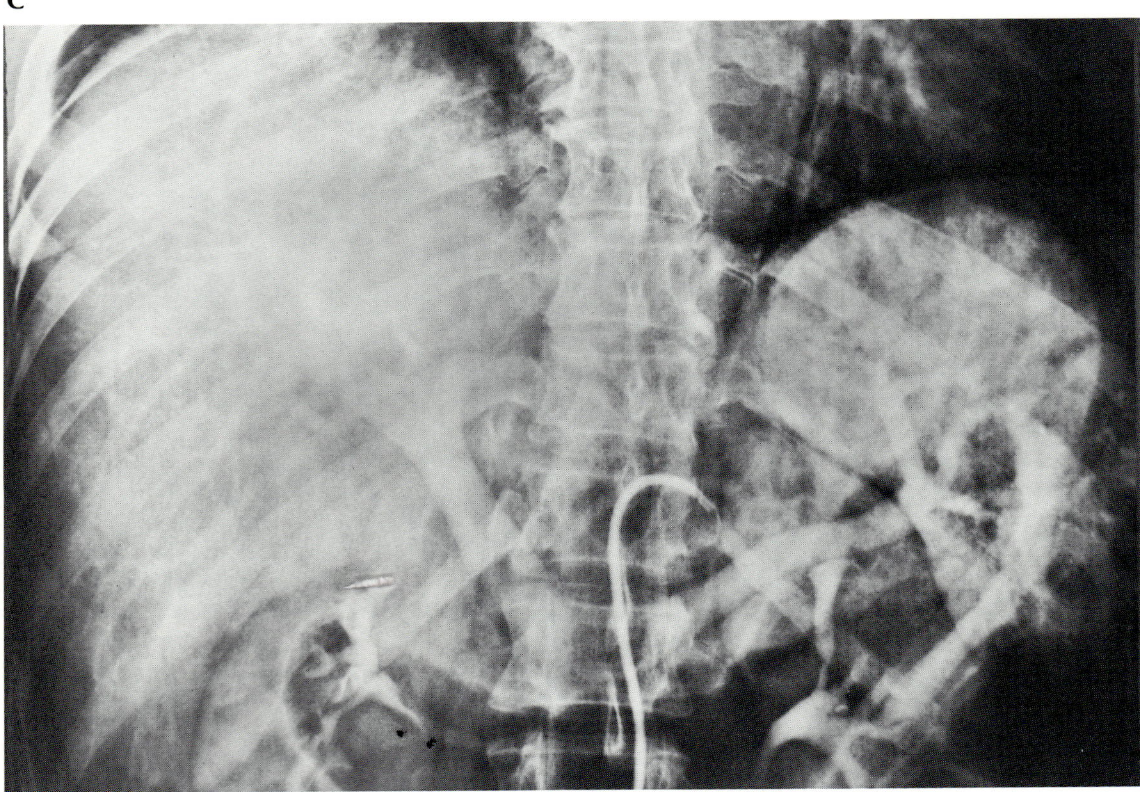

D

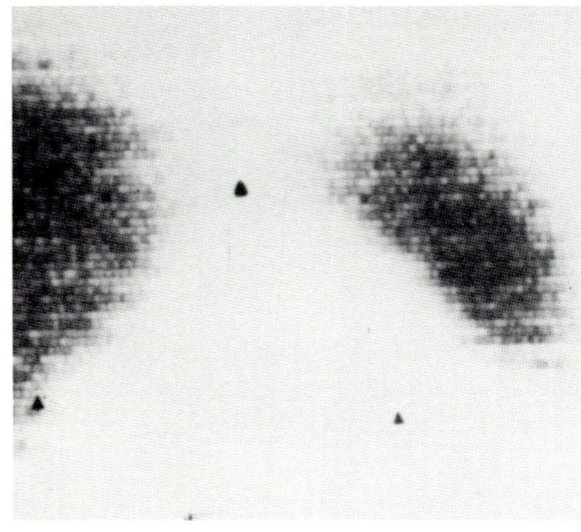

E

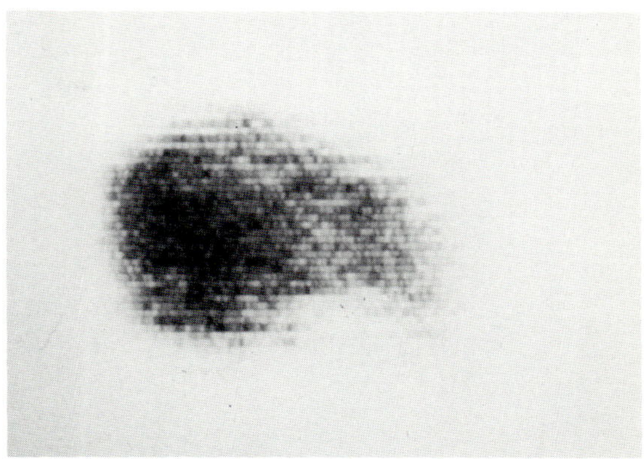

F

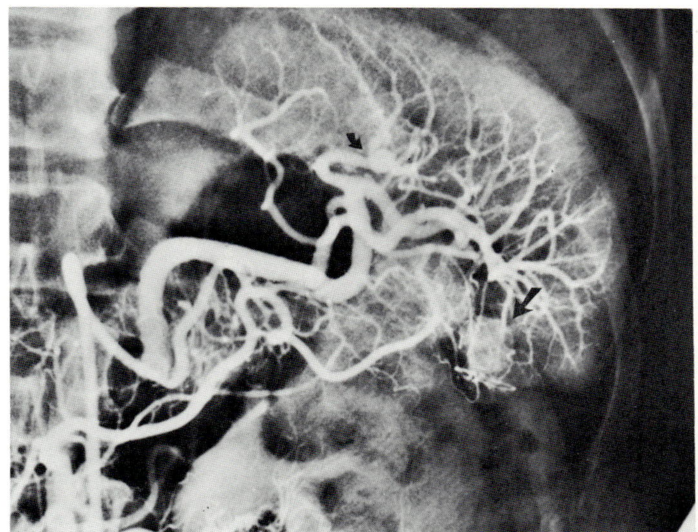

G

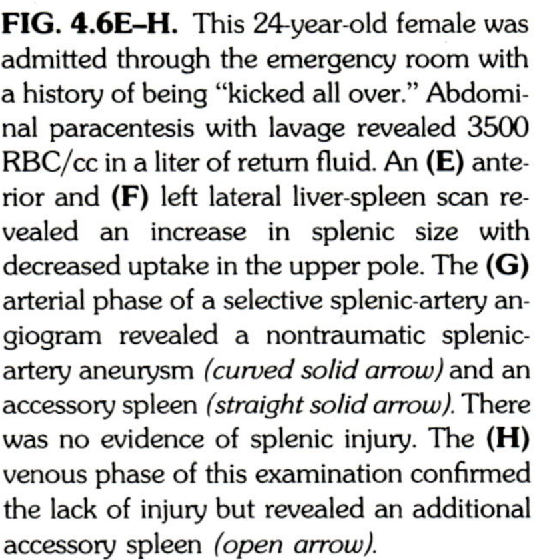

FIG. 4.6E–H. This 24-year-old female was admitted through the emergency room with a history of being "kicked all over." Abdominal paracentesis with lavage revealed 3500 RBC/cc in a liter of return fluid. An **(E)** anterior and **(F)** left lateral liver-spleen scan revealed an increase in splenic size with decreased uptake in the upper pole. The **(G)** arterial phase of a selective splenic-artery angiogram revealed a nontraumatic splenic-artery aneurysm *(curved solid arrow)* and an accessory spleen *(straight solid arrow)*. There was no evidence of splenic injury. The **(H)** venous phase of this examination confirmed the lack of injury but revealed an additional accessory spleen *(open arrow)*.

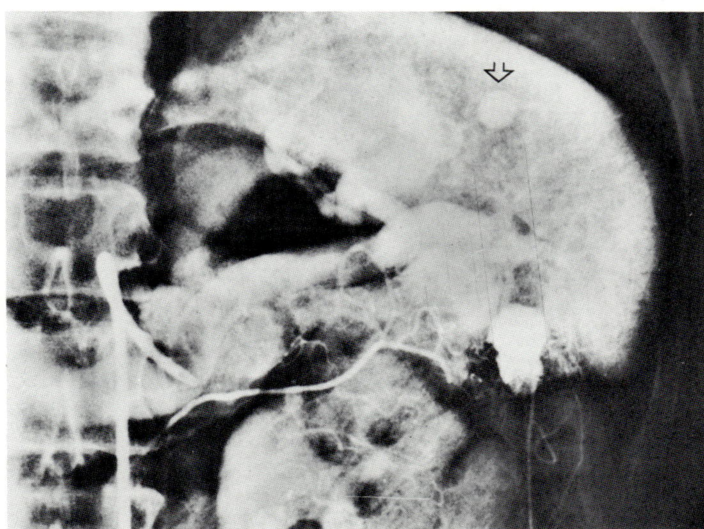

H

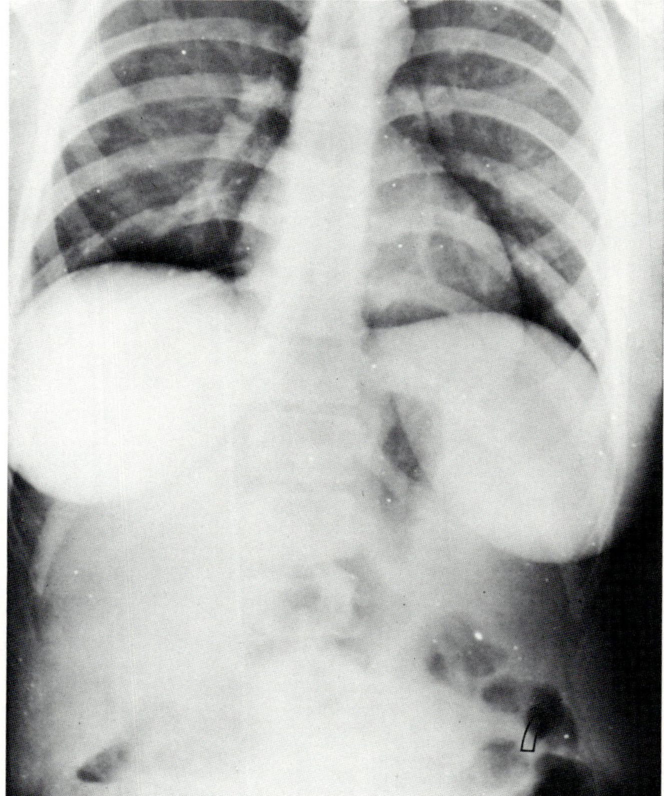

FIG. 4.7A–C. This 19-year-old female was admitted with a history of blunt trauma to the left upper abdomen. The **(A)** admission chest-abdomen examination reveals a LUQ soft-tissue mass that is displacing the stomach medially and depressing the splenic flexure. There is thickening of the proximal soft-tissue stripe of the left paracolic gutter *(curved open arrow)* consistent with the presence of free intraperitoneal fluid. No rib fractures are seen. The **(B)** left lateral decubitus and **(C)** Trendelenburg views of the abdomen with contrast (barium) in the stomach confirm the presence of a LUQ mass. A ruptured spleen was found at abdominal exploration.

A

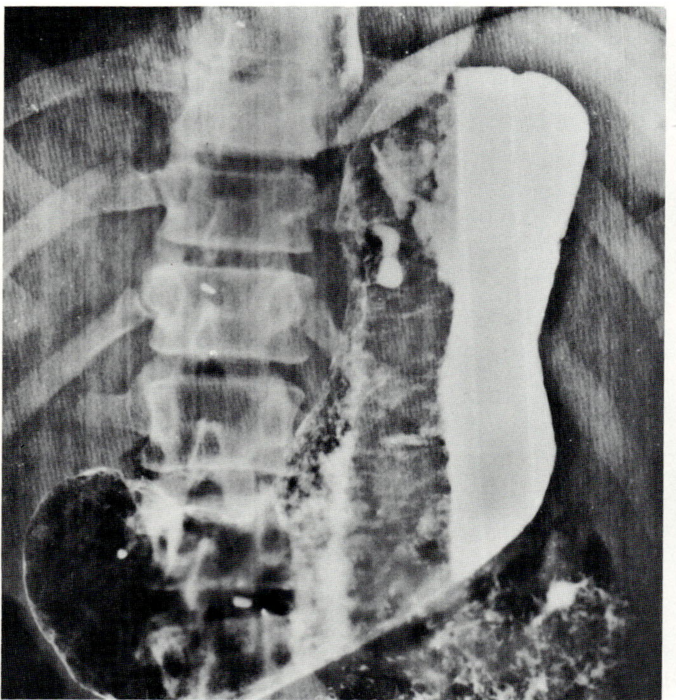

B

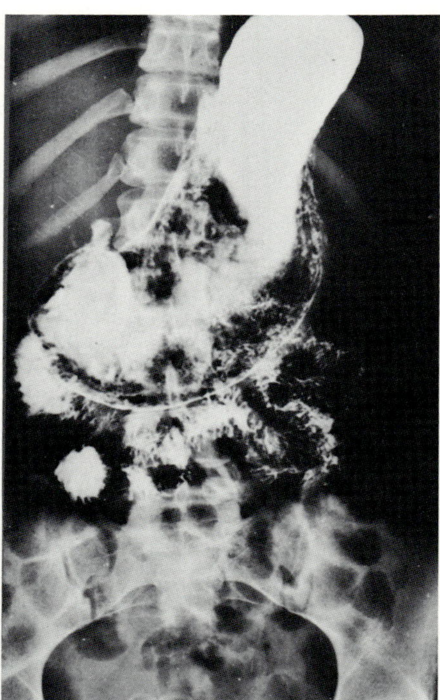

C

the regional surrounding tissues. It may also appear as a localized, well-defined collection of contrast indicating compartmentalization of the extravasation by surrounding hematoma or pseudoaneurysm formation (Fig. 4.8). In either case, the extravasated contrast material appears early in the arterial phase and remains until late in the venous phase.

2. Demonstration of venous shunts or early venous opacification (see Fig. 4.3). Assuming good angiographic technique and normal vascular anatomy, an angiogram can be divided into arterial, intermediate, and venous phases. Normally, arterial and venous channels are either not observed on the same film or are noted only after sufficient time has passed for the passage of contrast through the arterial, capillary, and venous channels. In the normal spleen, contrast does not appear in the splenic vein until 5–6 s after the injection of the contrast material. The demonstration of an opacified venous channel at 3 s or less after the injection of contrast is direct evidence of arterial-venous shunting even if the shunt cannot be demonstrated.
3. Mottled parenchymal phase. The intermediate phase of the splenic angiogram will, under normal conditions, demonstrate a homogenous accumulation of contrast within the confines of the splenic capsule. In splenic trauma, a common finding is the presence of a coarse, irregular, and relatively localized mottled parenchymal phase (irregular areas of relative radiolucency superimposed on the background of normal or increased intermediate-phase density). This finding is due to multiple, closely packed sites of arterial extravasation or disruption of sinusoids.

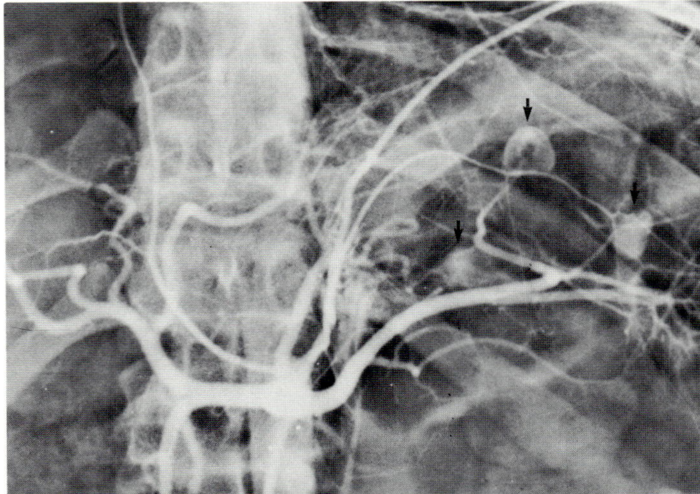

A

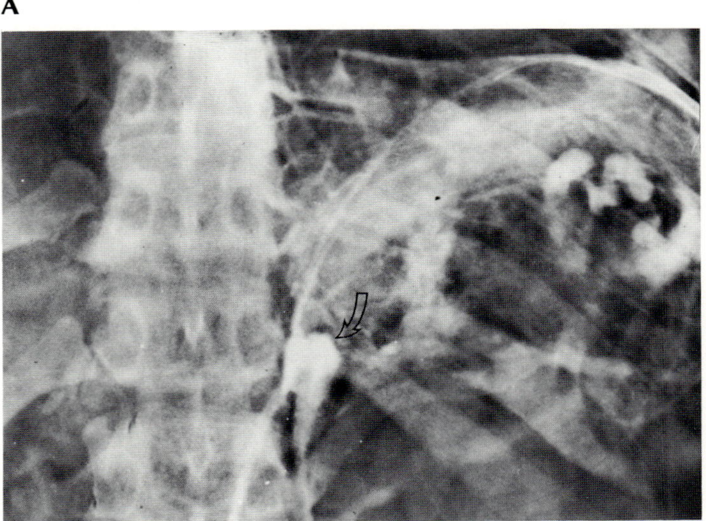

B

FIG. 4.8A and B. This 22-year-old male was admitted through the emergency room with the history of having fallen down four flights of stairs. Abdominal paracentesis with lavage revealed the presence of free intraperitoneal blood. A radionuclide scan of the spleen showed a 4–5 cm defect. Multiple left rib fractures were identified on his admission chest examination (see Figure 3.9). With a pressure injection of contrast for a flush aortogram, the tip of the flush catheter flipped into the left inferior phrenic artery. The **(A)** arterial phase of this injection revealed multiple sites of intrasplenic contrast extravasation *(solid arrows)*. The **(B)** intermediate phase of this injection shows contrast extravasation from the inferiophrenic artery *(curved open arrow)*, an area of relative lucency within this spleen, and multiple sites of intrasplenic contrast extravasation.

4. Amputation of vessels or the demonstration of intravascular thrombosis (Figs. 4.3,4.9). If a vascular channel abruptly ends without associated branching, it may ordinarily be assumed that reflex vasospasm, partial or complete transection of the vessel, or intravascular thrombosis is present. It must be appreciated, however, that other factors may be responsible. Thus, apparent abrupt termination of a vessel may require a repeat examination in a different projection in order to exclude acute angulation or other alteration in the course of the vessel. If a vascular thrombosis is the cause of an abrupt termination, one may occasionally note a filling defect within the vascular channel with an upstream convexity representing the head of the intravascular thrombosis.

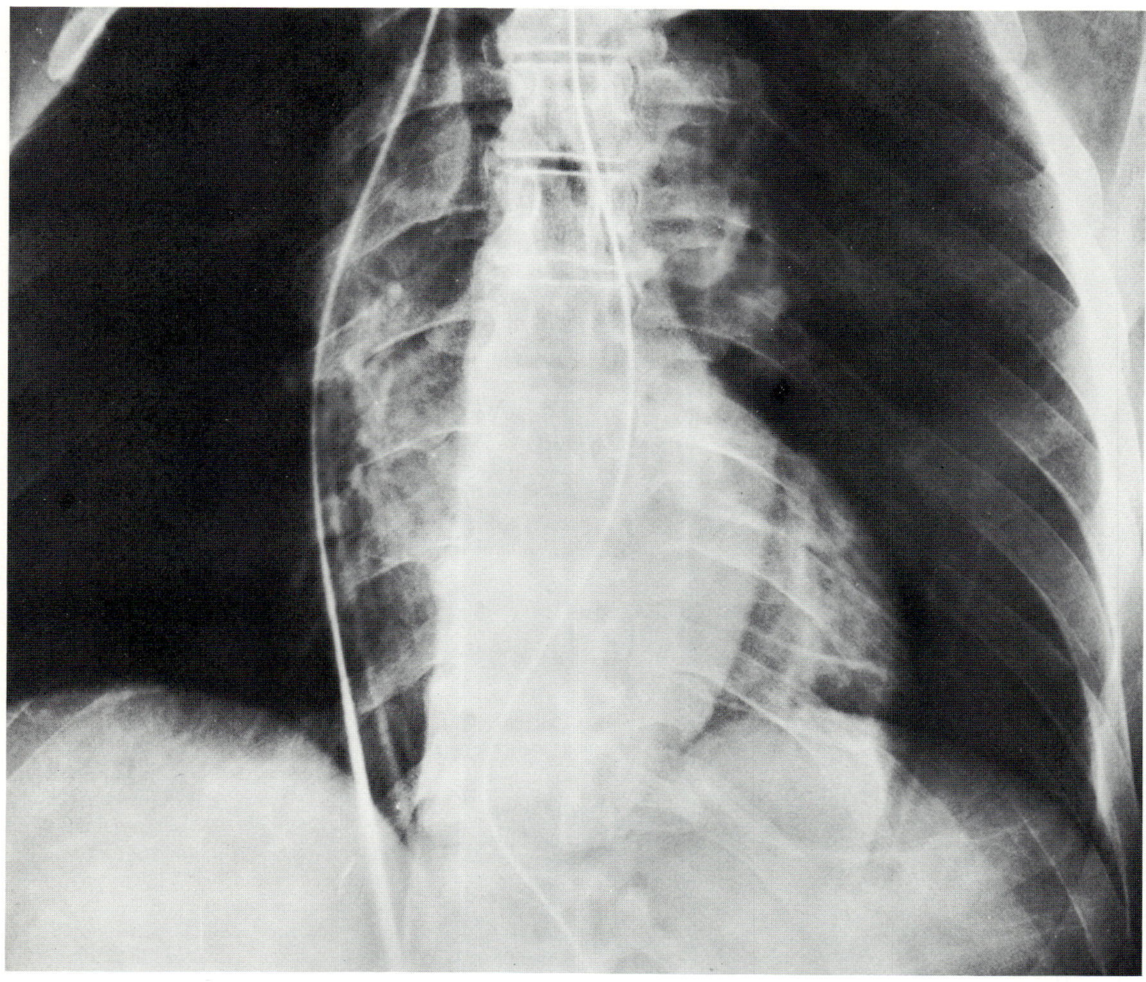

A

FIG. 4.9A–E. This 60-year-old male with a known history of alcohol abuse stated that on the evening prior to his admission he ingested a large quantity of alcohol, developed a sharp, lower abdominal bandlike pain, arose to vomit, and then collapsed. He was admitted the next day because of persistent LUQ pain. His **(A)** initial chest examination was interpreted to be normal except for cardiovascular changes due to hypertension. After 3 days in the hospital, the patient developed a left pleural effusion that was at first serosanguinous but then became purulent. His **(B)** frontal, erect examination of the chest now reveals blunting of the left costophrenic angle. A **(C)** left lateral decubitus view confirms the presence of a free left pleural effusion and reveals a previously unnoticed left 6th rib fracture *(curved open arrow)*. The **(D)** arterial phase of a celiac angiogram shows smooth encasement of the proximal splenic artery *(straight solid arrow)*. The intrasplenic branches of this artery are abruptly terminated with multiple sites of contrast puddling *(open arrows)*. The **(E)** venous phase of the study shows several, irregular defects *(solid arrows)* similar in size and location to defects noted on a previous isotopic scan of the spleen.

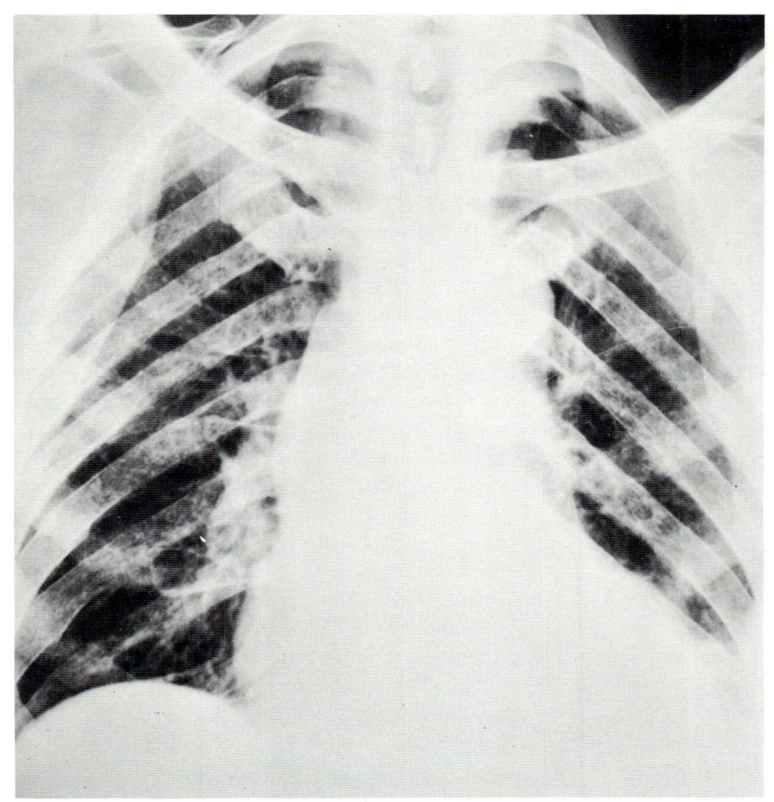

B

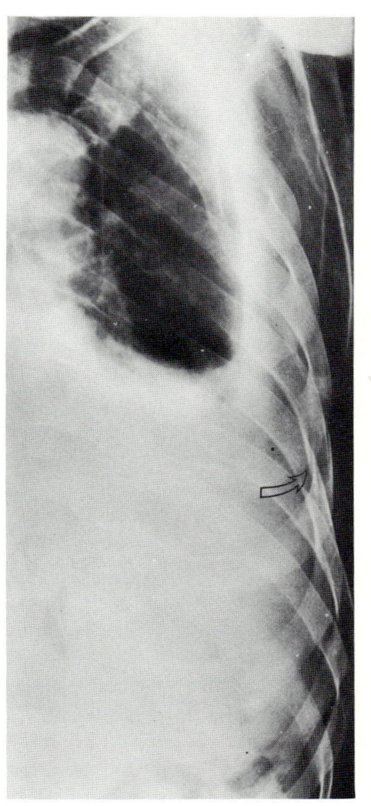

C

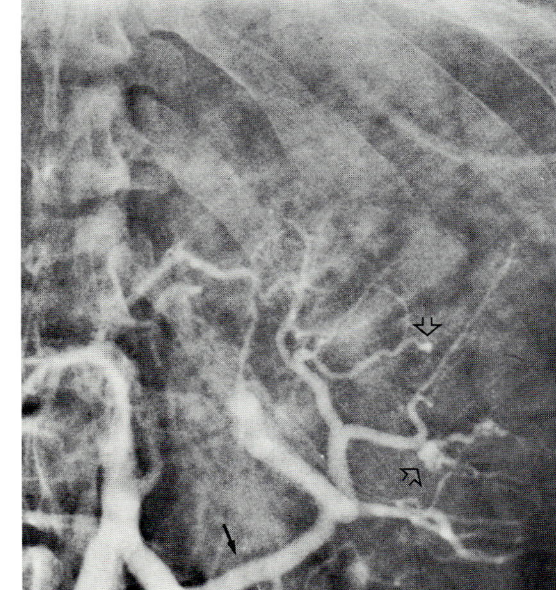

D

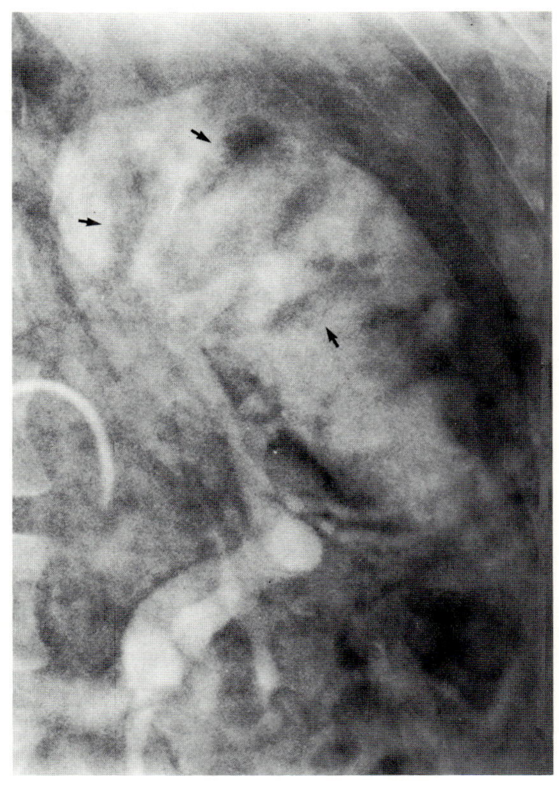

E

5. Bowing, stretching, or crowding of vessels (Figs. 4.3,4.9). Since an intrasplenic or subcapsular hematoma acts as a mass, an alteration in the course of adjacent vessels occurs resulting in bowing, stretching, and crowding of these vessels. Such vascular changes are highly reliable when present, particularly when surrounding a well-defined avascular area representing the splenic hematoma. If an avascular area about which these arterial changes occur cannot be defined, care must be taken not to overread such vascular findings. They may result from normal alterations of the splenic contour secondary to its relationship to other intraabdominal structures or the projection at the time of filming the angiogram.
6. Changes of the major splenic artery (Figs. 4.3,4.9). Injury to the spleen can result in reflex vasospasm of the splenic artery. However, this finding does not necessarily indicate the extent or degree of the splenic injury. Dislocation of the splenic artery from its normal course may be indicative of a splenic hematoma. On occasion, as blood dissects around the splenic pedicle, localized encasement of the splenic artery may be demonstrated.
7. Linear or wedge-shaped areas of radiolucency in spleen (Fig. 4.9). This finding may be indicative of the site of splenic laceration or of remote ischemia secondary to proximal arterial injury. Unfortunately, it is the most frequent cause of a false-positive angiographic diagnosis of splenic trauma. This may occur because in selective splenic angiography, all the vessels supplying the spleen, particularly those supplying its periphery, may not be filled with contrast. These areas of splenic parenchyma not opacified may then appear as radiolucent defects mimicking those produced by traumatic lesions. Therefore, it is wise to precede selective splenic angiography with a flush aortagram. If these same defects cannot be demonstrated on the flush aortagram, then they are probably artifactual in nature. The second major cause for confusion lies in the presence of fetal lobulation. When such lobulations exist, bands of connective tissue extend from the capsule into the splenic pulp. These relatively avascular septations will appear as linear filling defects on the intermediate and late phases of the splenic angiogram. It may be helpful to keep in mind that lacerations do not have distinct, sharp, smooth margins; that they are usually associated with other vascular and parenchymal findings; and that on occasion, frank contrast extravasation into the laceration may be demonstrated.
8. Splenic displacement from its normal anatomic location (Fig. 4.9). This is one of the most unreliable signs of splenic trauma. The classic location of the spleen is in the left upper quadrant beneath the left hemidiaphragm and abutting against the upper lateral abdominal wall. Unfortunately, a large number of individuals fail to show this classic localization because of congenital alterations of positioning and/or development, changes of location secondary to changes in positioning of the patient, normal alterations in the relationship between the spleen and the surrounding visceral structures (variations in filling of the stomach, variations in hepatic size, and alterations in the position of the splenic flexure with respect to the spleen, etc.), previous intraabdominal surgery, inflammatory disease, and other nontraumatic lesions. Osborn et al. [135] state that in only one situation is displacement of the spleen from the lateral thoracic wall a relatively reliable sign of injury to the spleen. This applies to the demonstration on the splenogram of a peripheral lenticular defect, with the margins of the spleen above and below this curved defect being closely applied to the upper lateral abdominal wall. This finding, when demonstrated, is indicative of a subcapsular hematoma.

Complications of Splenic Injury

Delayed Splenic Rupture

It is traditionally stated that one of the most frequent complications of either recognized or undiagnosed splenic trauma is delayed rupture. This entity, first recognized and described by Bodich in 1902, is observed in 14% to 33% of cases of splenic injury and accounts for one in five cases of splenic rupture [60,125]. Fortunately, the mortality in delayed splenic rupture is reported as 6.6% or less than for primary rupture.

Patients with delayed splenic rupture will demonstrate a quiescent interval between the initial injury and the appearance of symptoms of internal hemorrhage (Table 4.11). This time interval, which may be

TABLE 4.11. Relative incidence of acute and delayed splenic rupture

Author	No. of cases	Percentage of delayed rupture
Byrne	101	26.7
Zabinski and Harkins	111	14.5
Dobson	22	22.7
Bollinger and Fowler	24	33.3
Totals	258	21.4

Source: Bollinger JA, Fowler EF (1956) Traumatic rupture of spleen with special reference to delayed splenic rupture. Am J Surg 91: 561–570

as long as 36 to 48 h, has been called the "latent period of Baudet" [60,180]. Massive splenic hemorrhage occurring after this interval has been defined as "delayed rupture" [60,179]. Terry et al. [179] found that patients with delayed rupture had a latency period of less than 1 week in 50% of cases and less than 2 weeks in 75% of cases.

Although the exact etiology for this occurrence is uncertain, two explanatory theories [210] have been advanced. The first relates to breakdown of the hematoma. Following the initial injury with formation of subcapsular and/or subserosal hematoma, continued oozing of blood and fluid into the contused tissues takes place. The continued oozing and/or the mass effect of this oozing results in alterations of hemodynamics of the surrounding tissues, with subsequent ischemia and breakdown leading to intra- and retroperitoneal spillage of blood. The second theory suggests that a clot forming at the site of the initial injury becomes detached, resulting in hemorrhage into either the intra- or retroperitoneal area. Although McCort and others [109] suggest that subcapsular hematoma and minimal oozing from small-capsule lacerations are relatively rare occurrences in splenic injury, the statistics of delayed rupture, if correct, coupled with the theoretical explanations of its cause appear to refute McCort's premise.

Benjamin et al. [15] published a review of 320 patients with splenic trauma managed with diagnostic paracentesis and lavage. They question the traditional assertion that late rupture of the spleen has an 11% to 15% incidence. Only 6 patients (or 2% of their group) had surgery 2 or more days after injury. Only 1 patient in this group was truly asymptomatic. They suggest that most cases of delayed splenic rupture represent a delay in diagnosis. Their assertion is justified both by the common lack of precision in the diagnosis (Fig. 3.9) of blunt injuries and a tendency to clinically observe blunt-injury cases over a period of time (Fig. 4.9).

Current studies of splenectomy in children reported by LaMura et al. [82] and the nonoperative management of splenic trauma described by Joseph et al. [74] raise the question whether all patients with hemoperitoneum require exploratory laparotomy. In view of the fact that controlled bleeding from the spleen does not require immediate surgical intervention, intraperitoneal blood from a splenic tear is not an immediate indication for operation. Further studies are necessary to establish what degree of intraperitoneal bleeding mandates surgical intervention.

There are no radiologic findings (including angiography) that will predict delayed rupture. However, Bollinger and Fowler [19] have found that the accumulation of fluid at the left thoracic base 24 h after injury is highly suggestive of delayed rupture. It would appear that the safest course to follow is that of the immediate reevaluation of the patient for delayed splenic rupture, particularly in the presence of dramatic change in the patient's clinical status after a latency period following injury.

Pseudoaneurysm Formation

A pseudoaneurysm is formed by blood leaking from an injured vessel into the surrounding tissues. A hematoma is produced whose periphery becomes organized to form a fibrous capsule that is attached to the vessel wall at the site of the injury. Subsequent liquefaction of the center of the hematoma results in a residual space—the pseudoaneurysm. Four factors determine the size of the pseudoaneurysm: the size of the rent in the vessel, the patient's pulse pressure, the coagulability of the patient's blood, and the resistance of the surrounding tissues. A pseudoaneurysm can form in as little as 48 h after injury. It is more prone to rupture than a true aneurysm. A pseudoaneurysm may rupture into an adjacent venous channel, creating an arteriovenous fistula; it may alter hemodynamics by its mass effect, resulting in peripheral ischemia; and it may be converted into a mycotic aneurysm through bacterial infection. In addition, clot formation within the pseudoaneurysm can lead to peripheral embolization with ischemia and/or infarction [91] (Fig. 4.9).

Cyst Formation

A splenic cyst resulting from splenic trauma is in fact a pseudocyst representing the end stage in the evolution of a splenic hematoma [55]. As the hematoma becomes bordered by a fibrous capsular wall, liquefaction of its center occurs. The difference in osmolar factors inside the fibrous capsule wall compared with the outside results in continued accumulation of fluid within the cyst cavity. Rupture of the cyst or calcification of its wall can occur (see Fig. 3.1).

Splenosis

Splenic tissue has the capability of autotransplantation and can grow in ectopic sites following traumatic or surgically induced splenic injury [60,184]. This entity was recognized in 1883 and was designated *splenosis* by Buchbinder and Lipkoff in 1939. Such implants are usually asymptomatic and are discovered accidentally either during surgical procedures or on postmortem examination. However, such complications as intestinal obstruction due to mass formation may develop. Katzen and Levy [81] recently reported a case of splenosis simulating a fundal intramural gastric mass following surgery for a gastric leiomyoblastoma with splenic laceration occurring during the surgical procedure, necessitating a splenectomy. Plain-film radiologic studies may be suggestive but not definitive. Barium studies of the gastrointestinal tract may demonstrate an intramural lesion, simulating leiomyoma, metastatic disease, endometriosis, etc. Jacobson and DeNardo [72] have suggested the use of radionuclide scanning to aid in the diagnosis. Angiographic procedures may demonstrate contrast accumulation ("stain") at the site of seeding.

LIVER AND BILIARY TRACT

General Aspects of Injury

The liver is the second most frequently injured intraperitoneal organ, with a frequency of injury that is approximately one-half that of the spleen. Trauma to the liver comprises 5% to 10% of all injuries sustained as a result of blunt abdominal trauma. It is probably the most frequent injury identified at autopsy examination [109]. In children, the frequency of hepatic trauma is higher than in adults [149]. Hepatic trauma has a higher morbidity and mortality than does splenic injury. Injury to the liver from blunt trauma is considerably more dangerous than that produced with penetrating wounds. Elder, in 1887, reported a mortality rate of 66.8%, whereas McKesky et al., in 1957, reported a mortality of 67% [60]—no significant difference in a period of 70 years. The reason for this surprising lack of change in mortality lies in the significant blood loss associated with this injury (Table 4.12). Unless early control of hemorrhage is effected before

TABLE 4.12. Causes of prehospital death in victims with abdominal injury

	No. of cases	
Massive abdominal hemorrhage		
Liver	17	
Spleen	1	(23)
Major vessels	5	
Massive thoracic hemorrhage		
Aorta	23	
Heart	12	(47)
Lungs	12	
Head & spine injuries	12	
Drowned	1	
Aspiration	1	
Total	84	

Source: Foley RW, Harris LS, Pilcher DB (1977) Abdominal injuries in automobile accidents: Review of care of fatally injured patients. J Trauma 17(8): 611–615

there is exsanguination or irreversible shock, all the advantages of improved diagnostic and therapeutic measures are lost. The time-delay factor and mortality are summarized by Frey et al. [54]. The prognostic implication of hypotension in the presence of hepatic injury is dramatically illustrated by the experience encountered, i.e., 100% of the patients who died were in shock on arrival in the emergency room (Table 4.13). The more recent 15-year experience of Frey et al. [54] suggests that the once-dismal outlook for this injury is no longer justified. Whereas their overall mortality rate for the 15-year period extending from 1965 to 1970 averaged 26%, a breakdown in terms of 5-year intervals demonstrates a significant continued reduction in the mortality rate. In their study, the mortality ranged in the area of 50% from 1956 to 1960, 29% from 1961 to 1965, and 16% from 1966 to 1970. This mortality reduction was noted with all degrees of hepatic injury. With grade 1 injuries (a simple capsular tear), the mortality dropped from 33% to 0%; in grade 2 injuries (tears extending less than 1 cm into the liver), the mortality dropped from 37% to 14%; in grade 3 injuries (lacerations of 1–4 cm in depth, over 5 cm in length, associated with moderate bleeding that required direct suturing), the mortality dropped from 43% to 8%; and in grade 4 injuries (bursting injuries with multiple lacerations), the reduction in mortality was from 77% to 56%. Drezner, reporting in 1975 [44], agrees that the previous dismal prognosis for this lesion is not warranted. He indicates that the first significant reduction in mortality was reported by Manning et al. from their World War II experience, which showed an overall mortality for liver injury of 27%. The Vietnam experience indicated a mortality of 4.5% for hepatic injuries due to blunt trauma.

The accurate preoperative diagnosis of blunt hepatic injuries is made difficult by the frequent presence of associated multiple-system trauma. Corica and Powers [34] reported a series of 75 liver injuries in patients with blunt abdominal trauma. In 18.7% of the patients, there were no symptoms on initial presentation of the patient. In 26.6% of patients, localizing abdominal symptoms were present; in 41.3%, generalized abdominal symptoms were present. Corica and Powers made the correct diagnosis in 83.8% of patients by abdominal paracentesis. They also present a breakdown of various types of hepatic injury and cite mortality statistics (Tables 4.14 and 4.15, Fig. 4.10). The most commonly associated injuries are skeletal fractures, splenic rupture, pneumothorax, and trauma to soft tissues.

The frequent occurrence of hepatic injury in patients with penetrating abdominal trauma is evident in the figures reported in studies of both stab wounds

TABLE 4.13. Postcrash, preoperative evaluation of patients with hepatic injury

	1956–1960	1961–1965	1966–1970
Average time in minutes from accident to hospital			
Survivors	45	90	25
Deaths	100	45	28
Average time in minutes from emergency room to operating room in patients with 4+ hepatic injury			
Survivors	205	207	140
Deaths	183	148	112
Percent of patients in shock on arrival in the emergency room			
Survivors	40%	30%	35%
Deaths	80%	87%	100%
Number of patients undergoing abdominal tap/lavage			
Positive	9	10	46
False negative	4	1	2 (tap only)

Source: Frey CF, Trollope M, Harpster W, Snyder R (1973) A fifteen year experience with automotive hepatic trauma. J Trauma 13: 1039–1049

TABLE 4.14. Blunt liver injuries—Relationship between type of injury and mortality rate (75 cases)

Type of injury	No. of cases	% of total no. of cases	No. of deaths	Due to liver trauma: No. of deaths	Due to liver trauma: Mortality (%)
One laceration	33	44.0	12	1	3.0
Multiple lacerations	26	34.7	6	1	3.8
Stellate laceration	6	8.0	1	0	0
Bursting injury	7	9.3	5	3	42.9
Subcapsular hematoma	3	4.0	1	1	33.3
Total	75		25	6	

Source: Corica A, Powers SR Jr (1975) Blunt liver trauma: An analysis of 75 treated patients. J Trauma 15: 751–756

TABLE 4.15. Results of abdominal paracentesis in the diagnosis of intraabdominal hemorrhage; all patients had proven damage to the liver with bleeding

Abdominal paracentesis performed	No.	%
True positives 1st attempt	29	78.4
True positives 2nd attempt	2	5.4
Total true positives	31	83.8
False negatives	6	16.2
Four-quadrant tap	5	
Peritoneal lavage	1	
False positives	0	0.0

Source: Corica A, Powers SR Jr (1975) Blunt liver trauma: An analysis of 75 treated patients. J Trauma 15: 751–756

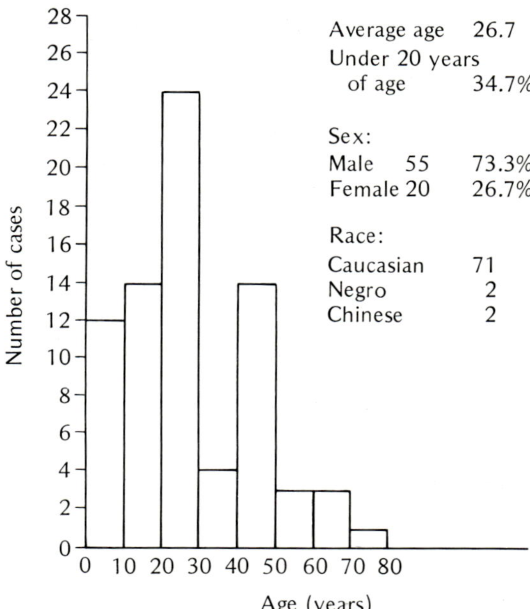

FIG. 4.10. Age distribution in 75 cases of blunt liver trauma, Albany Medical Center, 1969–1973. From Corica A, Powers SR Jr (1975) Blunt liver trauma: An analysis of 75 treated patients. J Trauma 15: 751–756

TABLE 4.16. Average number of injuries per year, 1939–1974 (1590 cases)

Time period	Average no. of liver injuries/year
1939–1954	18.7
1955–1961	48.5
1962–1970	47.5
1971–1974	130.5

Source: DeFore WW Jr, Mattox KL, Jordan GL, Beall AC Jr (1976) Management of 1590 consecutive cases of liver trauma. Arch Surg 111: 493–497

TABLE 4.17. Cause of liver injuries

Cause	No. of injuries (No. of deaths)				
	1939–1954	1955–1961	1962–1970	1971–1974	Total
Gunshot wound	140 (40)	172 (32)	226 (27)	322 (20)	860 (119)
Stab wound	136 (5)	125 (4)	129 (3)	100 (1)	490 (13)
Blunt trauma	24 (17)	43 (13)	73 (20)	100 (27)	240 (77)
Total	300 (62)	340 (49)	428 (50)	522 (48)	1590 (209)

Source: DeFore WW Jr, Mattox KL, Jordan GL Beall AC Jr (1976) Management of 1590 consecutive cases of liver trauma. Arch Surg 111: 493–497

TABLE 4.18. Associated injuries among 1590 patients over 36-year period

No. of associated injuries	No. of patients	Deaths	
		No.	%
None	596	26	4.4
1	457	35	7.7
2	278	47	16.9
3	130	33	25.4
4	81	33	40.7
5 or more	48	35	72.9

Source: DeFore WW Jr, Mattox KL, Jordan GL, Beall AC Jr (1976) Management of 1590 consecutive cases of liver trauma. Arch Surg 111: 493–497

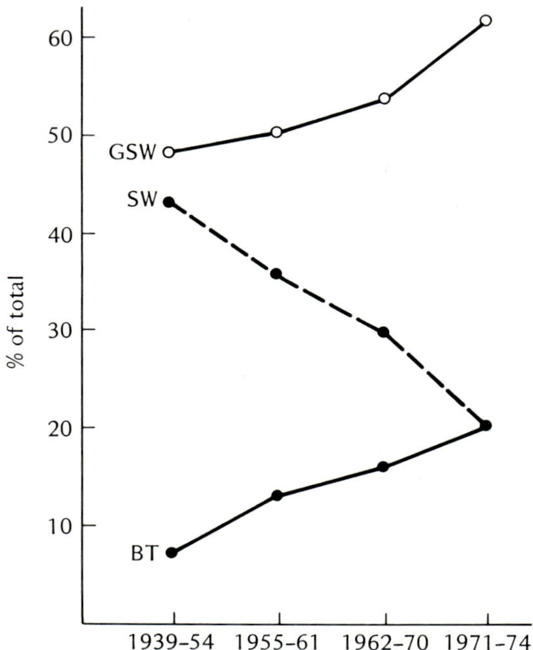

FIG. 4.11. Changing causes of liver injury by time period. GSW indicates gunshot wound; SW, stab wound: BT, blunt trauma. From DeFore WW Jr, Mattox KL, Jordan GL, Beall AC Jr (1976) Management of 1590 consecutive cases of liver trauma. Arch Surg 111: 493–497

and gunshot wounds. DeFore et al. [38] reviewed 1590 consecutive liver injuries from a variety of causes between 1939 and 1974. In addition to the increasing number of injuries to the liver over this period, there was a significant increase in hepatic lesions produced by gunshot wounds. DeFore's group also noted a declining overall mortality for all forms of liver trauma and a progressive correlation of increasing mortality with the number of associated organ injuries (Tables 4.16–4.18, Figs. 4.11 and 4.12). Frey et al. [54] also found associated injuries in 74% of surviving patients and in 94% of nonsurviving patients.

Mechanism of Blunt Injury

Blunt rupture of liver is caused by either direct or indirect forces. In the civilian population, the direct force is usually associated with an automobile accident. Other causes include blows, falls, and crush injuries. The direct force usually results in a stellate burst of the superior surface of the right lobe of the liver [60]. The right lobe is injured in about four-fifths of all blunt-trauma cases [109]. Indirect or contracoup injuries [60] are usually caused by falls from a height with the patient landing either on his feet or on his buttock. This type of trauma produces a bursting effect on the liver in its sagittal plane with occasional separation of liver fragments. In either situation, the most frequent result is massive free intraperitoneal bleeding.

A common mechanism for fatal vehicular-passenger injury is the ejection of the victim from the car onto the roadway or other surrounding solid objects. Trauma to the liver appears to follow a different pattern. Frey et al. [54] reported that of those patients

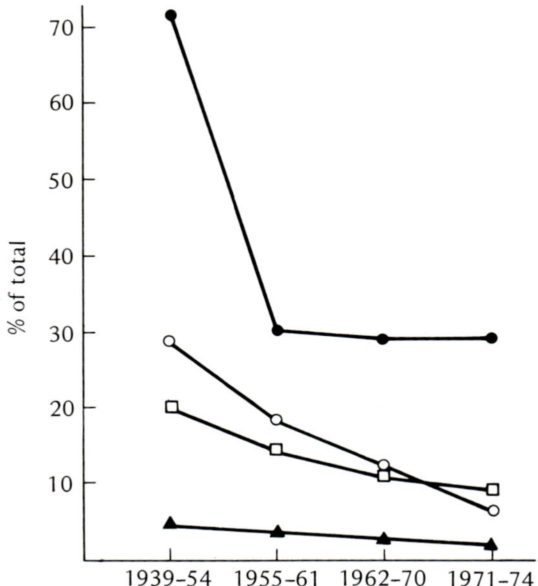

FIG. 4.12. Mortality with respect to wounding agent. *Solid circles,* blunt trauma; *clear circles,* gunshot wounds; *solid triangles,* stab wounds; *clear squares,* overall. From DeFore WW Jr, Mattox KL, Jordan GL, Beall AC Jr (1976) Management of 1590 consecutive cases of liver trauma. Arch Surg 111: 493–497

not surviving automobile accidents because of liver laceration, 82% were sitting in the driver's seat, 18% were in the passenger seat, and an insignificant number were ejected from the automobile. Of those patients who survived hepatic injury, 68% were in the driver's seat, 32% were in the passenger's seat, and only 6.8% were ejected from the car. These statistics indicate a high morbidity and mortality associated with the impact of the steering wheel against the patient.

Sonography

Ultrasonic examination of the traumatized patient can easily define the presence of free intraperitoneal fluid. In addition, localized or diffuse contour changes of the liver may be demonstrated and are easily separated from extrahepatic masses. Although it may be difficult to differentiate intrahepatic hematomas from other cystic masses, such as abscesses and necrotic tumors, the patient's history may be helpful in making such a distinction. The identification of subcapsular hematomas is extremely difficult because of the numerous artifacts produced by rib reverberations [10,43,58, 64,161,209].

Radiologic Studies

Because of the high frequency of massive hemorrhage and of associated intraabdominal and extraabdominal injuries, it is not unusual for the patient with hepatic trauma to have either an incomplete or no diagnostic radiologic workup. The type of patient who is usually evaluated has either had a minimal injury, has sustained a significant injury but is stabilized, or manifests a latent period between injury and the development of symptoms. A latent period is more commonly observed in splenic trauma but is not rare in hepatic injury.

The plain-film findings are essentially those of injury to associated supporting structures and intraabdominal organs. Radiologic changes relating to the liver are, of course, important.

Associated Injuries to Supporting Structures

A soft-tissue mass may be demonstrated at the site of the applied force. The outline of the right properitoneal fat and flank muscle may be obscured or absent due to a combination of dextrorotary scoliosis and hemorrhage. This combination results in shortening and widening of the silhouette of the right-flank soft tissues. In addition, 50% of patients will show fractures of the right lower ribs, and a high percentage of patients will demonstrate signs indicative of right diaphragmatic leaflet injury or rupture [80,107–110].

Associated Intra- or Extraabdominal Injury

Because of the nature of the forces producing hepatic trauma, there is a high frequency of injury to other intra- and extraabdominal structures. The signs associated with splenic, bowel, and right renal injury are frequently present. It is also not unusual to observe the manifestations of right pulmonary contusion, pneumothorax, or pleural effusion [9,80,107–110].

Plain-Film Signs of Hepatic Injury

The most frequent result of hepatic injury is massive intraperitoneal bleeding; thus, the most commonly demonstrated plain-film radiologic features are those indicative of free intraperitoneal fluid. In addition, localized bleeding into the subdiaphragmatic space without actual injury to the right diaphragmatic leaflet can result in marked elevation of the right hemidiaphragm. The accumulation of free or localized intraperitoneal fluid may result in obscuration of the liver silhouette, while intrahepatic bleeding can result in localized or diffuse enlargement of the hepatic density. Subcapsular hematomas may result in tumorlike swellings along the visualized liver margin [9,80,107–110].

Fluoroscopy

Fluoroscopic examination of the patient with hepatic trauma may be beneficial since alterations in motion of the right diaphragmatic leaflet are frequent. With diaphragmatic rupture, a paradoxical motion of the diaphragm is observed with an extremely high liver edge. A subdiaphragmatic hematoma will limit the motion of the diaphragm and may result in a normal or slightly lower position of the lower border of the liver. Splinting due to the trauma, without definite visceral or diaphragmatic injury, may simply result in an alteration in diaphragmatic motion with no significant change in the liver edge [109].

Angiography

The angiographic findings are essentially those described under the heading of splenic injury. It must be remembered that the response of a vessel to an insult, whether that vessel lies in the liver, spleen, small bowel, or pancreas, etc., is essentially the same and includes contrast extravasation, amputation of the vessels, displacement of vessels, mass effect, or any of the other previously mentioned signs. Angiography is helpful in determining the extent of injury and giving some clue as to whether the patient can be managed conservatively or is in need of an operative procedure. The following classification of liver injury is based on angiographic findings [1,3,18,19,87,88,91,107–110,124,145,146,172,185].

Subcapsular Hematoma (Figs. 4.13, 4.14). This is the least serious of the hepatic injuries, being due to a superficial rent in the surface of the liver confined by an intact capsule. The primary finding is that of an avascular mass on the periphery of the liver, optimally observed in the intermediate or venous phases of the angiogram. Stretching of vessels around the avascular area and, occasionally, an increase in contrast density about the rim of the mass are usually noted. If bleeding into the subcapsular compartment is continued, frank extravasation of contrast may be demonstrated, although uncommonly. Osborn et al.

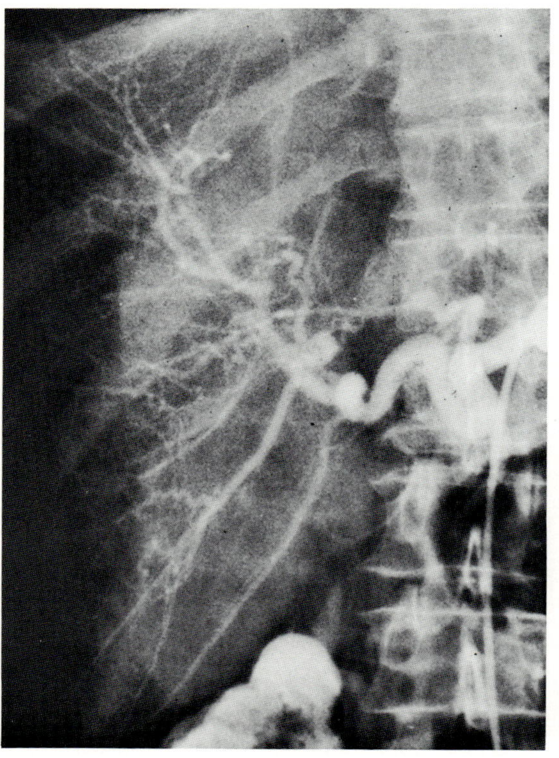

A

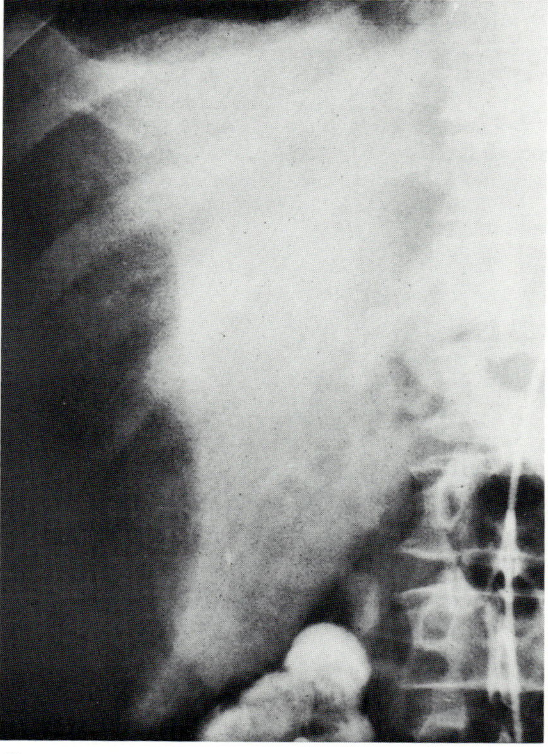

B

FIG. 4.13A and B. The **(A)** arterial phase of the hepatic angiogram of a victim of blunt abdominal trauma reveals bowing and stretching of the branches of the right hepatic artery. These branches fail to reach the right lateral abdominal wall. The **(B)** venous phase of this study shows an avascular, lucent area between the contrast-stained liver and the upper right lateral abdominal wall. These findings are consistent with a diagnosis of a subcapsular hepatic hematoma.

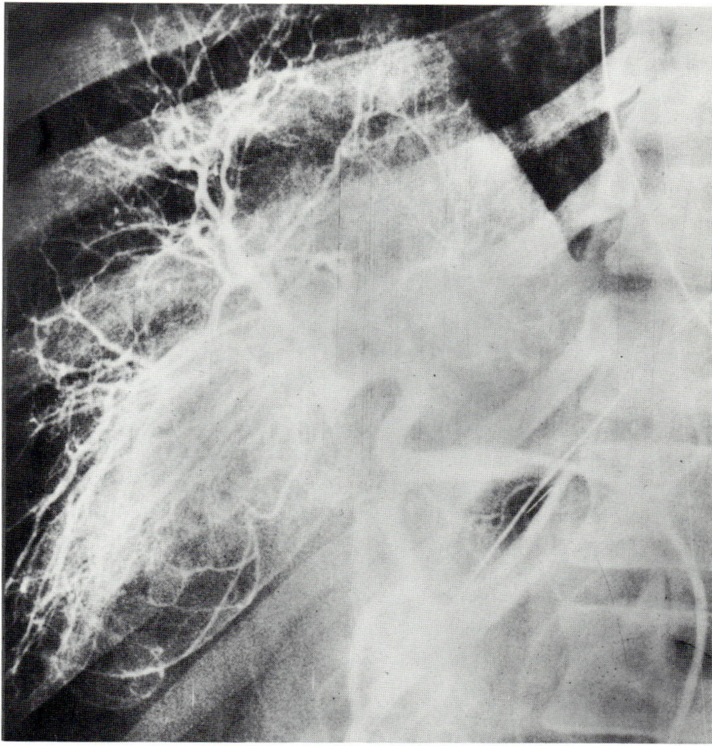

A

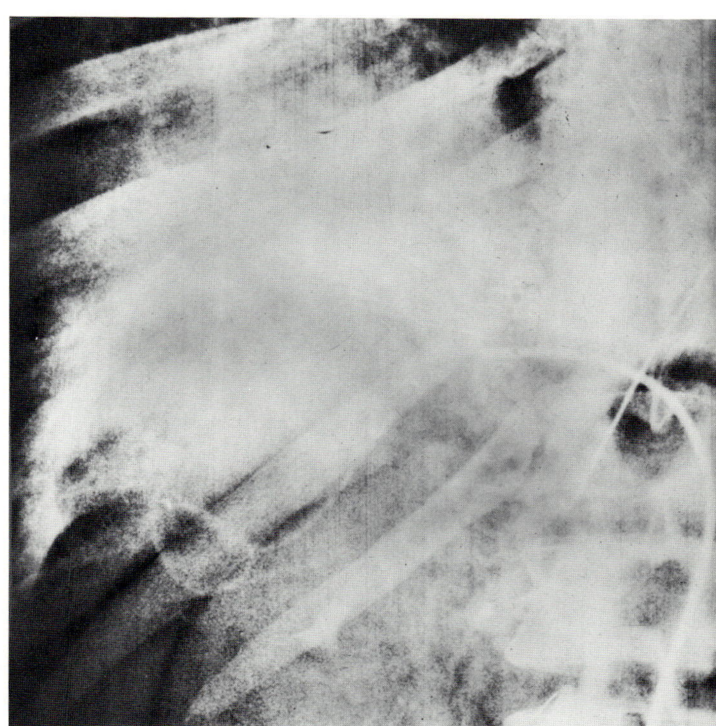

B

FIG. 4.14A and B. This young male patient with hemophilia was admitted with blunt abdominal trauma following an automobile accident. The **(A)** arterial phase of a selective common hepatic angiogram reveals separation of the right liver edge from the internal abdominal wall. This is confirmed on the **(B)** venous phase of the study. There is no evidence of contrast extravasation or other significant abnormality on either phase. Courtesy of Dr. Rogelio Moncada, Loyola University, Chicago, Ill.

[135] believe that a subcapsular hematoma can be differentiated from an intraperitoneal hematoma on the basis of angiographic findings. They state that the subcapsular hematoma will distort the hepatic artery and the liver outline, whereas the loculated intraperitoneal hematoma will not.

Parenchymal Rupture with Hematoma. A frank parenchymal rent may result in intraparenchymal bleeding. The typical angiographic findings relate to the presence of an avascular mass around which arteries and veins are observed to be stretched and bowed. Extravasation of contrast into the avascular mass may be demonstrated.

Parenchymal Contusion. Multiple small areas of disruption of the hepatic substance without a large hematoma are characteristic. Angiographically, patchy hypervascularity and irregular accumulation of contrast within the hepatic tissues are noted.

Laceration or Avulsion of Vessels. Definite tears of the arteries or veins result in extravasation of contrast or abrupt termination of vessels on angiography. Occasionally, as with splenic injury, a filling defect may be present in the lacerated vessel, indicating a thrombus.

Arteriovenous Fistula (Fig. 4.15). Total or partial transection of an artery and vein lying in close proximity to one another can result in a direct communication between them. In the liver, the most commonly encountered abnormal arteriovenous communication occurs between the hepatic artery and the portal vein. Such fistulae are initially clinically silent, but eventually they cause irreversible portal hypertension [84]. These traumatic malformations tend to develop very rapidly after the trauma. The close anatomic relationship between the hepatic artery and portal vein explains the high frequency of such fistulae as compared with shunts between the hepatic artery and hepatic vein. These two different types of shunts can be differentiated angiographically by following the course of the contrast from the artery into the venous system. If the contrast tends to flow centrally with improved visualization of the portal venous system, obviously the shunt is between the hepatic artery and portal vein. However, if the opacified venous structures ap-

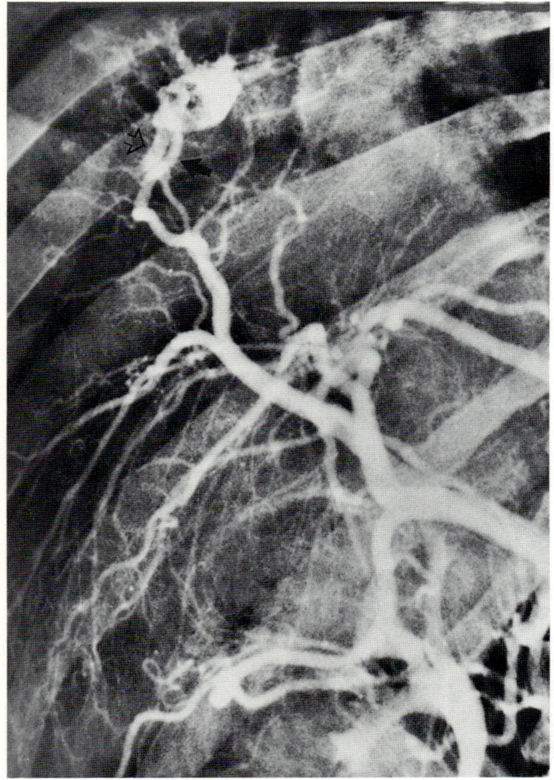

A

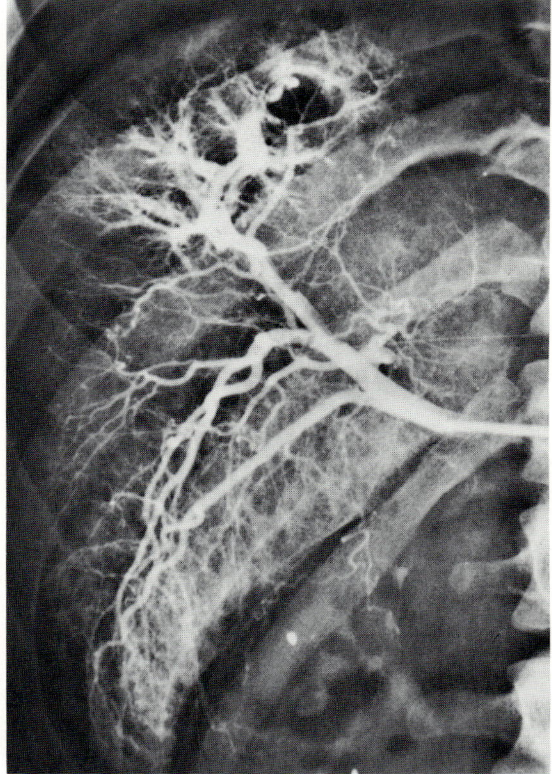

B

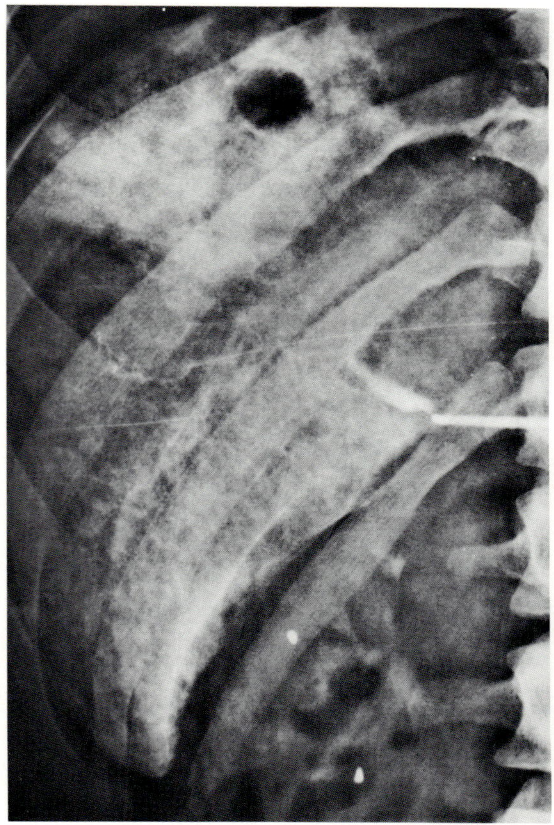

C

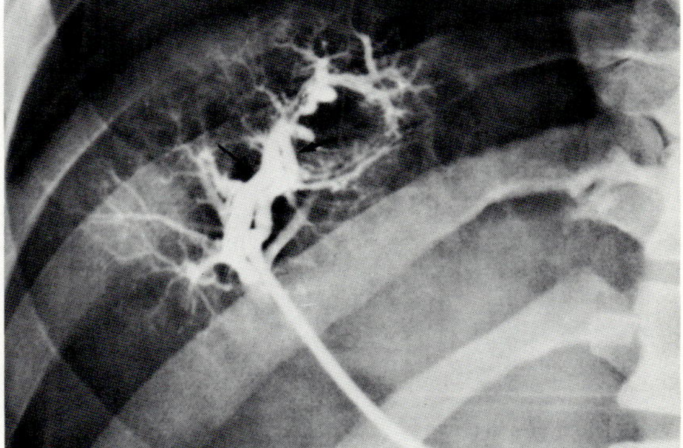

D

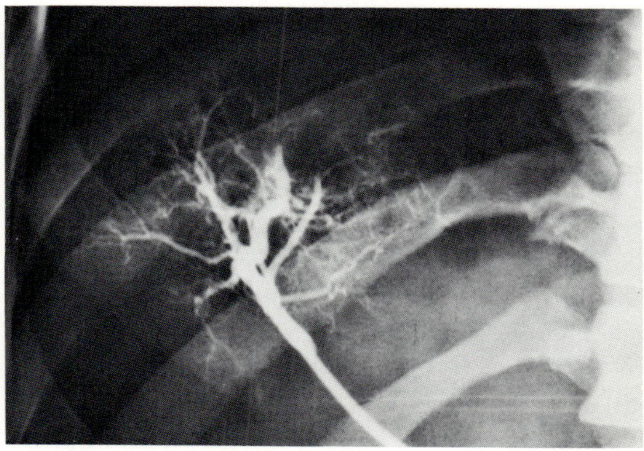

E

FIG. 4.15A–E. This 28-year-old male sustained multiple stab wounds to the chest and abdomen. At abdominal exploration, a laceration of the anterior surface of the liver was found and repaired. A radionuclide liver scan following this operation revealed a filling defect in the superior aspect of the right lobe at some distance from the laceration repair site. The **(A)** arterial phase from his initial hepatic angiogram shows a pseudoaneurysm arising from a peripheral branch of the right hepatic artery in association with a hepatic artery–*(solid arrowhead)* portal vein *(open arrowhead)* arteriovenous fistula. The patchy hypervascularity and irregular contrast accumulation about this site are consistent with contused tissue. The **(B)** arterial phase from a repeat angiogram performed 10 days after the first demonstrates "filling-in" of the pseudoaneurysm. The fistula is still patent, and the vascular structures comprising it appear to have enlarged. The **(C)** intermediate phase of this same study demonstrates an avascular area at the site of "filling-in" of the pseudoaneurysm. Patchy hypervascularity and irregular contrast accumulation is still present. The **(D)** subselective catheterization of the arterial branch leading to the area of abnormality demonstrates more clearly the site of arteriovenous fistulization (hepatic artery, *solid arrow;* portal vein, *open arrow*). Particles of gelfoam were embolized through the catheter resulting in occlusion of the fistula on the **(E)** postembolism contrast study.

pear to be converging toward the inferior vena cava and the right atrium, the shunt is between the hepatic artery and the hepatic vein.

Pseudoaneurysm with Hematobilia. Sandblom [160] in 1948, coined the term *traumatic hematobilia* for one of the least common forms of hepatic injury in which a central laceration of the liver establishes a communication between the bile ducts and the hepatic artery and/or vein or portal vein. Clinically, the entity is difficult to diagnose because the appearance of bleeding is often delayed for several weeks after surgery. The triad of abdominal pain suggestive of biliary colic, gastrointestinal bleeding, and a history of trauma is characteristic of hematobilia [109]. The onset of the pain is accompanied or followed by bleeding. This condition may develop after primary repairs have been instituted, and, if unrecognized, it has a very high mortality. On angiography, an avascular area is observed into which intrahepatic extravasation of con-

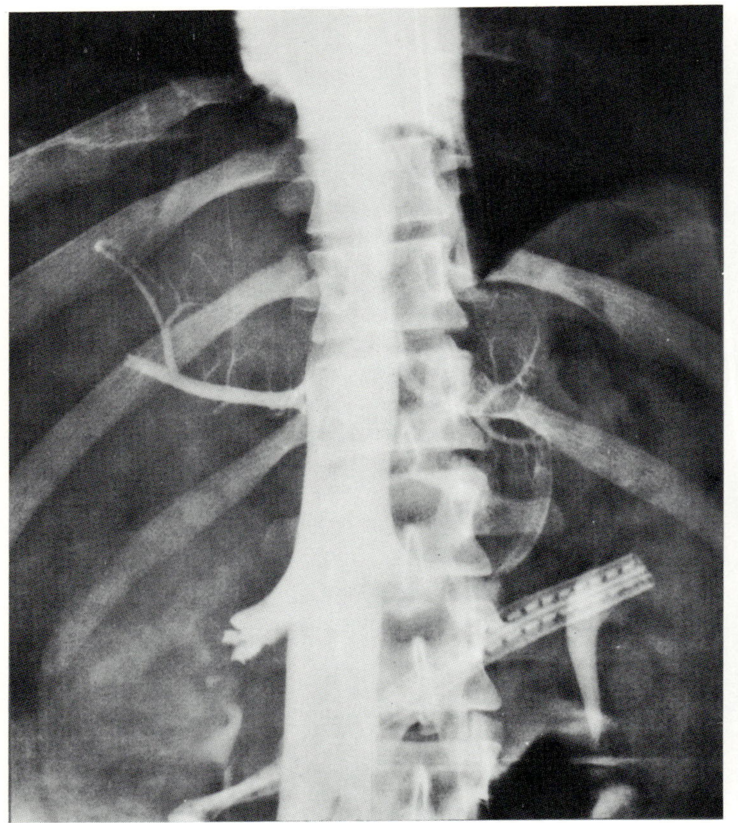

A

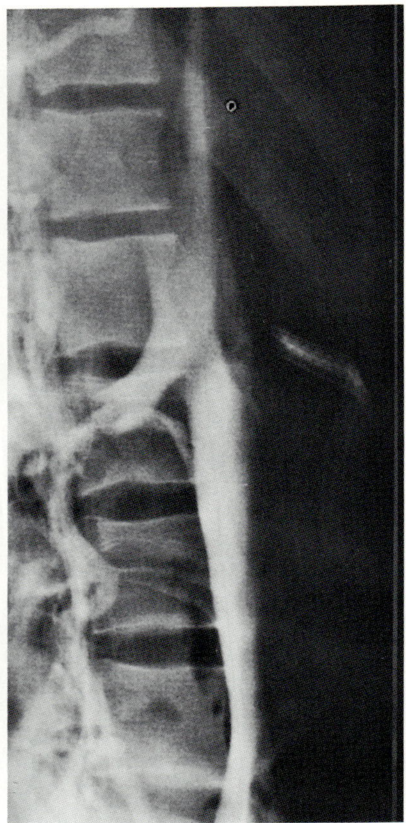

B

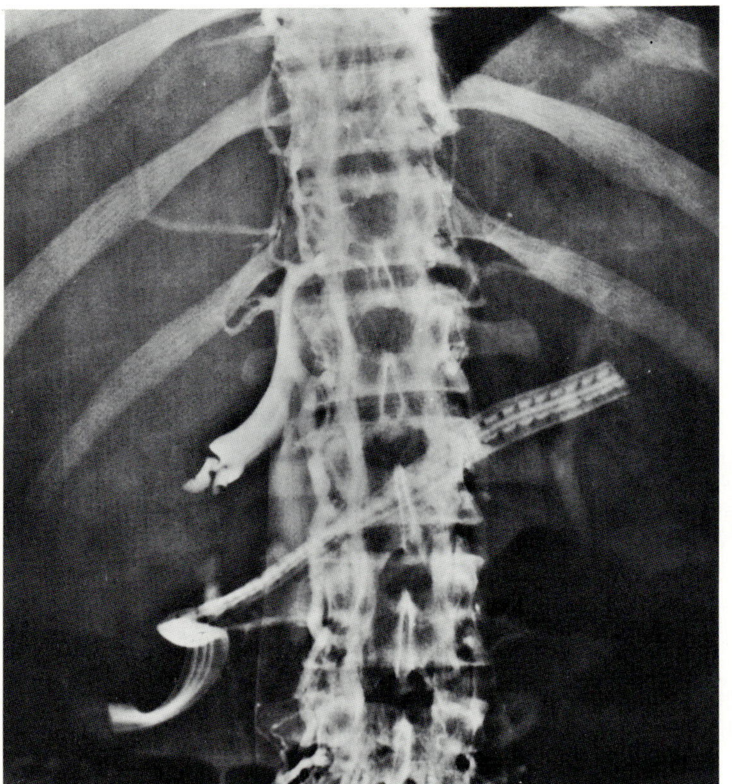

C

FIG. 4.16A–C. This 20-year-old male sustained blunt abdominal injury in an automobile accident resulting in a liver hematoma (see Figure 3.36A). The **(A)** frontal and **(B)** lateral projections from the early phase of his inferior vena cavogram reveal compression of the proximal, intrahepatic portion of the inferior vena cava without definite evidence of intravascular thrombosis. The **(C)** frontal projection from the intermediate phase of this study shows extensive filling of the paraspinal venous channels due to the partial obstruction to blood flow produced by the proximal caval compression.

trast occurs and an arterial-biliary or a venous-biliary fistula is demonstrated. The diagnosis can be confirmed by intraoperative cholangiography, during which the pseudoaneurysm may be opacified.

Posttraumatic Biliary Cyst. Laceration of one of the bile ducts with leakage of bile into the parenchyma of the liver can result in an avascular mass that cannot be differentiated from a hematoma. Angiographically, extravasation is usually absent, although stretching and bowing of vessels around the mass frequently are present. The rim of the mass may show an area of increased contrast density secondary to compression. The cysts will usually not fill during operative cholangiography.

Obstruction of Inferior Vena Cava. Because of the anatomic relationship of the inferior vena cava and the liver, significant enlargement of the liver can result in compression of this major vein. Hemorrhage from the liver around the course of the inferior vena cava can also result in obstruction by compression. It has been suggested, therefore, by some authors [87] that in any case of hepatic trauma, angiography must include evaluation of the inferior vena cava (Fig. 4.16).

Gallbladder

Injury to the gallbladder from penetrating or blunt abdominal trauma is relatively rare. According to Norgore [60], the earliest case reported was in 1388. Bullinger is credited with the first successful operation for this entity in 1898. The significance of recognizing trauma to the gallbladder was noted by Smith and Hastings [60] who, in 1954, reported that every patient operated upon for nonpenetrating rupture of the gallbladder after 1898 survived but that no patient had survived without an operation. Apparently, blood loss following such a perforation plays no major role in the incidence of survival. The most important feature appears to be the toxicity produced by the spillage of bile into the peritoneal cavity.

Extrahepatic Biliary Ducts

Laceration of the extrahepatic bile ducts rarely occurs in abdominal trauma. Laceration usually results from a direct penetration or blow to the upper abdomen with laceration or upward retraction of the liver and hepatoduodenal ligament, tearing the duct away from its fixed duodenal attachment [107]. The tears are either incomplete or complete, and the usual site for such tears is along the superior border of the pancreas. Jaundice, with acholic stools, is a constant late feature in rupture of the bile ducts but is relatively rare in instances of rupture or other significant trauma to the liver [109]. The optimal method of diagnosis of rupture of the gallbladder or extrahepatic bile ducts is through the use of transhepatic, endoscopic, retrograde cholangiography, or cholangiography during an operation.

Plain-film examination will demonstrate evidence of intraperitoneal free fluid secondary to gallbladder rupture and resulting peritonitis. Significant retroperitoneal accumulation of fluid occurs in instances of rupture of the common bile duct. Angiography is not diagnostic; however, it is conceivable that changes in the cystic arteries or variations in the wall of the gallbladder during the intermediate and late phases of an hepatic angiogram may aid in establishing the diagnosis.

INTESTINAL TRACT

General Aspects of Injury

The intestinal tract is the most frequently injured organ system in penetrating injuries to the abdomen from explosive devices, e.g., handguns, shotguns, fragments, missiles. Only the liver is more frequently lacerated by stab wounds. Intestinal-tract injury is third or fourth in order of frequency following blunt trauma. The reason for the intestinal tract's lower vulnerability to blunt trauma as compared to solid organs is that the attachments of bowel are less fixed, giving the intestinal structures considerable mobility [60, 146,182,195,198]. The lack of fixation is even more significant in the young, helping to explain why blunt intestinal injuries are encountered less frequently in this age group in contrast to older individuals. In addition, if the violent force is applied slowly rather than rapidly, the mobility and collapsibility of the intestinal tract allow segments of bowel to move away from the center of applied force, except at points of fixation [60].

The forces acting on a hollow viscus to produce injury are either tensile (that force which tends to pull apart or elongate an object), compressive (that force which tends to push objects together or shorten them), or shearing (that force which makes one part of an object slide over another immediately adjacent part). These forces, acting together or individually, create traumatic lesions by compressing the viscus against bone, bursting a distended loop, tearing the bowel or disrupting its mesentery, or by fracturing regional bony structures which then, in turn, act as tearing or puncturing agents [112]. The injuries that result are either intramural hemorrhage with or without obstruction, intraperitoneal perforation, retroperitoneal perforation, or a combination of intra- and retroperitoneal perforation. In addition, the vascular supply to these structures may be disrupted or thrombosed.

The studies of Williams and Sargeant [198] suggest that the shearing forces generated by compression of two opposing structures (usually the anterior abdominal wall and the lumbar spine or bony pelvis) are the major cause for injury to hollow viscus. In patients with abdominal trauma secondary to a vehicular accident, the steering wheel's impacting on the anterior abdominal wall represents the major source of the above-mentioned force [182]. Harrison and Debas [63] state that impact of the steering wheel is the main reason for injury to hollow viscus proximal to the ligament of Treitz, whereas seat belts are the most frequent cause of injury distal to this ligament.

Both large- and small-bowel blunt injuries can produce minimal initial findings with development of late manifestations such as perforation, obstruction from a hematoma, or leakage of bowel contents into either the intra- or retroperitoneal spaces. Evans reported three cases of traumatic rupture of the ileum as an isolated injury following abdominal trauma [49]. Symptoms and signs in those patients were delayed for between 5 and 12 h after injury. This delay was thought to be due to mucosal plugging of a laceration of the bowel wall. Spasm of circular muscles above and below the site of the injury may also play a part in this delayed clinical manifestation.

The human intestine ruptures at 7–8 lb of pressure per square inch when the pressure is applied to isolated segments. If distension is increased, the pressure necessary to cause rupture can be decreased. When bowel is ruptured, the serosa splits initially, followed by the mucosa, and then by the submucosa. Almost all lacerations of the bowel due to blunt injury are on the antimesenteric border.

Whether the force is secondary to impact of the steering wheel, seat belts, or some other cause, Counseller and McCormick, in a review of 1313 cases of injury to the gastrointestinal tract, found that approximately 80% of these injuries occurred between the duodenal-jejunal junction and the terminal ileum, and that approximately 10% each occurred in the duodenum and large intestine [60].

Historically, Aristotle was aware that rupture of the intestine could occur from nonpenetrating injury to the abdominal wall. Sacherus, in 1720, is credited with the first successful operation for rupture of the intestine; and Rambdohr, in 1730, is given credit for the first successful anastomosis for repair of a complete division of gut. The first reported case of rupture of the intestine in America is credited to Samuel Annan of Baltimore in 1837 [60].

Use of Contrast Agents for Diagnosis of Upper and Lower Gastrointestinal-Tract Traumatic Lesions

The question of whether to use water-soluble contrast or barium for evaluation of the gastrointestinal tract in patients with abdominal trauma is still undecided. In fact, the use of either contrast agent in this situation is open to controversy. Both advantages and disadvantages exist in using soluble contrast and barium. Personal experience and training generally dictate the decision. The authors believe that it is best to use water-soluble contrast media in all cases where perforation of bowel is suspected and to limit the use of barium to those situations where the possibility of perforation is not felt to exist.

Stomach

Although the stomach is often injured by penetrating forces, it is a thick-walled, mobile, collapsible organ and, therefore, rarely perforated by blunt abdominal trauma [182]. Contusion of the muscularis with formation of hematoma is more frequently encountered. Rupture of the stomach, although rare in adults, is frequently encountered in children [109]. When lacerations do occur, they are usually due to a high-velocity blow delivered to a localized area in the upper abdomen overlying a distended stomach [107]. The most frequent source for such a force is the impact of the steering wheel on the anterior abdominal wall. The frequency of gastric rupture from blunt trauma is less than 2%. The incidence in several series and a summary of typical cases are described in Tables 4.19 and 4.20.

TABLE 4.19. Incidence of gastrointestinal injury and stomach rupture in blunt abdominal trauma

	No. of cases		
Author	Blunt abdominal trauma	GI-tract injury	Stomach rupture
Allen	297	32 (14%)	3 (1.3%)
Fitzgerald	200	30 (15%)	2 (1.0%)
Rodkey	177	29 (16%)	3 (1.7%)
Morton	120	13 (11%)	2 (1.7%)
Clarke	107	19 (18%)	1 (0.9%)

Source: Yajko RD, Seydel F, Trimble C (1975) Rupture of the stomach from blunt abdominal trauma. J Trauma 15(3): 177–183

TABLE 4.20. Summary of cases of rupture of the stomach in closed abdominal trauma reported in the English-language literature, 1930–1973

Author	Date	Age	Sex	Operation	Result	Shock	Associated injury	Site and nature of stomach tear	Comments
Buchanan	1930	34	M	Yes	Survived	Yes	None	Greater curvature, 1 cm	Hit by piece of timber after a hearty lunch
Seeger	1930	3	M	Yes	Died	Not given	None	Fundus near cardia, "large"	Patient with encephalitis, seizures, vomiting, artificial respiration
Fancher	1932	31	M	Yes	Died	Yes	Extremities, ribs, hemothorax	Post. from cardia, 5 cm	Hit by automobile after large meal
Fancher	1932	29	M	Yes	Survived	Yes	None	Ant. pylorus, 2.5 cm	Thrown against steering wheel after drinking 2½ quarts malted milk
Wolf	1936	42	M	Yes	Survived	Not given	None	Ant. lesser curvature, near pylorus, 5 cm	Hit by mail sack
Casberg	1940	3	M	Yes	Survived	Yes	Spleen; gastric contusion	Greater curvature, 1 cm	Hit by automobile while in toy wagon
Erb	1940	37	F	No	Survived	Not given	None known	Posterior wall	Assaulted with kicks and blows to abdomen. Complicated by abscess and gastric fistula which closed spontaneously
Poer	1942	—	—	—	All died	—	Not given	Not given	Four cases, not described in detail, all fatal
de Villiers	1953	40	M	Yes	Died	Yes	None	Lesser curvature, 4 cm	Fell 12 ft after large meal, died in shock
Clarke	1954	31	M	Yes	Survived	Not given	Concussion; humerus, ribs, spleen	Ant. wall, 10 cm	Complicated by postoperative subphrenic abscess
Swartzbach	1954	5	M	Yes	Survived	Yes	Spleen, diaphragm, pneumothorax	Fundus, 10 cm	Run over by automobile
Pontius	1956	—	—	—	Survived	—	Not given	Not given	Not reported in detail, survived
Allen	1957	—	—	—	—	—	—	—	Three cases, not described
Franken	1957	11	M	Yes	Survived	No	None	Lesser curvature, across pylorus	Fell 6 ft, landing on feet after large meal. Three laparotomies; closure of gastric tear with omental patch; complicated by infection and fistula; finally had ant. gastrojejunostomy

(Continued)

TABLE 4.20. *(Continued)*

Author	Date	Age	Sex	Operation	Result	Shock	Associated injury	Site and nature of stomach tear	Comments
Morton	1957	—	—	—	—	—	—	—	Two cases, not described
Fitzgerald	1960	—	—	—	Both died	—	—	—	Two cases, both fatal, not described in detail
Mathieson	1962	—	M	Yes	Survived	—	Ruptured testis	Over pyloric antrum, 2.5 cm	Motorcycle accident
Demos	1964	67	M	Yes	Survived	Yes	None	Lesser curvature ant.	External cardiac compression and mouth-to-mouth resuscitation
Greig	1964	4	F	Yes	Died	Yes	None	Ant. pyloric area of body; 5 × 2.5 cm	Hit by car after evening meal
Greig	1964	34	M	Yes	Survived	Yes	None	Greater curvature ant., near fundus, 6 × 2.5 cm	Knocked off bicycle after drinking large quantity of beer
Greig	1964	47	M	Yes	Died	Yes	Liver, ribs, clavicle, scalp, flail chest, and pneumothorax	Ant. wall of body 7.5 cm	Thrown against steering wheel after eating lunch of bread, tongue, onions, cucumber, and beer. Died of "fat embolism"
Salberberg	1964	—	—	—	Died	—	—	—	Postmortem finding of stomach rupture following external cardiac compression
Valtonen	1964	85	F	Yes	Died	No	None	Lesser curvature, ant. below gastroesophageal junction, complete, 7 cm	Mouth-to-mouth resuscitation and sternal compression. Died of pulmonary embolism
Rodkey	1966	39	—	Yes	Died	Yes	Anoxic brain damage, respiratory failure, spleen, diaphragm, femur, tibia	Not given	Automobile accident
Rodkey	1966	—	—	—	Both survived	—	Not given	Not given	Two cases, not described in detail
Reynolds	1971	—	—	—	Both survived	—	Not given	Not given	Two cases, falls from heights, not described in detail
Yajko et al.	1971	45	M	Yes	Died	Yes	Ribs, abrasions, spleen	Lesser curvature, ant., 12–14 cm	Fell on abdomen after large meal in jump from train
Yajko et al.	1972	8	F	Yes	Survived	No	None	Anterior 12 cm	Auto—pedestrian

Source: Yajko RD, Seydel F, Trimble C (1975) Rupture of stomach from blunt abdominal trauma. J Trauma 15(3): 177–183

Radiologic Diagnosis

Plain films are generally of little help in diagnosing a gastric-wall contusion. If positive findings are present, they usually consist of significant prominence of the gastric folds or a localized bulge, representing the site of a hematoma, projecting into the gas-filled lumen of the stomach. Contrast studies aid in confirming the presence of prominent rugal folds or of a mural lesion. Laceration of the stomach will result in the presence of free intraperitoneal air in 80% of cases, and this air will usually be massive (Fig. 4.17). In addition, particularly if the stomach is distended by food and fluid, the plain films will show the radiologic evidence of free intraperitoneal fluid (Fig. 4.18). With perforation of the posterior wall of the stomach, changes suggesting loculation of air and/or fluid in the lesser peritoneal sac may be present. Studies with water-soluble contrast media will demonstrate the site of laceration by extravasation of contrast material. If angiography were to be performed on such a patient, it is speculated that localized or diffuse thickening of the wall of the stomach would be demonstrated in those patients who have sustained simple contusions, and extravasation of contrast or amputation of vessels would be observed in those patients with frank lacerations. Such studies, as far as the authors can determine, have not been performed.

Duodenum

A series of 131 duodenal wounds was reported by Morton in 1968. Eighty-nine percent of the injuries were the result of penetrating trauma. The causes and anatomic locations of the injuries are presented in Tables 4.21–4.23 and Figs. 4.19–4.21 [63]. Woolley et al. [205] reported eight patients with duodenal hematomas, four of these patients were the victims of child

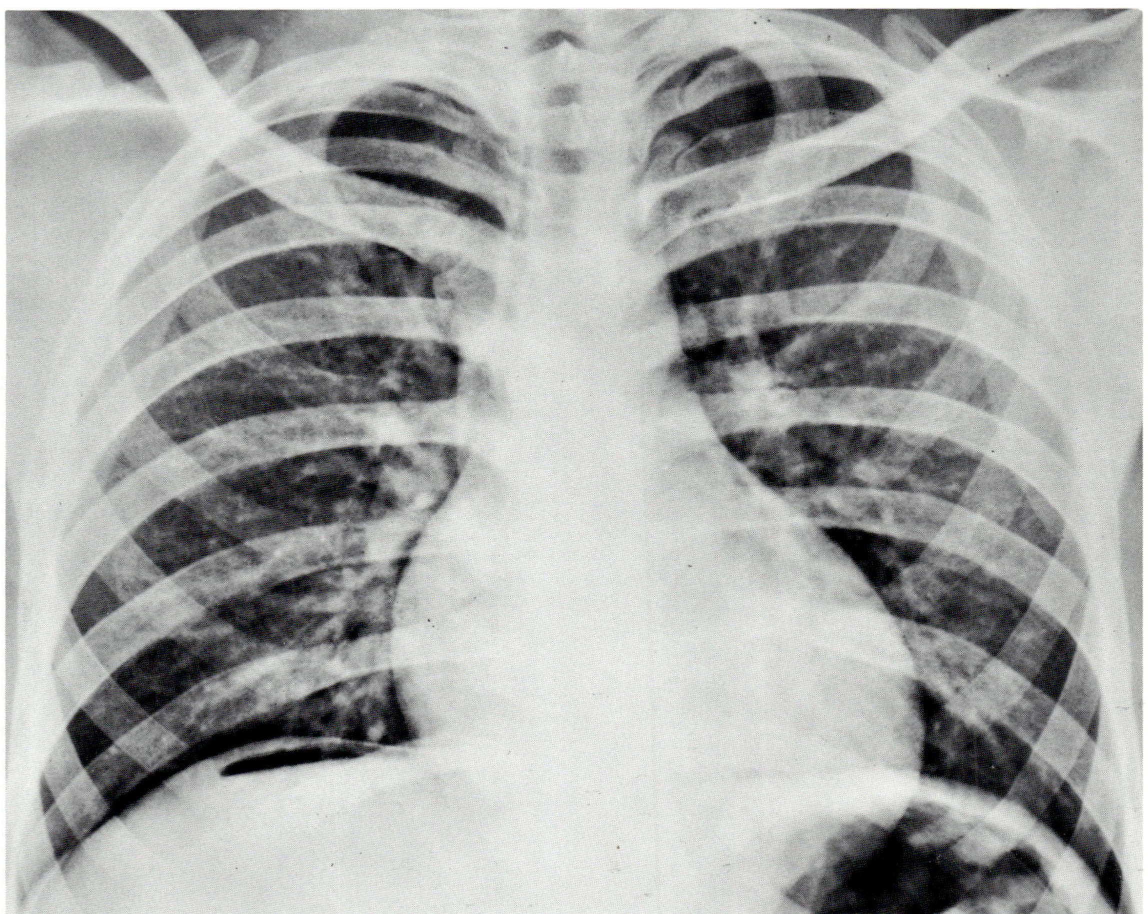

FIG. 4.17. The erect chest examination of this 23-year-old male victim of blunt abdominal trauma reveals free intraperitoneal air consistent with hollow-viscus laceration. At exploration, a gastric laceration was found and repaired.

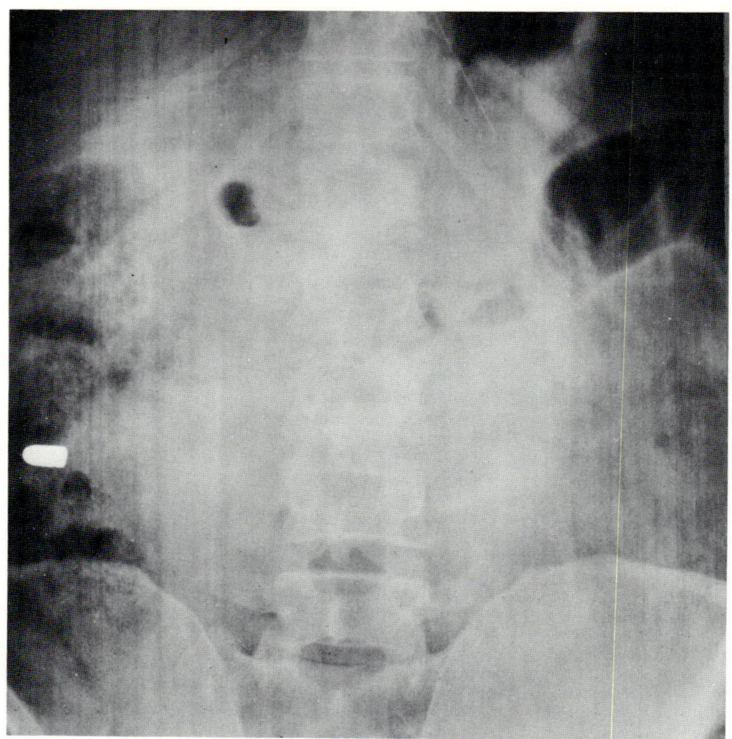

A

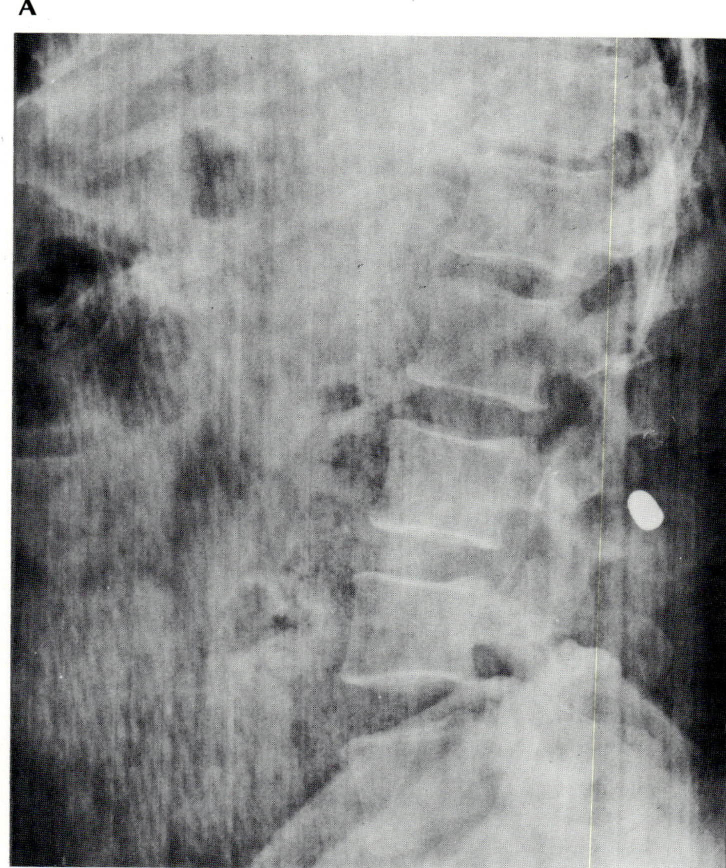

B

FIG. 4.18A and B. This male patient was admitted following an abdominal gunshot wound. At surgical exploration, lacerations of the stomach, jejunum, and colon were found and repaired. The **(A)** AP supine view of the abdomen reveals the bullet in the RLQ but does not show any evidence of free intraperitoneal air. Free intraperitoneal fluid is present. The **(B)** lateral projection places the bullet in the soft tissues of the right lower back.

TABLE 4.21. Mechanisms of injury in 131 patients with duodenal wounds

Mechanism	No. of patients		%	
Penetrating	117		89	
Knife		22		17
Bullet		87		66
Shotgun		8		6
Blunt	14		11	
Total	131		100	

Source: Morton JR, Jordan GL (1968) Traumatic duodenal injuries: Review of 131 cases. J Trauma 8(2): 127–137

TABLE 4.23. Causes of death in 28 patients with duodenal injury

Cause of death	No. of patients
Hemorrhage and shock	14
Posttraumatic renal insufficiency	5
Intraabdominal infection	4
Duodenal fistula[a]	2
Stress ulcer with subsequent uremia	1
Massive chest injury	1
Unexplained cause	1

[a] Both cases represent duodenal perforations that were missed at the time of surgery.

Source: Morton JR, Jordan GL (1968) Traumatic duodenal injuries: Review of 131 cases. J Trauma 8(2): 127–137

TABLE 4.22. Mortality rates according to mechanisms of injury in duodenal wounds

Type of injury	No. of patients		Mortality No.		Mortality %
Penetrating	117		26		22
Knife		22		0	0
Bullet		87		20	23
Shotgun		8		6	75
Blunt trauma	14		2		14
Total	131		28		21

Source: Morton JR, Jordan GL (1968) Traumatic duodenal injuries: Review of 131 cases. J Trauma 8(2): 127–137

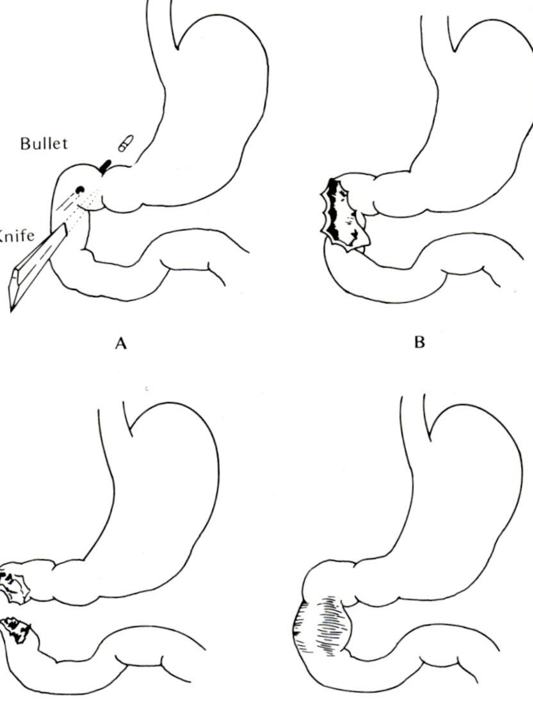

FIG. 4.19A–D. An illustration of some of the duodenal wounds resulting from penetrating and blunt trauma. **(A)** Simple lacerations, **(B)** severe lacerations, **(C)** complete transections, **(D)** contusions. From Morton JR, Jordan GL Jr (1968) Traumatic duodenal injuries. J Trauma 8(2): 127–137

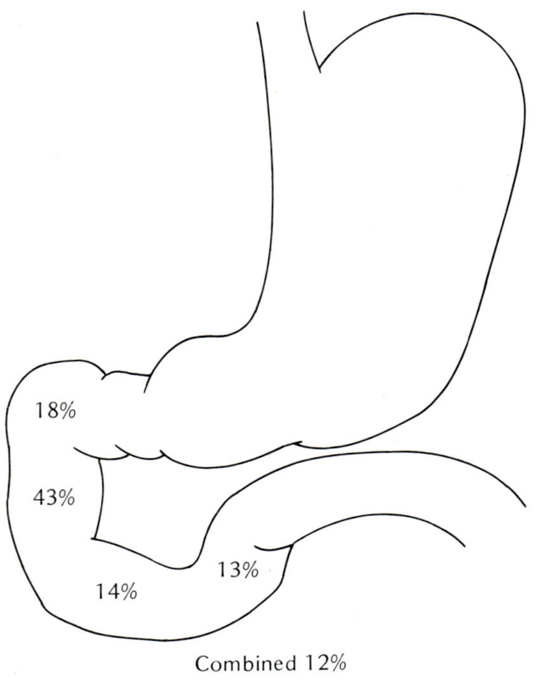

FIG. 4.20. The incidence of wounds encountered in the four portions of the duodenum. Including those wounds involving more than one portion, the second portion was involved in almost 50% of 131 patients. From Morton JR, Jordan GL Jr (1968) Traumatic duodenal injuries. J Trauma 8(2): 127–137

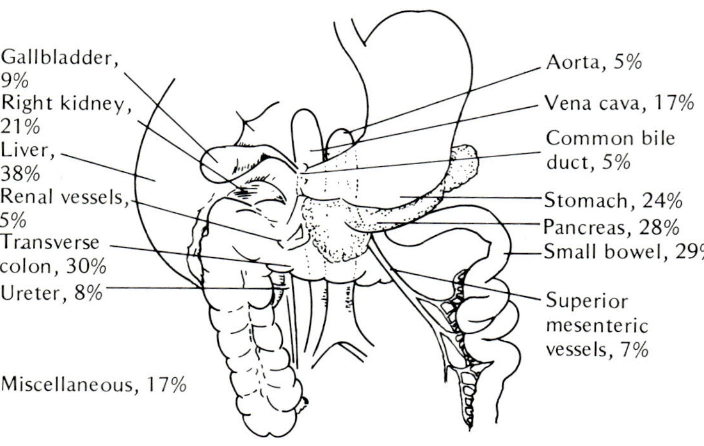

FIG. 4.21. An illustration demonstrating injuries to nearby organs and vessels. Note the high incidence of hepatic, pancreatic, and vascular injury. From Morton JR, Jordan GL Jr (1968) Traumatic duodenal injuries. J Trauma 8(2): 127–137

TABLE 4.24. Demographic data on eight patients with duodenal hematoma

Case	Sex/Age (yr)	Race	Family structure	Type of trauma
1	M/1.9	Caucasian	Parents married, living together, patient adopted at 5 days of age	Battered by parent
2[a]	M/2.5	Black	Parents divorced, mother has custody	Battered by parent
3[a]	M/1.7	Spanish American	Parents married, living together	Fell against tricycle handlebar
4	M/1.9	Spanish American	Natural father in Mexico, patient lives with mother and stepfather	Fell from rocking horse (suspected battering but not proved)
5	M/5	Spanish American	Parents married, living together	Fell from tree on doghouse
6	F/2.6	Spanish American	Mother married, but not to patient's father	Battered by mother's boyfriend
7[a]	M/4	Caucasian	Parents divorced, mother living with boyfriend	Battered by mother's boyfriend
8	M/5.3	Caucasian	Parents married, living together	Fell on bicycle handlebars

[a] Associated with bowel perforation.

Source: Woolley MM, Mahour GH, Sloan T (1978) Duodenal hematoma in infancy and childhood: Changing etiology and changing treatment. Am J Surg 136: 8–14

TABLE 4.25. Historical and physical findings on eight patients with duodenal hematoma

Case	Symptoms	Interval between trauma and symptoms	Interval between trauma and admission	Physical findings
1	Vomiting	3 days	5 days	Dehydration, multiple bruises, abdominal tenderness, fear, irritability
2[a]	Anorexia, abdominal pain, vomiting	?	2 days (?)	Dehydration, apathetic, generalized abdominal tenderness
3[a]	Vomiting, abdominal pain	1–2 h	32 h	Lethargic, shock (blood pressure 70/50), abdomen silent and diffusely tender
4	Vomiting	2.5 days	5.5 days	Lethargic, dehydrated, bruised on abdomen, right-upper-quadrant tenderness
5	Vomiting	12 h	2 days	Generalized abdominal tenderness
6	Vomiting, hematemesis	36 h	2.5 days	Pale, withdrawn, abdominal tenderness, many bruises
7[a]	Abdominal pain, vomiting	3–4	15 h	Diffuse abdominal tenderness, distension, bruises, febrile, acutely ill
8	Vomiting, abdominal pain	9 h	24 h	Epigastric tenderness

[a] Associated with bowel perforation.

Source: Woolley MM, Mahour GH, Sloan T (1978) Duodenal hematoma in infancy and childhood: Changing etiology and changing treatment. Am J Surg 136: 8–14

abuse. They emphasized the changing etiology of this condition in children (Tables 4.24, 4.25). Approximately two-thirds of duodenal injuries from adult blunt trauma are secondary to vehicular accidents and, of this group, two-thirds of the injuries are due to the impact of the steering wheel on the anterior abdominal wall [107]. The fixed position of the duodenum directly over the spine establishes this portion of the intestinal tract to be most susceptible to injury [107].

Blunt trauma to the duodenum has had considerable attention in the literature. Diagnosis may be difficult. Most patients have been involved in high-speed auto collisions, and many of the patients are under the influence of alcohol. Lucas and Ledgerwood reported 36 patients from the Detroit General Hospital [98]. Of these, 28 had complete perforation of the duodenal wall and 8 had contusions, hematomas, or tears of the seromuscular surface. The patients with tears had transverse, full-thickness disruption of the antimesenteric border. In 19 patients, there was associated pancreatic injury; 22 of the 36 had no intraperitoneal injury. The delay in management of these patients was considerable because of failure to make the diagnosis early. Treatment was delayed more than 12 h in 19 patients and more than 24 h in 10 of the 19. Talbot and Shuck reported eight cases of retroperitoneal duodenal injury [177]; seven of the eight had trauma due to the steering wheel of an automobile and three of these died. They emphasized the unreliability of early physical findings and the need for frequent, ongoing physical examination of these patients (Table 4.26, Fig. 4.22). Three of their eight patients had serum amylase elevations. The authors stated that there must be careful search for duodenal injury at the time of laparotomy, since duodenal injury is overlooked in 10% to 20% of cases with a resultant morbidity of 77%.

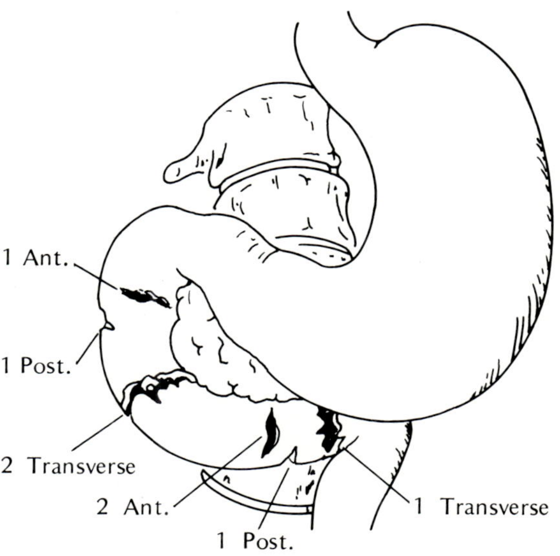

FIG. 4.22. The location of retroperitoneal duodenal injury due to blunt abdominal trauma. From Talbot WA, Shuck JM (1975) Retroperitoneal duodenal injury due to blunt abdominal trauma. Am J Surg 130: 654–666

TABLE 4.26. Diagnostic maneuvers in blunt duodenal trauma

Case	Age (yr) and sex	Physical examination	X-ray films	Peritoneal aspirate	Serum amylase	Time before exploration
I	17, M	Late abdominal rigidity	Normal	Negative	Normal	24 h
II	21, M	Late abdominal rigidity	Normal		Normal	30 h
III	37, M	Equivocal	Retroperitoneal air		Elevated	7 h
IV	39, M	Equivocal	Normal	Negative	Normal (urine	72 h
V	39, F	Equivocal, later tender abdomen	Retroperitoneal air; Gastrografin showed leak	Negative	Elevated	48 h
VI	46, M	Shock, abdominal distension				Immediate exploration
VII	18, M	Tender abdomen	Postoperatively, Gastrografin showed leak		Elevated	Immediate exploration; reoperation 3 days later
VIII	44, M	Equivocal	Normal	Positive blood		12 h

Source: Talbot WA, Shuck JM (1975) Retroperitoneal duodenal injury due to blunt trauma. Am J Surg 130: 654–666

Intramural Hematoma

Traumatic intramural hematomas of the bowel are usually observed in children, with boys showing a marked preponderance [122,203]. Such injuries have their highest incidence in the duodenum and ileocecal areas [203] and may represent the most common lesion secondary to trauma in the upper segments of the small bowel [108]. The blood loss produced by such lesions is usually negligible. However, a strategically located hematoma may obstruct the duodenum and even the common bile duct, resulting in jaundice [108].

RADIOLOGIC DIAGNOSIS

Plain-film examinations are usually nonspecific. Obstructive or nonobstructive distension of the duodenum and stomach proximal to the lesion may be present, and the right psoas margin may be obliterated either because of associated scoliosis or because of retroperitoneal hemorrhage associated with a duodenal-wall lesion. Occasionally, a soft-tissue mass representing the intramural hemorrhage may be demonstrated [203] (Fig. 4.23).

Contrast studies with water-soluble agents or barium usually demonstrate a short segment of duodenal involvement approximately 10–20 cm in length. Proximal to this lesion, thickening and coarsening of the mucosal folds may be noted. A mass, apparently widening the lumen of the duodenum, may be observed. The widening is really from the serosal-to-serosal surface of the duodenum, while the mucosal-to-mucosal diameter of the lumen is actually narrowed. Evidence of incomplete obstruction of the duodenum, proximal to the mass, is usually apparent. The valvulae conniventes at the level of the soft-tissue mass are crowded together, producing a coiled-spring appearance. These findings usually subside within 1 week and disappear within 1 month [25,50,104,107–110,122,203].

Felson and Levin [50] and Wiot [203] feel that the combination of mass, coarsening, and coiled-spring appearance of the mucosal folds of the duodenum is pathognomonic for an intramural duodenal hematoma. However, a prolapsing gastric mass, e.g., a gastric polyp with a long stalk, can produce intussusception in the duodenal sweep mimicking an intramural hematoma.

Retroperitoneal Perforation

Retroperitoneal perforation of the duodenum represents approximately 10% of all traumatic intestinal perforations [59,122,127,170,183]. The most common injury is a 30% to 70% transverse, full-thickness disruption along the antimesenteric border of the second and third portion of the duodenal sweep [92,98,182]; 50% of these retroperitoneal ruptures are associated with significant trauma to the head of the pancreas [127].

According to Griswald and Collier [60], gastrointestinal perforations are overlooked at operations because of superficial observation, inadequate exposure, and lack of persistence on the part of the surgeon. The percentage of missed retroperitoneal duodenal perforations has been reported to be as high as 33% to 50%. These statistics are significant when it is realized that retroperitoneal duodenal perforations have a mortality rate of from 75% to 90% when inadequately treated [127,183].

While Sperling and Rigler, as far back as 1937, are believed to have reported the first case diagnosed radiographically [60], a continued delay in diagnosis persists because of the lack of appreciation of significant but subtle abdominal findings on physical examination and erroneous radiologic interpretation. Lucas and Ledgerwood [98], in reviewing patients with blunt abdominal trauma from 1960 to 1975, found that 90% of the group had nonspecific signs of retroperitoneal injury within 12 h. These nonspecific signs included scoliosis and obliteration of the right psoas. However, more than 50% of these patients had diagnostic radiologic findings of retroperitoneal air.

RADIOLOGIC DIAGNOSIS

As noted previously, nonspecific radiologic signs are scoliosis, with convexity to left and obliteration of the right psoas muscle. Specific findings include the demonstration of retroperitoneal air and evidence of retroperitoneal bleeding.

Gas (air) or fluid extravasated into the retroperitoneal area can: (a) dissect around the right kidney and then upward toward the diaphragm into the posterior mediastinum or downward along the psoas muscle or both, (b) dissect into the transverse mesocolon and into the base of the mesentery of the small bowel, and (c) dissect into the peritoneal cavity. Dissection of air along these pathways accounts for the primary radiologic features consistent with duodenal perforation. Bubbles, streaks, or pockets of air may outline the right kidney or even both kidneys. Air may be visualized along the border of one or both psoas muscles and may dissect upward under the diaphragm or may gravitate into the pelvis. Mediastinal and/or cervical emphysema may result. Emphysema in the right flank may follow lateral dissection. Free intraperitoneal air may also be demonstrated. These same pathways may be outlined by contrast studies with water-soluble media that will delineate spillage into the retroperitoneal area and the other structural pathways just described (Fig. 4.24).

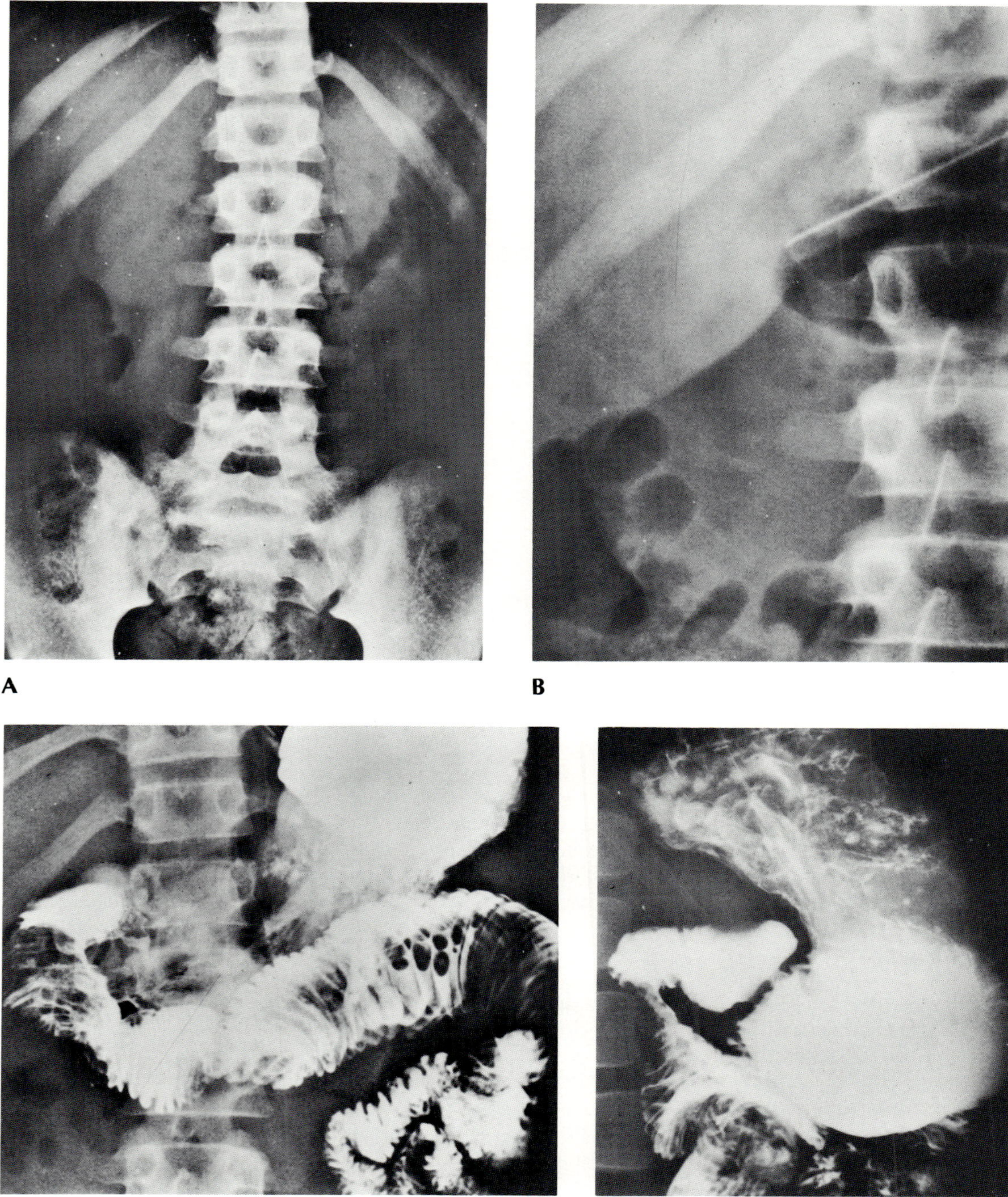

FIG. 4.23A–D. This $10\frac{1}{2}$-year-old female, without a definite history of trauma, was admitted to the hospital with a 2-day history of abdominal pain and fever. After a clinical diagnosis of acute appendicitis was made, the patient went to surgery and a normal appendix was delivered. Postoperatively, the patient drained excessive amounts (1000 cc in a few hours) of bile-stained gastric juice through an indwelling nasogastric tube. A review of her **(A)** admission abdominal examination reveals levoscoliosis of the lumbar spine with a soft-tissue mass to the right of L1–3. A **(B)** close-up view of the RUQ confirms the presence of this mass. **(C)** AP and **(D)** oblique views from a subsequent upper GI series demonstrates an intramural duodenal hematoma.

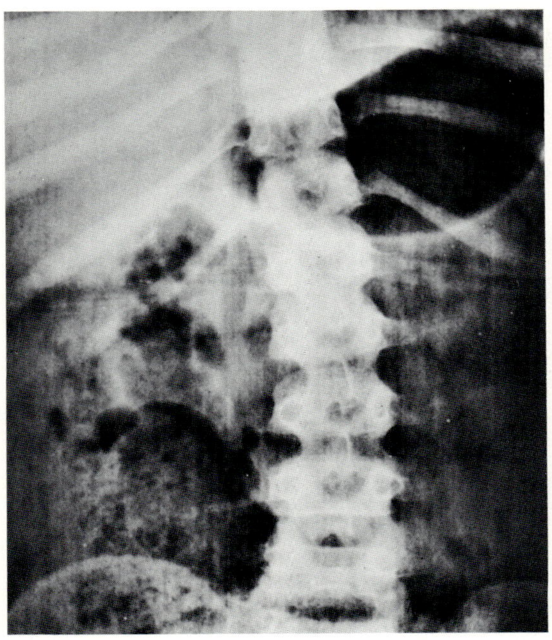

A

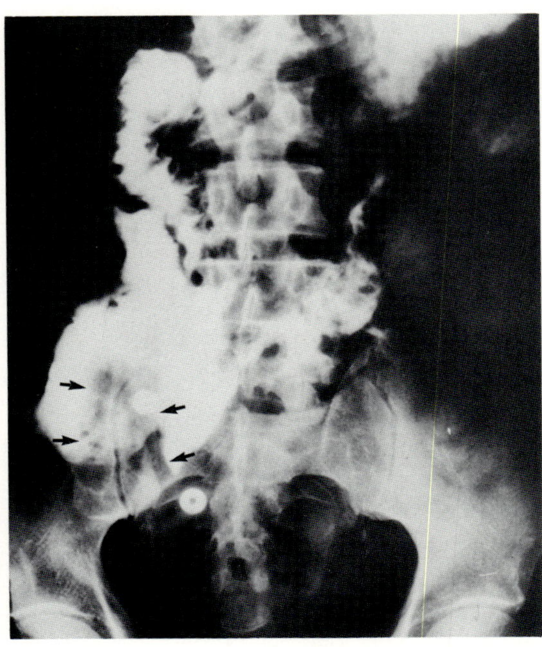

B

FIG. 4.24A and B. This male patient was admitted to the hospital with blunt abdominal injury following an automobile accident. The **(A)** AP supine view of the abdomen reveals a mottled collection of radiolucency to the right of the lumbar spine that is consistent with retroperitoneal air. An **(B)** AP view from the upper GI series of a patient with a similar injury reveals extravasation of water-soluble contrast into the anterior pararenal space to outline the ascending colon *(short arrows).*

Intraperitoneal Perforation

This injury is the least common of the duodenal traumatic lesions. Plain-film examination may demonstrate the presence of free intraperitoneal air and/or fluid. Contrast studies with water-soluble media will often show spillage of contrast into the peritoneal cavity.

Small Bowel

Injury to the small intestine (full thickness) by penetrating or blunt trauma should produce the classic clinical picture of peritonitis. Contamination of the peritoneal cavity by intestinal injury represents the prototype for visceral trauma and should result in physical findings typified by rigidity, generalized or localized guarding, tenderness, rebound tenderness, and absent bowel sounds. The physical findings in penetrating trauma with significant injury to intraabdominal organs compared with penetrating injury without injury to organs are documented in the section on physical diagnoses (p. 45). Cerise and Scully reported the clinical features in a series of 20 patients with blunt trauma to the bowel [30] (Tables 4.27–4.29].

DiVincenti et al. [40], in a series of 518 patients with blunt abdominal trauma, described 60 patients with injury to hollow viscera. The predominant areas of involvement were jejunum, ileum, colon, and rectum (Table 4.30).

The subject of blunt injuries to the small intestine in children was reviewed by Kakos et al. [75]. They reported 2 deaths in a series of 26 patients. Of the injured patients, 35% had complications requiring prolonged hospitalization. There were 17 perforations, 8 duodenal hematomas, and 1 mesenteric avulsion. Kakos et al. [75] noted that delay in diagnosis was a critical problem. Obtaining an accurate history was difficult, and only after the severity of the injury was fully appreciated could an accurate story of injury be elicited. The upper gastrointestinal series was diagnostic in 8 patients with duodenal hematomas. Plain films of the abdomen were helpful in only 40% of patients with perforations. Serum amylase elevations were noted in 11 of 26 patients, and in only 2 of these patients was pancreatitis present.

Two primary small-bowel lesions are associated with blunt abdominal trauma: intramural hematoma and perforation [109]. In both, the jejunum is most frequently involved [71,182]. The plain films (see Fig. 4.23) and studies with contrast media show findings that are similar to those for duodenal hematoma.

TABLE 4.27. Blunt trauma to the small intestine: Site of rupture of the small bowel

	No.	Totals
Duodenum		
Part 1	2	
Part 2	3	
Junction of parts 2 and 3	1	
Part 3	2	
Junction of parts 3 and 4	1	
Part 4	3	
		12
Jejunum		
Within 10 cm of ligament of Treitz	4	
Other	2	
		6
Ileum	2	2
Total		20

Source: Cerise EJ, Scully JH (1970) Blunt trauma to the small intestine. J Trauma 10(1): 46–50

TABLE 4.28. Blunt trauma to the small intestine: Associated injuries

Injury	No.
Abdominal	
Laceration of spleen	4
Laceration of liver	2
Trauma of pancreas	2
Laceration of mesenteric vein	1
Perforation of sigmoid	1
Rupture of rectus muscle	1
Total	11
Extraabdominal	
Fracture of ribs	4
Hemothorax	3
Laceration of face	3
Fracture of face	2
Fracture of humerus	1
Fracture of tibia	1
Total	14

Source: Cerise EJ, Scully JH (1970) Blunt trauma to the small intestine. J Trauma 10(1): 46–50

TABLE 4.29. Blunt trauma to the small intestine: Clinical findings

	No.
Abdominal pain and tenderness	20
Guarding	19
Decreased or absent bowel sounds	13
Hematemesis	8
Free air under diaphragm	4
Abdominal paracentesis	
Positive	4
Negative	1

Source: Cerise EJ, Scully JH (1970) Blunt trauma to the small intestine. J Trauma 10(1): 46–50

TABLE 4.30. Ruptured hollow viscera due to blunt trauma seen in 52 patients

	No. of cases	Deaths
Stomach	6	3
Duodenum	6	0
Jejunum	22	3
Ileum	10	1
Colon and rectum	12	4
Gallbladder	3	1
Common bile duct	1	1

Source: DiVincenti FC, Rives JD, LaBorde EJ, Fleming ID, Cohn I Jr (1968) Blunt abdominal trauma. J Trauma 8: 1004–1013

Intraperitoneal Perforation

The hallmark of intraperitoneal perforation on plain films is the demonstration of free air. Unfortunately, in less than 50% of patients with small-bowel perforation will free air be demonstrated [92,182]. The reasons for this have been mentioned previously. Contrast studies with water-soluble agents may demonstrate the site of perforation via extravasation into the peritoneal cavity. The importance of making the diagnoses must be stressed. Intestinal injuries, excluding those to the retroperitoneal duodenum, should have a favorable prognosis of greater than 90% if appropriate treatment is instituted promptly.

Angiography is usually not indicated in the diagnoses of perforation of bowel. If an angiogram is performed, the findings to be anticipated include arterial distortion or spasm, slowing of the arterial flow localized to the region of trauma, and arterial occlusion and extravasation [135].

Colon and Rectum

Colonic injuries have received increasing attention recently owing to their frequency and the controversy over the appropriate techniques for surgical management (Tables 4.31–4.34 and Figs. 4.25,4.26). The diagnosis of colonic rupture and secondary peritonitis can be made by clinical and radiologic examinations in most instances. However, infraperitoneal and retroperitoneal rectal and colonic injuries tend to be subtle and may be difficult to diagnose.

TABLE 4.31. Incidence of colon injuries

	1927–1942	1943–1958	1959–1974
Age (yr)	30	31	27
Sex (M:F)	5:1	4:1	8:1
Race (B:W)	3:1	2:1	5:1

Source: LoCicero J, Tajima T, Drapanas T (1975) A half century of experience in the management of colon injuries: Changing concepts. J Trauma 15(7): 575–579

TABLE 4.33. Colon injury: Associated injuries

	1927–1942 No. pts. (%)	1943–1958 No. pts. (%)	1959–1974 No. pts. (%)
Colon only	79 (40%)	51 (28%)	100 (25%)
Colon with associated injuries	118 (60%)	132 (72%)	293 (75%)
Totals	197	183	393

Source: LoCicero J, Tajima T, Drapanas T (1975) A half century of experience in the management of colon injuries: Changing concepts. J Trauma 15(7): 575–579

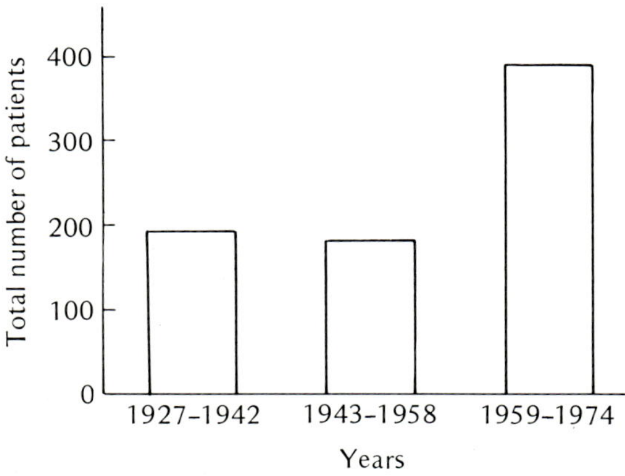

FIG. 4.25. Colon injuries, Charity Hospital, 1927–1974. From LoCicero J, Tajima T, Drapanas T (1975) A half-century of experience in the management of colon injuries: Changing concepts. J Trauma 15(7): 575–579

Schrock and Christiansen [163] reviewed 147 patients with perforating injuries to the colon admitted to the San Francisco General Hospital between 1960 and 1970. Eighty-five percent of the patients were between the age of 11 and 50 years. There were 84 gunshot wounds, 43 stab wounds, 10 shotgun wounds, 4 with blunt trauma, 3 rectal foreign bodies, 2 enema perforations, and 1 proctoscopic injury. The distribu-

TABLE 4.32. Site of colon injury

	1927–1942	1943–1958	1959–1974	Totals
Cecum and colon	47	38	68	153
Transverse colon	54	68	161	283
Left colon and sigmoid	58	66	112	236
Rectum	17	11	47	75
Undetermined	21	0	5	26
Totals	197	183	393	773

Source: LoCicero J, Tajima T, Drapanas T (1975) A half century of experience in the management of colon injuries: Changing concepts. J Trauma 15(7): 575–579

TABLE 4.34. Colon injury: Mortality

	1927–1942 No. pts. (%)	1943–1958 No. pts. (%)	1959–1974 No. pts. (%)
Primary repair alone	0	3 (1.6%)	4 (1%)
Repair and proximal colostomy	0	18 (10%)	12 (3%)
Exteriorization	133 (67.5%)	3 (1.6%)	20 (5.1%)
Totals	133 (67.5%)	24 (13.1%)	36 (9.2%)

Source: LoCicero J, Tajima T, Drapanas T (1975) A half century of experience in the management of colon injuries: Changing concepts. J Trauma 15(7): 575–579.

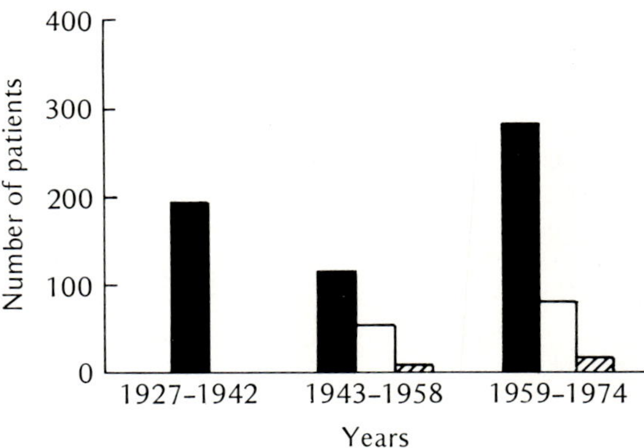

FIG. 4.26. Colon injuries: Mechanism of injury. *Solid bars,* gunshot; *clear bars,* stab; *striped bars,* blunt. From LoCicero J, Tajima T, Drapanas T (1975) A half-century of experience in the management of colon injuries: Changing concepts. J Trauma 15(7): 575–579

tion of the injuries was 49 right colon, 44 transverse colon, 53 left colon, and 13 cases involving the extraperitoneal rectum and anus. Schrock and Christiansen's experience related the prognosis to the number and extent of associated injuries, the presence of shock, and the degree of fecal contamination. They described the morbidity associated with anorectal injuries as "awesome." Complications were severe and hospitalization was often prolonged. The early and accurate diagnosis of anorectal injuries must be emphasized in view of the urgent need for therapeutic intervention.

Injuries to the colon following blunt abdominal trauma occur less frequently than injuries to the small bowel. It is estimated by McKenzie et al. [112] that traumatic lesions of the colon account for only 3% to 5% of individuals experiencing blunt abdominal trauma. The distribution and type of blunt injury to the colon is presented by Howell et al. in a review of 25 cases [69] (Table 4.35, Fig. 4.27).

As expected for blunt abdominal trauma, the automobile is the underlying causative factor in the majority of cases. It appears that the increasing frequency of such lesions is due to the widespread use of lap-type seat belts [195]. The force required to produce colonic injury is usually considerable, with a high incidence of extraabdominal as well as other intraabdominal injuries [112]. The colonic lesions produced may be separated into the categories of (a) mesenteric laceration, (b) intramural hematoma, and (c) bowel-wall laceration.

Mesenteric Laceration

This type of colonic lesion is the most common with blunt abdominal trauma [195]. It is usually a relatively minor injury associated with hematoma and a viable bowel. Rarely, laceration of major vessels occurs with significant blood loss and subsequent ischemia of bowel. According to Killen [195], venous thrombosis occurs more frequently than does major arterial injury.

TABLE 4.35. Type of colon injury resulting from blunt trauma in 19 patients

Hemorrhagic contusion	13
Partial laceration	4
Perforation	4
Transection	2
Necrosis	2
Total injuries	25

Source: Howell HW, Bartizal JF, Freeark RJ (1976) Blunt trauma involving the colon and rectum. J Trauma 16: 624

No specific plain-film findings are diagnostic of colonic trauma, although with a significant retroperitoneal hematoma, changes consistent with fluid in the retroperitoneal tissues may be observed. If the lesion goes undiagnosed for a significant period, resulting in ischemia, the plain films may show thickening of segments of bowel wall due to infiltration of blood and other fluids into the soft-tissue spaces, a "thumb printing" pattern, rigidity of affected loops, and later a formless loop pattern. A longstanding traumatic lesion may result in narrowing of the involved segment of the bowel with distension of proximal loops indicating varying degrees of bowel obstruction.

Contrast studies, using water-soluble agents or barium, will generally confirm the plain-film findings. Angiography is usually not utilized in establishing the diagnosis. However, if angiography is performed, the arterial changes would be similar to those described for other hollow-viscus lesions. If the injury is to the venous structures, slowing and localized stasis of arterial flow in conjunction with nonvisualization of normally expected venous channels may be observed. Thickening of the bowel wall in the affected area may also be demonstrated on the intermediate and venous phases.

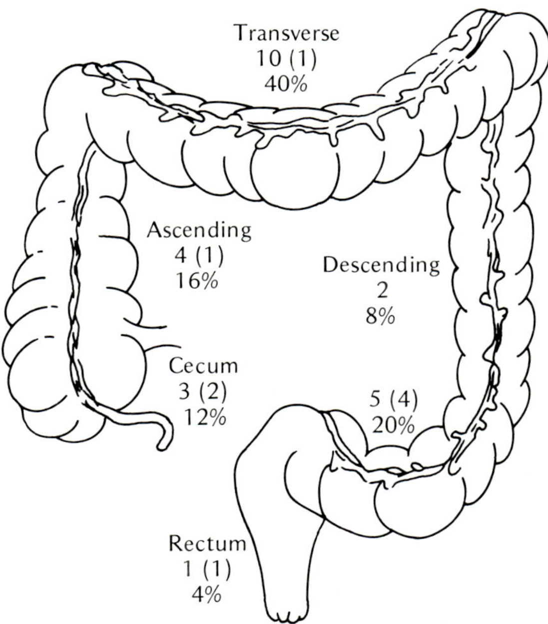

FIG. 4.27. Location, incidence, and severity of 25 colon injuries in 19 patients who sustained blunt trauma (parentheses denote severe injury). From Howell HW, Bartizal JF, Freeark RJ (1976) Blunt trauma involving the colon and rectum. J Trauma 16: 624

Intramural Hematoma

This lesion is usually asymptomatic unless the bowel is obstructed. With obstruction, the usual findings consistent with intestinal obstruction will be present in the segments of bowel proximal to the lesion. Contrast studies of the colon will demonstrate features essentially similar to those observed in duodenal or other small-intestinal hematomas.

Colonic Laceration

The pattern of distribution of injuries of the colon has been presented by Howell et al. and by LoCicero et al. (Table 4.32, Fig. 4.27). Lacerations are of three types: (a) seromucosal tears that involve the serosa and muscularis with an intact mucosa (apparently the mucosa and the muscularis mucosa are the most resistant to blunt abdominal trauma); (b) complete tears, which usually occur along the antimesenteric border of the colon; and (c) complete transection, which is rare. Such perforations may occur immediately after the traumatic episode, or perforation may occur days to weeks after the traumatic event. Acute perforations, when they take place, are usually in the transverse colon, whereas delayed perforation occurs more frequently in the cecum and sigmoid colon [107, 195].

It is stated that intraperitoneal perforation of the colon inevitably produces free intraperitoneal air. If significant spillage of fluid and blood develops with the perforation, the radiologic signs of free intraperitoneal fluid will be observed. Since the ascending and descending colon are retroperitoneal structures, perforations in these areas can present as either retroperitoneal lesions, intraperitoneal lesions (if perforation results in laceration of the overlying peritoneum), or a combination of both. Since the ascending and descending colon lie in the anterior pararenal space, perforation of these colonic segments results in the collection of air and fluid in this compartment. The hallmark of the presence of gas in this space is mottled

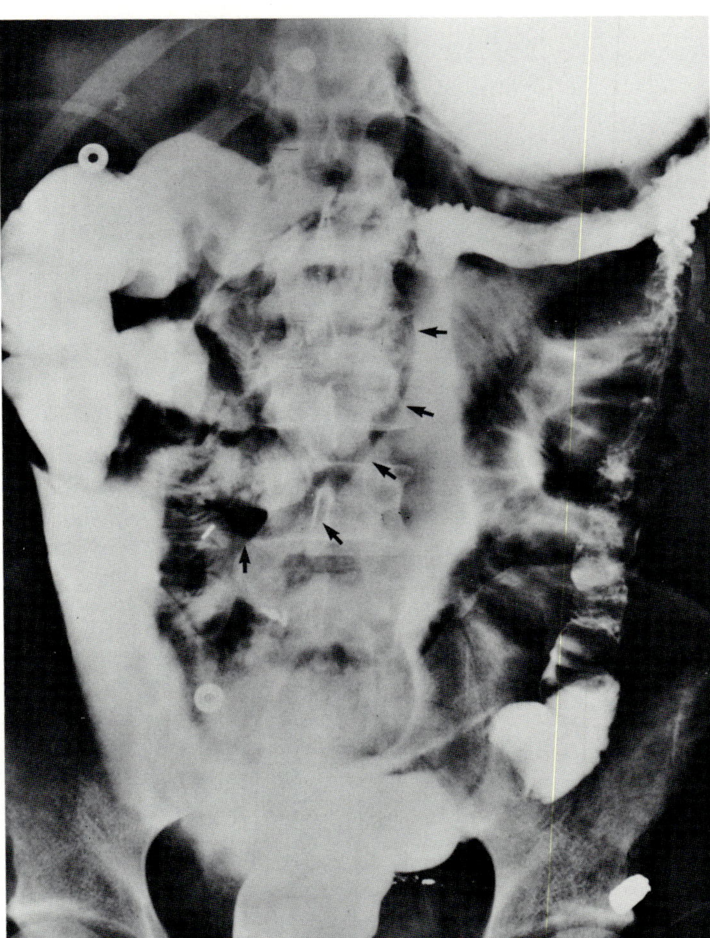

FIG. 4.28. This patient received a gunshot wound to the right buttock. A contrast enema using water-soluble material reveals contrast extravasation into the peritoneal cavity from a rent in the rectosigmoid area. The contrast outlines small-bowel loops and the small-bowel mesentery *(small arrows)*. The small metallic densities (bullet fragments) lead to the final position of the bullet and suggest its course. Courtesy of Dr. Subbarao.

or linear radiolucent area that often lies along established fascial planes, showing little change with alteration in the patient's position. Because of the contaminated material spilled into this compartment, a retroperitoneal abscess is frequent. For the same reason, intraperitoneal spillage is frequently associated with the chemical and radiologic signs of peritonitis. The ingestion of water-soluble contrast media or its instillation into the rectum should demonstrate the site of perforation by spillage of contrast into the retroperitoneal space or into the peritoneal cavity or both (Fig. 4.28).

Rectal Injury

Injury to the rectum is usually associated with blunt trauma to the buttocks and severely comminuted pelvic fractures with protruding sharp, bony fragments. Specific radiologic signs establishing the diagnosis are absent.

The diagnostic clue clinically to rectal injury is the occurrence of rectal bleeding or a positive digital rectal examination for blood in the stool. Careful examinations of the rectum both digitally and endoscopically must be performed in patients who are suspected of having a rectal injury. Contrast studies are of help in the diagnosis of colonic injury but are of limited aid in rectal injury.

Mesenteric Injury

Traumatic lesions of the mesentery usually accompany other visceral injuries, particularly those of the small and large bowel. In general, three types of injuries are sustained: (a) localized hematoma, (b) free bleeding, and (c) venous occlusion. These traumatic lesions have been discussed previously under the headings for small- and large-bowel injuries. Their greatest importance is not in loss of blood from acute extravasation, but rather in hemodynamic alterations produced by such loss or stasis of blood. The two most significant complications are ischemic necrosis and posttraumatic bowel stenosis. With ischemic necrosis as a late complication, air may be noted in the bowel wall owing to mucosal necrosis. Posttraumatic stenosis may result, with late complications of incomplete and complete bowel obstruction. In a case report by Moore and Moore, a patient is described with lower gastrointestinal hemorrhage and abdominal pain as a result of blunt abdominal injury, causing mesenteric vascular trauma. Injury to the superior mesenteric vessels was demonstrated by preoperative arteriography [119].

RETROPERITONEUM

The problem of retroperitoneal hemorrhage in patients with blunt abdominal trauma was reviewed by Nick et al. [128]. In their series of 285 patients with blunt injuries to the abdomen, 65 patients had retroperitoneal hemorrhage. They emphasized the high percentage of patients with blunt injury who have associated retroperitoneal injury. In their series, 75% of the patients had extraabdominal trauma and 40% had intraperitoneal injuries. Radiologic examination, serum amylase determinations, and urine analysis are the tests of significant value in the diagnosis of retroperitoneal injury. The subtle nature of this injury and difficulties associated with the decision for or against laparotomy are reviewed by these authors.

Pancreas

Trauma to the pancreas is not common in occurrence with either penetrating or blunt injury. However, the diagnostic problems and subtlety related to injury of this organ has caught the attention of many over the years. A number of good reviews of pancreatic injury with detailed presentations of etiology, diagnostic considerations, and complications are available.

An experience with pancreatic trauma in 418 cases between 1940 and 1977 was reported from Texas by Graham et al. (Tables 4.36, 4.37). The incidence of penetrating injury declined over the period of study with an increase in blunt injury. Graham et al. reported a far greater overall percentage of cases with penetrating injury associated with pancreatic trauma than did Bach and Frey in 1971[8] (Tables 4.38–4.41) and White and Benfield in 1972 [196] (Tables 4.42–4.44).

The mortality rates vary somewhat in the reported series—from 10% to 20% depending on the etiology of the trauma (Table 4.37). All of the reported reviews stress the frequency of complications (Table 4.42).

TABLE 4.36. Comparison of pancreatic injury by incidence in two groups

Type of injury	Percentage of patients	
	1940–1967	1968–1977
Penetrating	83.5	75.0
Gunshot wounds	50.7	59.2
Shotgun wounds	5.0	4.2
Stab wounds	27.8	11.6
Blunt	16.5	25.0

Source: Graham J, Mattox K, Jordan G (1978) Traumatic injuries of the pancreas. Am J Surg 136: 744–748

TABLE 4.37. Comparison of mortalities in two groups according to type of pancreatic injury

Type of injury	Mortality 1940–1967	1968–1977
Penetrating	19.6	15.2
Gunshot wounds	23.9	15.4
Shotgun wounds	28.5	46.1
Stab wounds	10.2	2.8
Blunt	8.7	16.9
Total	17.8	15.6

Source: Graham J, Mattox K, Jordan G (1978) Traumatic injuries of the pancreas. Am J Surg 136: 744–748

TABLE 4.38. Etiology of pancreatic injury

Injury	Agent	No. of patients	Mortality
Penetrating	Bullet	7	2
			(20%)
	Shotgun	3	0
Blunt	Steering wheel	29	5
			(20%)
	Other	5	2
Total		44	9 (20%)

Source: Bach RD, Frey CF (1971) Diagnosis and treatment of pancreatic trauma. Am J Surg 121: 20–29

TABLE 4.39. Serum amylase determinations performed in patients with pancreatic injuries

Interval from accident to first determination (h)	No. of patients	No. of patients with normal serum amylase levels
1–5	19	7
5–48	5	1
>48	9	0
Not drawn	11	—

Source: Bach RD, Frey CF (1971) Diagnosis and treatment of pancreatic trauma. Am J Surg 121: 20–29

TABLE 4.40. Results of nonoperative treatment in six patients with pancreatic injuries

Injury	Interval (days) from accident to celiotomy	Diagnosis to celiotomy	Complications Preoperative	Postoperative	Deaths
Transection	18	17	1	1	
Transection	60	30	1	3	
Transection	90	31	2	0	1
Transection	60	30	1	0	1
Pseudocyst	90	90	1	1	
Pancreatic pseudocyst	60	30	4	5	1

Source: Bach RD, Frey CF (1971) Diagnosis and treatment of pancreatic trauma. Am J Surg 121: 20–29

TABLE 4.41. Nature of pancreatic injury determined at operation or autopsy

Pancreatic injury	No. of patients	Type of injury Blunt	Sharp	Deaths
Contusion	9	6	3	0
Laceration	11	6	5	2
Transection	16	14	2	4
Exact nature of injury unknown				
Pancreatic abscess	1	1	0	1
Pseudocyst	3	3	0	0
Pancreatitis				
Acute hemorrhagic	2	2	0	2
Chronic	2	2	0	0
Total	44	34	10	9

Source: Bach RD, Frey CF (1971) Diagnosis and treatment of pancreatic trauma. Am J Surg 121: 20–29

TABLE 4.42. Pancreatic trauma (1965–1971)

Organ	Associated injuries in 49 of 63 patients Blunt (14/27)	Penetrating (35/36)
Stomach	0	18
Liver	7	15
Spleen	5	13
Duodenum	6	8
Colon	0	11
Major vessels	0	16
Other	4	20
Total	22	101
	Complications in 37 of 63 patients	
	Blunt (18/27)	Penetrating (19/36)
Prolonged pancreatitis	12	5
Pancreatic fistula	2	1
Pancreatic pseudocyst	2	0
Subphrenic abscess	2	3
Other	3	11
Total	21	20

Source: White PH, Benfield JR (1972) Amylase in the management of pancreatic trauma. Arch Surg 105: 158–163

TABLE 4.43. Mortality after pancreatic trauma (1965–1971)

	No. of patients	Died	%
Blunt trauma	27	1	3.7
Penetrating injury	36	5	13.8
Total	63	6[a]	

[a] All were multiple-trauma victims, and the overall mortality was 9.5%.

Source: White PH, Benfield JR (1972) Amylase in the management of pancreatic trauma. Arch Surg 105: 158–163

Northup and Simmons directly related the mortality in their series to the number of associated injuries [130]. As expected, a direct correlation existed between mortality of over 40% with four or more associated injuries (Fig. 4.29).

Mechanism of Injury

Injury to the pancreas secondary to blunt abdominal trauma is relatively uncommon because of the protected anatomical position of the pancreas in the abdomen. When injury does occur, the mechanism is usually a crushing blow to the upper portion of the abdomen, a light blow to the upper segment of the abdomen with the blow being delivered while the traumatized individual is in acute flexion, or injury produced by sustained and severe flexion of the trunk [109]. Since the force that produces injury is usually severe, a high incidence (77%) of associated injuries occurs [60,202]. It is the combination of pancreatic and associated injury that is responsible for the high mortality when steering-wheel impact is the causative factor. Wilson et al. [202] have noted that the mortality rate with steering-wheel injury is approximately 56%, as compared with a mortality of 29% for other forms of blunt trauma that injure the pancreas.

Types of Injury

Contusion of the pancreas is probably the most common effect of blunt injury, often leading to traumatic pancreatitis, representing 2.3% to 5% of all cases of acute pancreatitis [60]. Selective dorsal pancreatic and gastroduodenal angiography may be definitive in establishing the diagnosis of traumatic pancreatitis by demonstrating punctate leaks of contrast medium [84].

A second major form of injury is pancreatic laceration, the first reported case of which appeared in the St. Thomas Hospital report in 1827. Garré is credited with the first reported cure achieved by suture of a ruptured pancreas. When fractures of the pancreas occur, they are usually beneath or to the left of the

TABLE 4.44. Urinary diastase levels in pancreatic trauma (1965–1971)

Diastase level when nasogastric tube removed	No. of patients	Prolonged pancreatitis	%
>7200 Somogyi units/24 h	14	11	78.5
<7200 Somogyi units/24 h	28	1	3.5

Source: White PH, Benfield JR (1972) Amylase in the management of pancreatic trauma. Arch Surg 105: 158–163

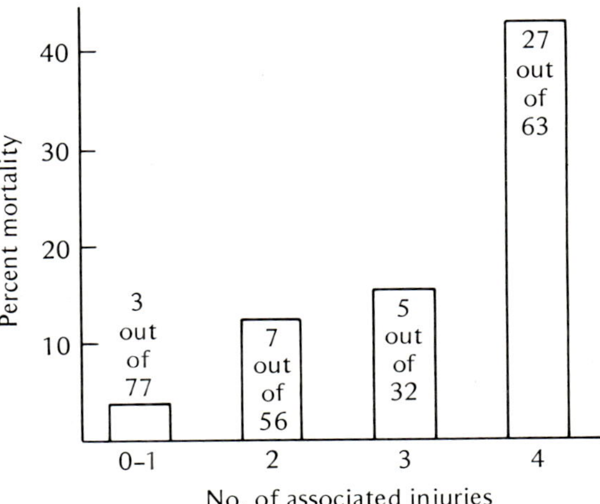

FIG. 4.29. Effect of associated visceral injury on the mortality rate following pancreatic trauma. As the number of associated injuries increased, the mortality rate increased markedly. From Northrup WF, Simmons RL (1972) Pancreatic trauma: A review. Surgery 71(1): 27–43

superior mesenteric artery [42,60]. Associated vascular injuries or rupture of a hollow viscus constitute the major causes of death. Whereas the mortality rate ranges from 12% to 55% (with an average of 20%), the combination of pancreatic laceration with rupture of a hollow viscus, e.g., the duodenum, substantially increases the mortality rate [42].

Radiologic studies may be helpful in the diagnosis of laceration of the pancreas and in defining the associated injuries. Selective angiography of the major vessels supplying the pancreas may reveal extravasation of contrast and/or early venous opacification. Edema and hemorrhage may be reflected by encasement or splaying and displacement of the dorsal pancreatic and transverse pancreatic arteries. Regional vessels such as the splenic artery and vein and the pancreaticoduodenal artery may be stretched, splayed, or displaced by intrapancreatic hematoma. The intermediate and late phases of the angiographic study may show areas of decreased parenchymal opacification and avascularity at sites of hematomas [84]. Additional contrast studies of the duodenum, liver, spleen, and ascending and transverse colon are warranted when a traumatic pancreatic lesion is identified.

Complications are observed in approximately one-third of cases of pancreatic injury [42,60,107] and are associated with prolonged morbidity and even late mortality. Although the onset of complications is usually early, within a few hours after injury, the recognition of these complications months to years later is not unusual. These complications include (a) delayed massive hemorrhage, (b) acute pancreatitis and fat necrosis, (c) hypocalcemic tetany and psychotic behavior patterns (d) sepsis and multiple abscesses, (e) subdiaphragmatic abscess, (f) internal and external pancreatic fistulae, (g) pseudocysts due to a collection of secretions in the lesser omental bursa, (h) chronic relapsing pancreatitis due to excessive scarring and fibrosis with pancreatic calcification, (i) diabetes, and (j) chronic steatorrhea [60].

Vascular System

Management of traumatic injury to major vessels had a limited history until the era of rapid transport of patients. Rich and Spencer [148] have extensively reviewed vascular trauma, including abdominal blood vessel injuries, stressing the experience in Vietnam. They have emphasized that diagnostic efforts in vascular trauma are limited by the critical condition of the patient on arrival at a surgical-care facility. Major vascular trauma is characterized by a profound state of shock, and except in the case of tamponade and thrombosis little time for diagnostic procedures exists.

Most of the major abdominal vascular injuries are sustained as a result of penetrating trauma, both in military and civilian life. Low-velocity gunshot wounds to the aorta and vena cava were reported by Mandal and Boitano in 1978 [99], including a review of the recent literature (Tables 4.45–4.47, Figs. 4.30–4.32).

TABLE 4.45. Anatomic location and frequency of inferior vena cava, aorta, and combined injuries from low-velocity gunshot wounds

Location	IVC[a]	Aorta	IVC[a] and aorta
Suprarenal			
Retrohepatic	3	1	0
Infrahepatic	3	1	0
Infrarenal	4	2	4
Totals	10	4	4

[a] IVC = inferior vena cava.

Source: Mandal AK, Boitano MA (1978) Reappraisal of low-velocity gunshot wounds of the aorta and inferior vena cava in civilian practice. J Trauma 18(8): 580–585

TABLE 4.46. Low-velocity gunshot wounds of the aorta and inferior vena cava: Associated injuries

Injury	No.
Major vascular injuries	
Portal vein	3
Renal artery	2
Renal vein	2
Common iliac artery	4
Common iliac vein	2
Total vascular injuries	13
Nonvascular injuries	
Liver	6
Small bowel	6
Duodenum	4
Stomach	4
Colon	4
Kidney	2
Fracture of lumbar vertebra	2
Pancreas	1
Spleen	1
Gallbladder	1
Diaphragm	1
Central nervous system	1
Peripheral nervous system	1
Total nonvascular injuries	34

Source: Mandal AK, Boitano MA (1978) Reappraisal of low-velocity gunshot wounds of the aorta and inferior vena cava in civilian practice. J Trauma 18(8): 580–585

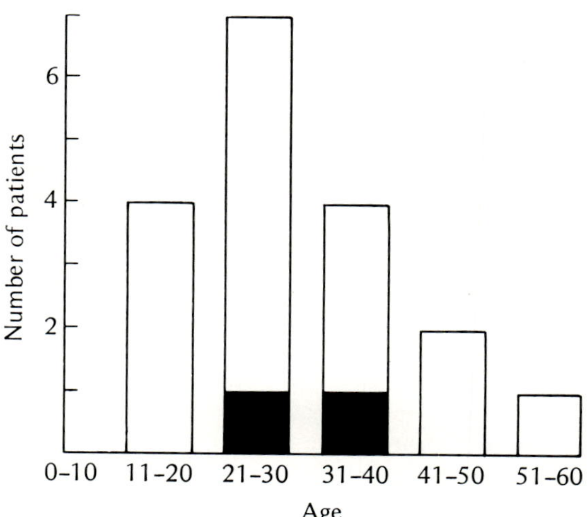

FIG. 4.30. Gunshot wounds of the aorta and inferior vena cava; incidence distribution by sex and age. *Clear bars,* male (16); *solid bars,* female (2). The age ranges from 14 to 53; the average age is 33. From Mandal AK, Boitano MA (1978) Reappraisal of low-velocity gunshot wounds of the aorta and inferior vena cava in civilian practice. J Trauma 18(8): 580–585

TABLE 4.47. Summary of literature review of low-velocity gunshot wounds[a]

Author (year)	Duration of study (years)	IVC[b] No. of pts.	IVC[b] No. of deaths (%)	Aorta No. of pts.	Aorta No. of deaths (%)	Aorta and IVC No. of pts.	Aorta and IVC No. of deaths (%)
Suprarenal							
Starzl (1962)	5	4	1 (25%)				
Mattox (1974)	4	17	10 (59%)	24	14 (58%)		
Lim (1974)	5			10	7 (70%)	2	2 (100%)
Fullen (1974)		5	3 (60%)				
Burns (1975)	5	8	3 (38%)				
Aderoju (1976)	9	3	1 (33%)				
Total		37	49%	34	62%	2	100%
Infrarenal							
Starzl (1962)	5	5	(0%)				
Lim (1974)	5			3	1 (66%)	2	2 (100%)
Aderoju (1976)	9	4	1 (25%)				
Total		9	11%	3	66%	2	100%

[a] See text of article for reports that have been excluded from the table.

[b] IVC = inferior vena cava.

Source: Mandal AK, Boitano MA (1978) Reappraisal of low-velocity gunshot wounds of the aorta and inferior vena cava in civilian practice. J Trauma 18(8): 580–585

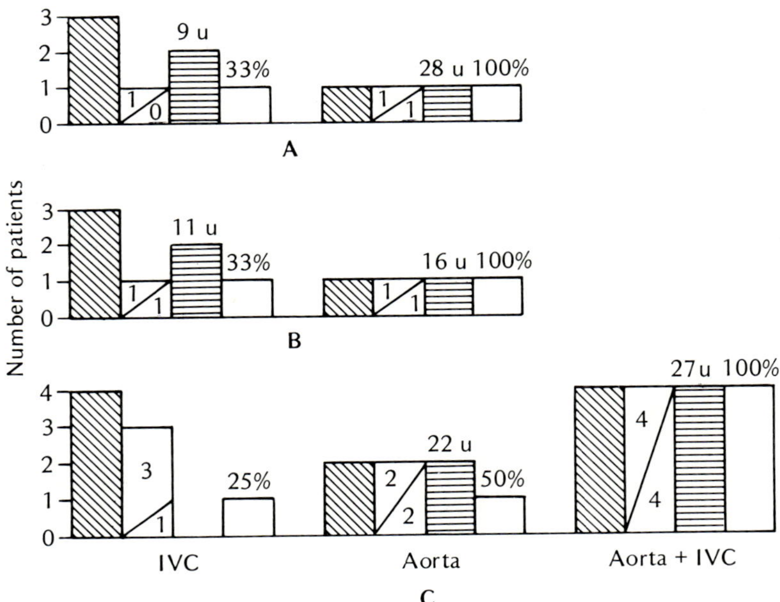

FIG. 4.31. Gunshot wounds of the aorta and inferior vena cava; mortality. Correlation with shock, cardiac arrest, and active bleeding. **(A)** Suprarenal retrohepatic, **(B)** suprarenal infrahepatic, **(C)** infrarenal. ▧ Number of patients, ◸ number of patients in shock, ◺ number of patients with cardiac arrest, ▤ number of patients with active bleeding (average units of blood), □ number of deaths (%). From Mandal AK, Boitano MA (1978) Reappraisal of low-velocity gunshot wounds of the aorta and inferior vena cava in civilian practice. J Trauma 18(8): 580–585

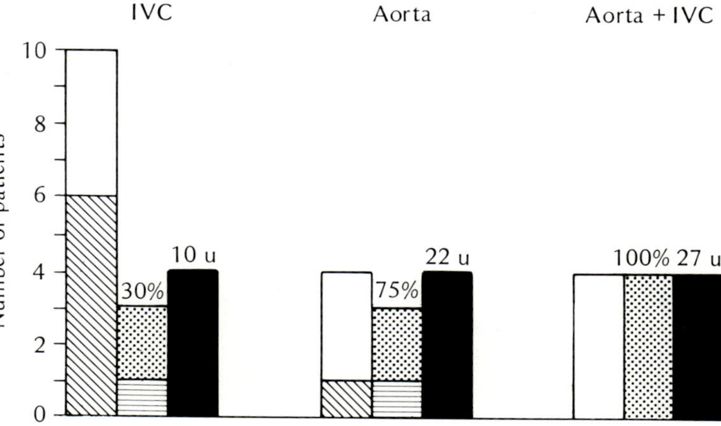

FIG. 4.32. Gunshot wounds of the aorta and inferior vena cava; mortality. Correlation with associated vascular injuries. □ Number of patients, ▧ number of patients with associated vascular injuries, ▩ number of deaths (%), ▤ number of deaths in patients with associated vascular injuries, ■ number of patients with active bleeding (average units of blood). From Mandal AK, Boitano MA (1978) Reappraisal of low-velocity gunshot wounds of the aorta and inferior vena cava in civilian practice. J Trauma 18(8): 580–585

The forces that produce injury to the solid and hollow viscera of the abdomen also act on the vascular structures supplying these viscera. The injuries sustained may be categorized as follows: (a) acute arterial insufficiency with disruption; (b) arterial insufficiency due to stretching, angulation, compression, or spasm; and (c) delayed arterial insufficiency due to the development of pseudoaneurysms and arteriovenous (AV) fistulae [11].

The end result of vascular trauma, particularly arterial trauma, varies according to the mode of injury. In general, penetrating injuries usually result in transection (either total or partial), formation of AV fistulae, or intramural hematomas. On the other hand, blunt abdominal trauma most frequently leads to thrombosis of the injured vessel. However, if the concussive force is great enough or if an associated fracture produces vascular laceration, blunt abdominal trauma can result in findings similar to those produced by penetrating injuries [91].

Total Transection

With total transection of a vessel the major problem is bleeding. The prognosis for such injuries is dependent on the size of the vessel, whether the vascular structure is an artery or a vein, and the location of the vessel. With larger vessels, such as the aorta or the inferior vena cava, total transection usually results in rapid exsanguination. Allen and Blaisdell [6] in evaluating injuries to the inferior vena cava, found that 50% of patients who sustained this injury died before they reached the hospital and 40% of those who lived to reach the hospital subsequently died either from exsanguination or from complications from their injuries. If the vessel is small, particularly if it is a vein and confined, bleeding continues until the pressures resulting in the bleeding are balanced by the pressures of the surrounding tissues and/or other hemostatic influences come into play.

Radiologic plain-film studies in transection of a vessel may demonstrate fluid (blood) within the peritoneal cavity, a soft-tissue mass consistent with a hematoma, diffuse or localized alteration in the size of affected viscera, or ischemic changes in the viscera peripheral to the site of transection. If angiography is performed, frank extravasation of contrast may be demonstrated, or complete block of vascular flow with a filling defect in the transected vessel may be demonstrated. The filling defect, having a convex proximal border, represents an intraluminal thrombosis. Collateral vessels bridging the site of transection may be opacified. If peripheral ischemia or infarction develops, areas of lucency in the intermediate phase of the angiogram may be demonstrated.

Partial Transection and Pseudoaneurysm Formation

With partial transection one of the hemostatic influences, vascular retraction, is compromised. The tendency for severe bleeding exists because the site of laceration cannot retract into surrounding soft tissues where vasoconstriction and thrombosis can occur. The development of a hematoma often results. In time, the hematoma develops a peripheral cap of fibrous tissue, centrally liquefies, and develops an endothelial lining resulting in a pseudoaneurysm.

Plain-film studies in patients with partial transection and pseudoaneurysm demonstrate a soft-tissue mass with or without calcification (Fig. 4.33). Angiography will show an extraluminal sac of variable size, usually in continuity with the transected vessel. The actual size of the pseudoaneurysm is not always reflected in the size of the contrast-filled sac because of eddy currents and adherent clot, which may also produce variations in the degree and extent of the opacification of the pseudoaneurysmal sac (Fig. 4.34).

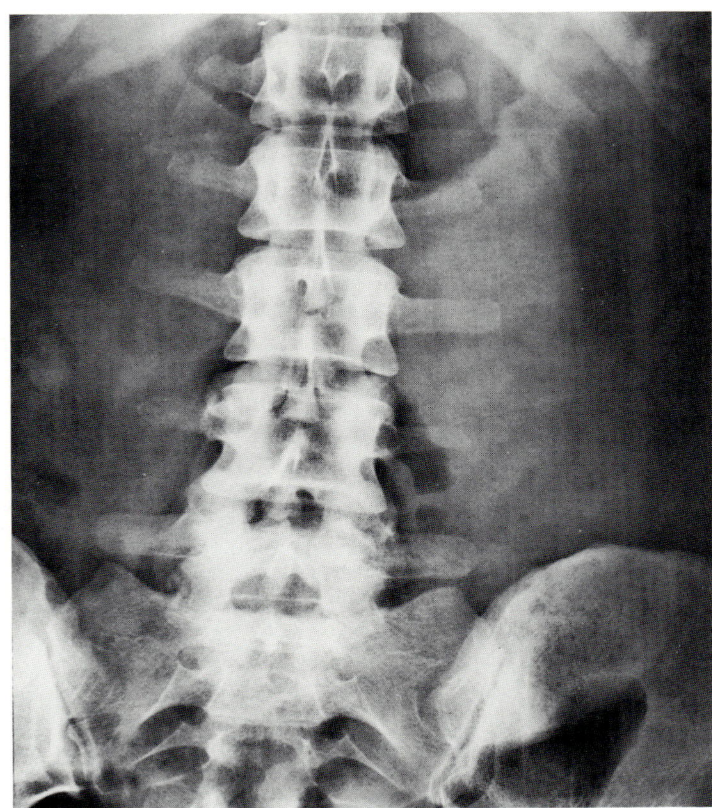

FIG. 4.33. This 21-year-old female was stabbed in the left midabdomen. An AP supine examination of the abdomen reveals a mild levoscoliosis of the lumbar spine and loss of the left psoas and renal silhouettes consistent with the presence of a retroperitoneal-fluid collection. At exploration, a left retroperitoneal hematoma with a through-and-through laceration of the abdominal aorta and a laceration of the 4th portion of the duodenum were found.

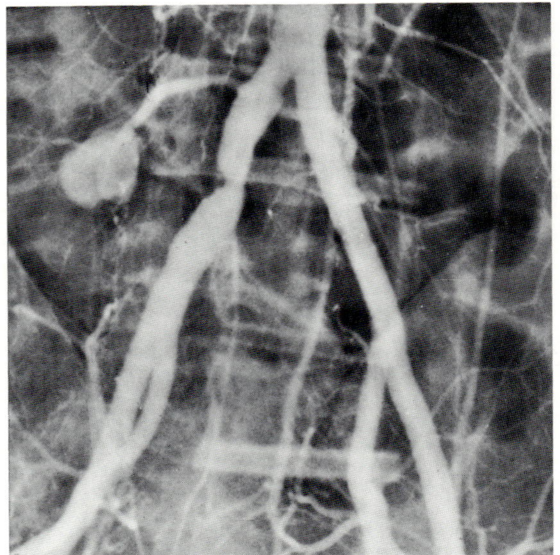

A

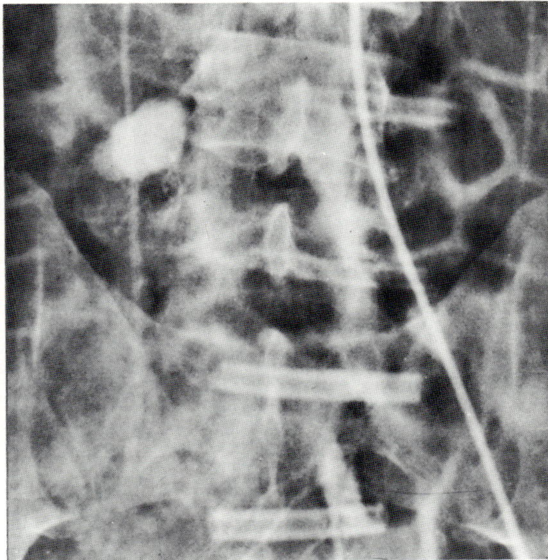

B

FIG. 4.34 A and B. This middle-aged male was admitted to the hospital with a stab wound in the right lower back. At exploration, lacerations of the inferior vena cava and right common iliac artery were found and repaired. Two days after surgery, bright-red blood was found draining from the stab wound. This bleeding stopped spontaneously only to recur 4 days later. The **(A)** arterial phase of a flush aortogram reveals narrowing of the right common iliac artery at the site of previous repair and a pseudoaneurysm of the distal right 4th lumbar artery. The **(B)** intermediate phase shows persistence of the contrast extravasation confirming the arterial injury.

Traumatic Arteriovenous Fistula

Two types of traumatic arteriovenous (AV) fistula exist: the aneurysmal varix and the varicose aneurysm. The former is a direct communication between an artery and a vein; the latter is also a direct communication, complicated by the presence of pseudoaneurysm. Superficial injuries are likely to cause AV fistulae at anatomic sites where an artery and vein lie in close proximity. Deeper wounds have a tendency to produce varicose aneurysms. Whatever the type, the fistula results in a left-to-right shunt with an increase in venous return, cardiac output, pulse pressure, and cardiac rate. If the shunt is large enough, high-output cardiac decompensation may result. Angiography will opacify the fistula and will demonstrate significant vascular and hemodynamic changes around the fistula. The artery proximal to the fistula dilates, and collaterals develop bridging the site of the fistula. The flow in this proximal artery is increased but the direction of flow is normal. Distal to the fistula the artery usually is normal in size, but collaterals from the proximal vessel are outlined. The direction of flow is usually normal but may be reversed depending on the size of the fistula and duration of the lesion. The vein proximal to the fistula is dilated with the demonstration of dilated collateral venous channels. The direction of flow in this vein is normal, but the rate of flow is increased and venous congestion is usually present. Distal to the fistula, if venous valves are present, they may become incompetent, resulting in dilation and tortuosity of the vein. Reversal of flow in the vein may also occur, particularly when the valves either fail or are absent. Angiography will demonstrate the fistula with early venous filling and enlargement of the feeding artery and emptying vein. Plain-film studies may show edema of the surrounding soft tissues, foreign bodies in the area of the fistula, calcifications in vascular walls, and, with chronic AV fistulae peripheral osteoarthropathy [14,84].

Traumatic Dissection

In this entity, the forces causing the abdominal trauma result in partial disruption of and bleeding into the wall of the affected vessel. The severity of the bleeding will determine whether partial or complete obstruction of the lumen of the vessel will result. Usually an intimal tear will be present. The dissection can extend and progress to involve a significant portion of the affected artery and/or its branches proximal or distal to the site of injury. The primary concern is the peripheral ischemia, which may be produced by proximal narrowing and even occlusion of the affected vessel.

Plain-film examination demonstrates a vascular channel wider than normal. If intramural calcification of the affected vessel is present, an increase in soft-tissue density between the lateral border of the intramural calcification and the lateral margin of the vessel wall is observed, reminiscent of the radiologic features frequently delineated in nontraumatic dissection of the thoracic aorta. Angiography may demonstrate an intraluminal mass (hematoma), or, if an intimal tear is present, the contrast may enter the wall of the affected vessel, producing the effect of a double lumen.

Genitourinary Tract

Kidneys

The kidneys, positioned deep in the abdomen, are protected posteriorly by the ribs and medially by the spine and are cushioned by the muscle mass and fat of the retroperitoneum and posterior abdominal wall. Despite this protected location, the kidneys are among the most frequently injured abdominal organs in the individual exposed to blunt trauma. The kidneys are also frequently injured (2% to 31%) in patients with penetrating abdominal wounds (Table 4.50). During the past half century, the increase in renal trauma has paralleled the increase in automotive and industrial accidents with 75% to 90% of renal injuries associated with the automobile, falls, or athletic injuries [82]. While approximately 80% of renal injuries are the result of blunt abdominal trauma, in two-thirds of cases the kidney is the only organ that is significantly damaged [140].

Both the normal anatomy of the kidneys and the presence of preexisting renal abnormalities help to explain their unusual vulnerability to trauma. The kidneys differ from other organs in that the vascular pedicle is the primary point of intraabdominal fixation. The kidneys have been likened to a weighted pendulum swaying about the fixed attachment of the renal arteries to the aorta. As a result, horizontal and vertical acceleration and deceleration injuries can produce tearing of the renal arteries from the aorta and or the renal veins from the inferior vena cava.

The presence of any renal abnormality will increase the vulnerability of the kidney to traumatic injury. Cass and Ireland [28] reported a 14.5% incidence of preexisting lesions in their series of renal injuries, and Richardson et al. [149] found that one-half of renal injuries occurred in abnormal kidneys. Hydronephrosis is the most significant preexisting renal lesion. Lowsley and Kerwin [96] state that the hydronephrotic kidney is six times more likely to rupture if subjected to external violence than a normal kidney; Cass and Ireland [28] have reported that more than 50% of patients with preexisting renal lesions had hydronephrotic kidneys (Tables 4.48–4.52).

TABLE 4.48. Genitourinary injuries—January 1, 1961–December 31, 1965

Renal			116	Urethra		23
Nonpenetrating		93		Avulsions of bladder neck (female patients)	2	
Contusions	82.8%			Bulbous urethra	9	
Major lacerations	12.9%			Membranous urethra	9	
Shattered kidneys	4.3%			Perineal hematomas	3	
Penetrating		23				
Ureter			0			
Bladder			38	Penis		32
Contusions		5				
Extraperitoneal rupture		17		Scrotum		19
Intraperitoneal rupture		11				
Combined intraperitoneal and extraperitoneal rupture		5		Testicle		23
				Total		251

Source: Waterhouse K, Gross M (1969) Trauma to the genitourinary tract: A 5-year experience with 251 cases. J Urol 101: 241–246

TABLE 4.49. Associated injuries with renal trauma in children

	Classification of renal injury				
Associated injury	Contusion	Laceration	Rupture	Pedicle injury	Total
Number of children with associated injuries	39	11[a]	1	3[a]	54[a]
Fractured ribs	6	2	1		9
Ruptured diaphragm		2			2
Lacerated spleen	14	6		1	21
Lacerated liver	3	3	1	2	9
Bowel perforation	3	1		2	6
Fractured skull	6	1	1		8
Fractured spine	1	2			3
Fractured pelvis	5				5
Fractured extremities	15	2	1		18
Other (head injury, pancreas, vascular)	12	2		1	15
Deaths	2	1	1	1	5

[a] One child had bilateral injuries: laceration (right kidney) and renal pedicle injury (left kidney).
Source: Cass AS, Ireland GW (1974) Renal injuries in children. J Trauma 14(8): 719–722

TABLE 4.50. Comparison of studies of renal injuries in children

	Mertz	Persky	Javadpour	Morse	Present study
Number of injuries	70	65	110	80	82
Etiology					
Falls and blows	70%	69%	36.5%		27%
Traffic accidents	23%	29%	26.5%	N.K.	65%
Penetrating	3%	2%	31%		8%
Other	4%		6%		
Classification					
Contusion		74%	26%	78%	80%
Laceration		14%	59%	19%	15%
Rupture	N.K.[b]	12%	7%	3%	1%
Pedicle injury			8%		4%
Associated injuries	30%	N.K.	25%	40%	67%
Preexisting anomalies	21.5%	25%	10%	10%	2%
Surgical treatment[a]					
Rate	33%	12%	25%	20%	16%
Nephrectomy	13%	12%	7%	8.5%	5%
Operations preserving renal tissue	20%	N.K.	18%	11.5%	11%

[a] Excluding preexisting renal anomaly.
[b] N.K. = not known.
Source: Cass AS, Ireland GW (1974) Renal injuries in children. J Trauma 14(8): 719–722

TABLE 4.51. Clinical manifestations in 59 cases of renal trauma

	No.	%
Hematuria	59	100
Gross	34	57
Microscopic	25	43
Shock	2	3.3
Pain and tenderness, right flank	35	59
Pain and tenderness, left flank	24	41
Coma	1	2
Muscle guarding	9	15
Multiple lacerations or contusions	8	13
Associated fractures	8	13
Head injuries	5	8
Palpable mass	2	3.3
Ruptured spleen	2	3.3
Subdural hematoma	1	2
Pneumothorax	1	2

Source: Emanuel B, Weiss H, Gollin P (1977) Renal trauma in children. J Trauma 17(4): 275–278

Children experience a higher incidence of renal trauma than do adults. The ptosis inherent to children's kidneys and the immature development of Gerota's fascia are factors contributing to the vulnerability of the excretory system of children. In children, renal injuries were more common than splenic rupture and four times more common than trauma to the pancreas, lung, heart, or major vessels. In considering the genitourinary system only, renal injury are 10 times more common than injury to the urinary bladder and 100 times more common than trauma to the ureter or urethra.

The incidence of renal injury described in several large series substantiates the greater vulnerability of the child's kidney. In the series by Linke et al. from the University of Rochester [89], 75% of patients with renal trauma had involvement of a second organ system. However, in the pediatric age group, the incidence of involvement of a second organ drops to 40%. As in other forms of abdominal trauma, the male child is more commonly injured than the female child. Campbell [24] reports a male-to-female ratio of 4:1, with 50% of the patients less than 30 years of age. This sex-related difference reflects the decreased exposure of the female in our society to trauma.

The force of impact required to injure the kidney is frequently severe enough to produce injuries to other intraabdominal structures. The incidence of injuries associated with renal trauma is reported as 20% to 30%; fractures of the lower ribs and transverse processes of the lumbar spine and lacerations of the liver and spleen are most frequently encountered.

Penetrating injuries to the genitourinary tract are increasing in incidence. Scott et al. [165] reported on 181 patients with injuries (Tables 4.53–4.56). Tynberg

TABLE 4.52. Correlation of etiology of renal injury with age of patients

Age	Auto accident	Hit by car	Sports accident	Direct blow	Fall	Totals
<5 yr	2	0	0	0	2	4
5–10 yr	10	6	2	1	10	29
11–15 yr	15	1	7	1	2	26
Totals	27	7	9	2	14	59

Source: Emanuel B, Weiss H, Gollin P (1977) Renal trauma in children. J Trauma 17(4): 275–278

TABLE 4.53. Penetrating renal injuries: Injuries of the vascular pedicle, 29 patients

Type of injury	No. patients	Nephrectomy	Repair	Deaths
Artery and vein	10	9	1	5
Vein only	13	3	10	0
Artery only	6	1	5	2
Total	29	13	16	7

Source: Scott R Jr, Carlton CE Jr, Goldman M (1969) Penetrating injuries of the kidney: An analysis of 181 patients. J Urol 101: 247–253

TABLE 4.54. Penetrating renal injuries: Analysis of 41 patients without hematuria

Type of injury	No. patients	%
Pedicle injury	13	32
Major parenchymal	10	24
Minor parenchymal	18	44
Total	41	100

Source: Scott R Jr, Carlton CE Jr, Goldman M (1969) Penetrating injuries of the kidney: An analysis of 181 patients. J Urol 101: 247–253

TABLE 4.55. Predominant pyelographic findings in 121 patients with penetrating injuries of the kidney

Interpretation	Patients	%
Normal pyelogram	41	34
Obliteration psoas or renal shadow	34	28
Decreased visualization	21	17
Nonvisualization	13	11
Extravasation	12	10
Total	121	100

Source: Scott R Jr, Carlton CE Jr, Goldman M (1969) Penetrating injuries of the kidney: An analysis of 181 patients. J Urol 101: 247–253

TABLE 4.56. Injury of abdominal viscera; 181 patients with penetrating injury

Associated injury	No. patients	%
Liver	80	42
Colon	43	24
Spleen	44	23
Stomach	41	23
Chest	35	18
Pancreas	31	17
Small intestines	24	13
Duodenum	21	12
Vena cava	11	6
Portal vein	7	4
Gallbladder	7	4
Aorta	5	3
Superior mesenteric artery	4	2
Others	10	6

Source: Scott R Jr, Carlton CE Jr, Goldman M (1969) Penetrating injuries of the kidney: An analysis of 181 patients. J Urol 101: 247–253

TABLE 4.58. Symptoms and hematuria in 60 cases of renal injury associated with penetrating abdominal wounds

		Hematuria		
	Shock	None	Microscopic	Gross
Type I	4	7	19	12
Type II	9	2	4	11
Type III	5	1	0	4
Total	18 (30%)	10 (17%)	23 (38%)	27 (45%)

Source: Tynberg PLH, Hoch WH, Persky L, Zollinger RM (1973) The management of renal injuries coincident with penetrating wounds of the abdomen. J Trauma 13(6): 502–508

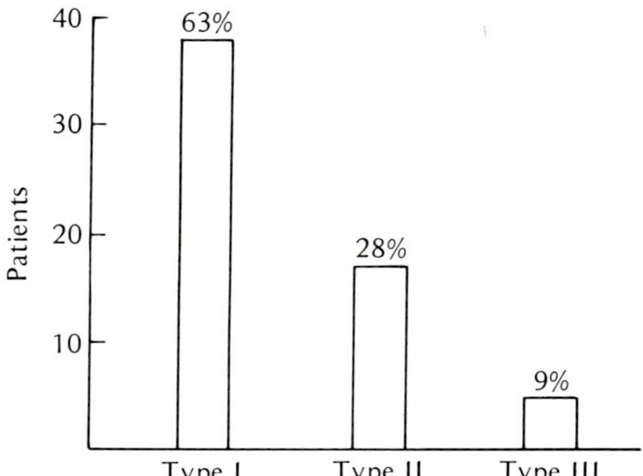

FIG. 4.35. Distribution of renal injuries. From Tynberg PLH, Hoch WH, Persky L, Zollinger RM (1973) Management of renal injuries coincident with penetrating wounds of the abdomen. J Trauma 13(6): 502–508

TABLE 4.57. Etiology in 60 cases of renal injury associated with penetrating abdominal wounds

	Gunshot wound	Stab	Total
Type I, parenchymal damage only	29	9	38
Type II, collecting system damage	15	2	17
Type III, fracture or vascular pedicle injury	5	0	5
Total	49 (82%)	11 (18%)	60

Source: Tynberg PLH, Hock WH, Persky L, Zollinger RM (1973) The management of renal injuries coincident with penetrating wounds of the abdomen. J Trauma 13(6): 502–508

TABLE 4.59. Results of excretory urography in 60 cases of renal injury associated with penetrating abdominal wounds

	IVP omitted	Normal	Abnormal
Type I	13	13	12 {5 poor visualization; 7 hematoma}
Type II	5	1	11 {6 poor visualization; 4 extravasation; 1 hematoma}
Type III	3	0	2 poor visualization
Total	21 (35%)	14 (23%)	25 (42%)

Source: Tynberg PLH, Hock WH, Persky L, Zollinger RM (1973) The management of renal injuries coincident with penetrating wounds of the abdomen. J Trauma 13(6): 502–508

et al. [187] reviewed penetrating injuries of the genitourinary tract coincident with penetrating wounds of the abdomen. They described the presenting symptoms in 60 cases and categorized the injuries according to the severity of the trauma. As expected, the more severe injuries were in patients presenting in shock and with gunshot wounds (Tables 4.57–4.59, Figs. 4.35–4.37).

Diagnostic Evaluation

After thorough initial diagnostic evaluation of the patient with injury of the genitourinary, appropriate measures must be used to stabilize the patient's condition. Often, as with all other forms of abdominal trauma, the prognosis in such patients is dependent on their clinical status immediately following the traumatic episode. In some patients, continuing life-threatening hemorrhage will mandate immediate surgical intervention. However, most patients are able to undergo a logical diagnostic workup proceeding from

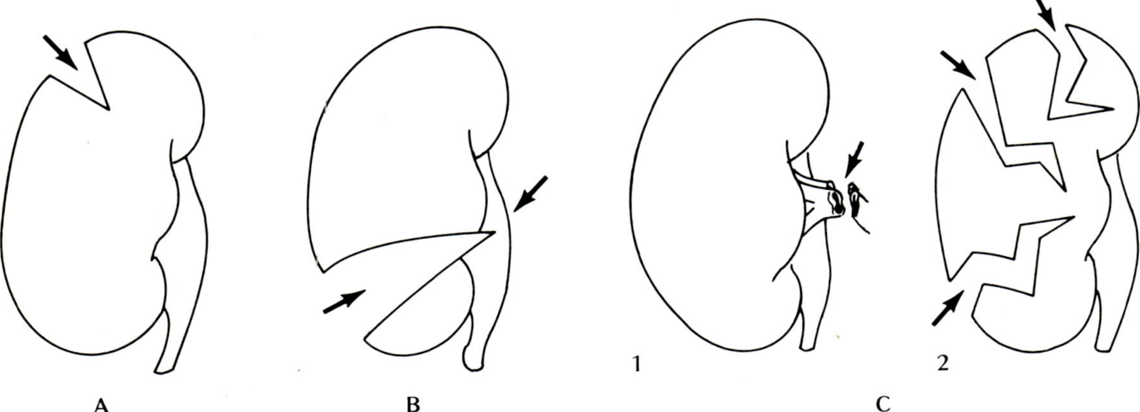

FIG. 4.36. Classification of renal injury after Carlton and Scott. **(A)** Type I: Parenchymal damage. **(B)** Type II: Damaged parenchyma and collecting system. **(C)** Type III: **1,** Vascular disruption; **2,** Kidney fracture. From Tynberg PLH, Hoch WH, Persky L, Zollinger RM (1973) Management of renal injuries coincident with penetrating wounds of the abdomen. J Trauma 13(6): 502–508

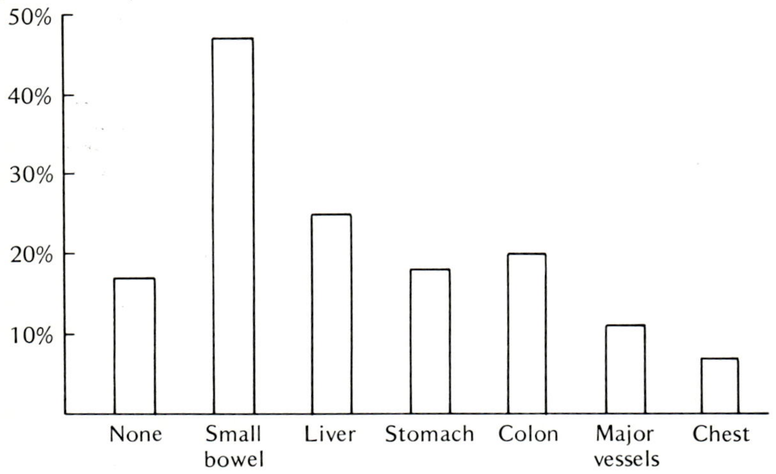

FIG. 4.37. Injuries of intraabdominal organs associated with renal injury. From Tynberg PLH, Hoch WH, Persky L, Zollinger RM (1973) Management of renal injuries coincident with penetrating wounds of the abdomen. J Trauma 13(6): 502–508

the least-invasive procedure to more complex studies until a diagnosis is established.

It should be appreciated that definitive assessment of the urinary tract must begin with a history and physical examination. However, in the severely injured patient, the first and only clue to the presence of trauma to the genitourinary tract may be an abnormal urine. Obtaining a urine specimen as a required baseline of study in such patients cannot be overemphasized. If the patient can void voluntarily, the likelihood of urethral injury is diminished. If the patient cannot void, or is unconscious, a Foley catheter should be inserted gently through the urethra into the bladder. Care must be taken that the catheterization does not worsen an unsuspected urethral injury. The presence of an intact bony pelvis decreases the likelihood of urinary bladder injury, especially if the traumatic forces were not applied to a distended bladder. Fracture or dislocation of the bony pelvis mandates an excretory urogram and retrograde cystogram to rule out bladder and/or urethral injury.

CLINICAL SIGNS AND SYMPTOMS

Hematuria is the most common clinical feature in renal trauma. It may consist of contamination of the urine specimen with free red blood cells, clots or casts. Cylindrical casts containing solid blood elements are highly suggestive of upper-urinary-tract bleeding. It must be stressed that the absence of hematuria does not exclude the possibility of a traumatic lesion of the urologic system. The absence or intermittent occurrence of blood elements in the specimen of urine under such circumstances can be explained by the swelling of the renal parenchyma which follows the injury, resulting in increased intraparenchymal tension with decrease in renal function. Such pathologic changes may result in hematuria initially, with rapid clearing of subsequent urine specimens, and the total absence of any blood within the urine. The traumatic incident may primarily or secondarily result in obstruction of the outflow tract of the kidney, either by clots present in the upper tract or by clots or other solid tissue passed distally and producing obstruction. Involvement of the renal parenchyma may occur without communication with the collecting system. Total transection of the ureter in severe trauma may be encountered. The amount of blood demonstrated in the urine is not a reliable index of the severity of the injury. If only one kidney is injured, the blood passing into that collecting system may be diluted in the bladder by uncontaminated urine passing from the uninvolved side.

Massive extravasation of blood into the urologic tract, the retroperitoneal soft tissues, or the peritoneal cavity in a traumatized patient may be evidence of a serious renal injury. In the presence of a severely shattered kidney and an intact Gerota's fascia, massive hemorrhage may be controlled owing to the tamponade effect of the intact fascia. If the patient is carefully managed with adequate bed rest, continued until the urine is microscopically clear, secondary hemorrhage is not likely to occur (Fig. 4.38). The passage of large amounts of blood in the urine is highly suggestive of laceration of the renal parenchyma and of the pelvocalyceal system. The presence of free blood in the peritoneal cavity in association with a renal injury may indicate a tear in Gerota's fascia and escape of blood from the retroperitoneal space. Evidence of massive hemorrhage is obviously an indication that additional diagnostic information is necessary to define the type and extent of renal injury.

Flank pain or tenderness to palpation may indicate injury to the abdominal wall or the lower ribs. Pain associated with crepitation on palpation of the posterior ribs indicates the presence of a fracture and means a substantial force was applied to produce the injury. Flank pain may be localized to the point of injury or may radiate as in renal colic. Radiating pain is common in parenchymal injuries with capsular distension or with the passage of a thrombus down the ureter on the side of the injury.

Palpation of a mass through a flank or through the anterior abdominal wall may indicate a significant extravasation of blood or urine into the retroperitoneal space. Although the detection of a mass does not define its etiology and composition, its presence may be the only indication of severe retroperitoneal injury. Palpation of such a mass necessitates study of the urinary tract in order to establish an accurate diagnosis. This is particularly important when the mass appears to be increasing in size with the patient under observation.

RADIOLOGIC DIAGNOSIS OF RENAL TRAUMA

In terms of accuracy in demonstrating the details and extent of injury, routine and specialized radiologic techniques are unrivaled in their value in the diagnosis of trauma to the genitourinary tract. Drezner [44] and Kaufman and Brosman [76] have reported a 50% to 80% positive correlation between excretory urogram and renal trauma. The excretory urogram was diagnostic in 75% of patients with renal injury. Williams and Zollinger [99] agreed that radiologic evaluation of the traumatized patient is particularly helpful in the diagnosis of urinary-tract injuries.

The modalities most frequently used are plain films of the abdomen, excretory urography, renal isotope scan, ultrasonography, and angiography. The previously popular retrograde pyelography has been almost eliminated as a diagnostic tool in the traumatized patient because of the recent introduction of angiography and sonographic scanning. The reduction in retrograde pyelographic procedures is fortunate since the potential of retrograde seeding of infection may outweigh the value of the information that can be obtained by this procedure. However, in institutions not equipped to perform the more sophisticated radiologic procedures, retrograde pyelography may prove useful, especially in cases of nonvisualization of the kidney on excretory urography or to exclude rupture of the pelvocalyceal system or ureter.

Plain Films. The findings most frequently demonstrated on plain films relate to injury of the associated supporting structures, e.g., fractures of ribs and transverse process of lumbar vertebrae. In addition, scoliosis of the spine to the side of injury with an associated loss of the ipsilateral psoas margin is suggestive of significant abdominal trauma. The diagnostic significance of these two radiologic findings is greatly enhanced if they are observed in association with ipsilateral renal enlargement (either localized or diffuse), loss of the renal outline, alteration of the renal axis, and displacement of the kidney from its normal position.

Intravenous Pyelography. The use of large doses of contrast media (1.5 cc/kg of 75% to 76% Hypaque or Renografin in the adult and 2 cc/kg in children) with routine tomographic cuts of the kidneys will result in high-quality pyelographic examinations and a high yield of diagnostic information [82,150].

The infusion of contrast may be by bolus or drip. In severely injured patients, the intravenous drip offers the advantage of a readily available infusion line should the patient's deteriorating state require the rapid infusion of blood or other fluids. The examination cannot

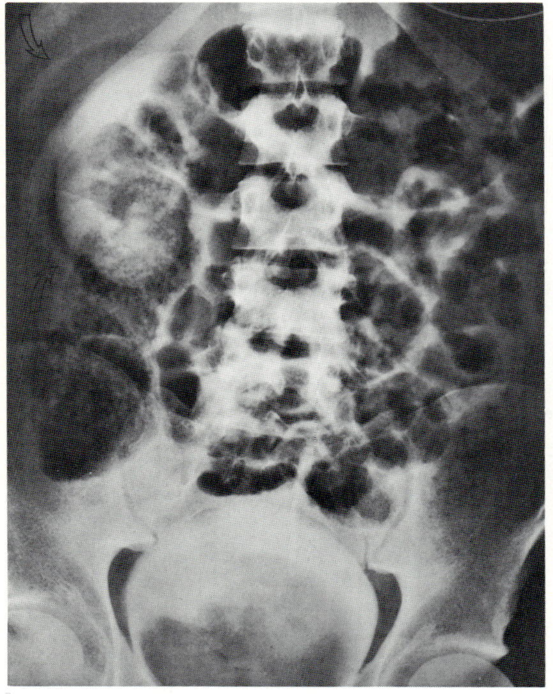

A

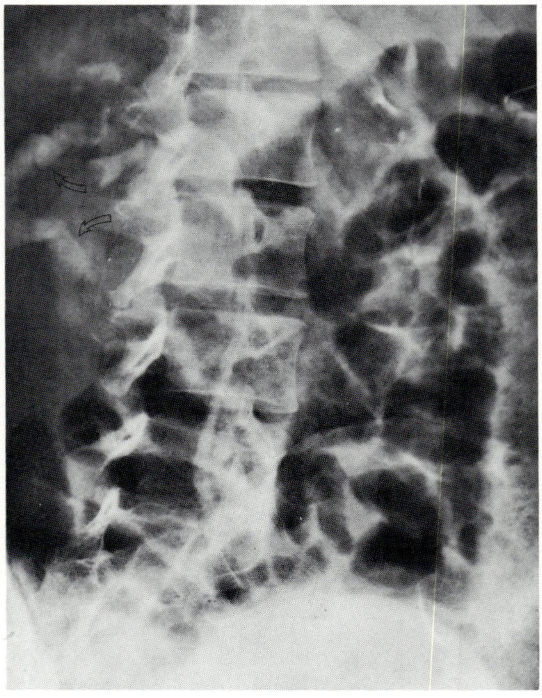

B

C

FIG. 4.38 A–C. This 21-year-old male was stabbed in the right flank. The **(A)** 20-min AP film from his initial excretory urogram reveals a prolonged, dense nephrogram of the right kidney, faint contrast extravasation from this kidney *(open arrows),* and an irregular filling defect (a blood clot) in the bladder. The **(B)** left posterior oblique view from this examination confirms and more clearly defines the contrast extravasation *(open arrows)* from the right upper pole. An abdominal exploration revealed lacerations of the right lobe of the liver and upper pole of the right kidney, which were repaired. **(C)** Excretory urographic evaluation of the right kidney 13 days after surgery reveals deformity of the right upper pole collecting system with a filling defect (clot) within it. There is no evidence of contrast extravasation.

be considered complete unless there is satisfactory visualization of the ureters and bladder. The drip technique seems to provide the best visualization of the ureters. Filled and postvoiding bladder films in frontal, oblique, and possibly lateral projections must be obtained to exclude extravasation of contrast either into the bladder wall or into the perivesical soft tissues.

Nonvisuálization of one or both kidneys on excretory urography does not necessarily indicate severe renal injury in the traumatized patient. Prior renal disease, unilateral absence of a kidney (either congenital or acquired), or acute renal shutdown secondary to posttraumatic reflex vasospasm may be present. Thus, failure to visualize the kidney or ureters on excretory urography requires further diagnostic evaluation. Decrease in nephrographic or pyelographic density and attenuation of the pelvocalyceal system may occur because of a combination of interstitial edema and decreased renal blood flow secondary to the trauma (Fig. 4.39). A decrease in renal size may

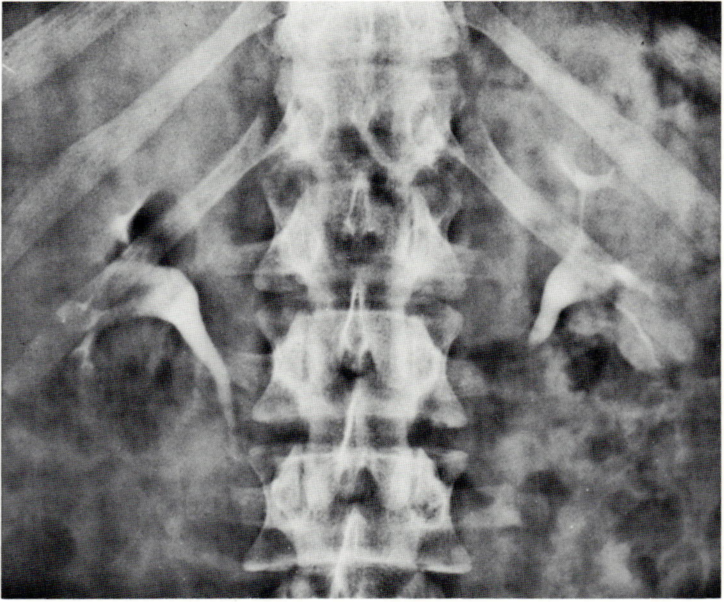

A

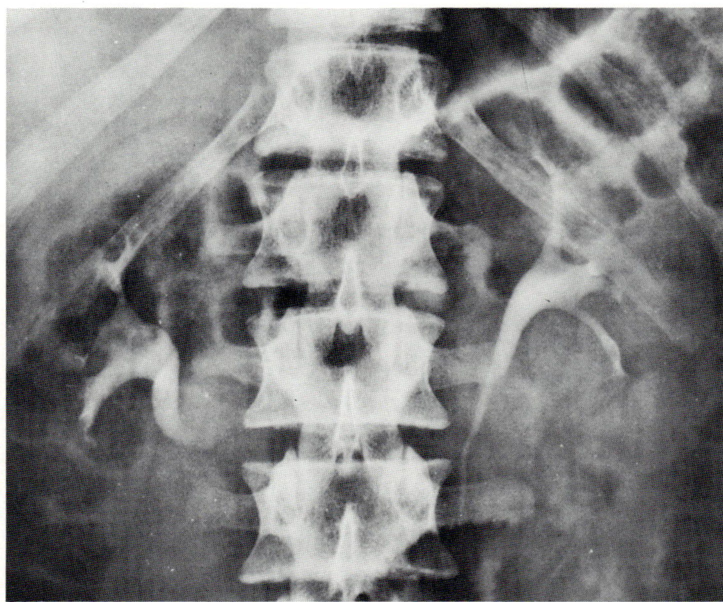

B

FIG. 4.39 A and B. This 16-year-old male sustained blunt abdominal trauma with rupture of the spleen, requiring splenectomy. His **(A)** preoperative excretory urogram shows spasm of the left upper and lower pole collecting systems consistent with renal contusion. The **(B)** postoperative excretory urogram shows persistence of these findings, particularly in the left lower pole, but with some internal improvement.

be secondary to previous inflammatory (chronic pyelonephritis, glomerulonephritis, etc.) or noninflammatory (preexisting renal vascular disease or renal infarction, renal hypoplasis, etc.) disorders.

Posttraumatic thrombosis of the renal artery is being reported with increasing frequency [14,61,86,121]. The left renal artery is more frequently involved than the right. Renal-artery thrombosis may occur as a result of decrease in perfusion of the kidney from hypotension and hypovolemia, perirenal pedicle compression, and arterial spasm. The early diagnosis of posttraumatic renal artery thrombosis is mandatory if the kidney is to be salvaged.

Diffuse but moderate enlargement of the kidney may be secondary to the accumulation of edema fluid and is not necessarily indicative of a significant renal lesion. However, the intact renal capsule may prevent significant enlargement of the renal silhouette despite extensive kidney injury with intraparenchymal extravasation of blood and urine. Marked enlargement of the kidney frequently follows trauma to the renal vein, resulting in gross laceration and destruction of the vein or in the formation of thrombus within it. Localized enlargement of the kidney is suggestive of either focal injury or localized accumulation of subcapsular blood or urine.

Following trauma, focal nephrographic defects are highly suggestive of areas of ischemia. Fissures in the nephrogram raise the possibility of either ischemia or renal fracture. Caution must be used in the interpretation of such radiologic findings, since they may be due to other unrelated pathologic disorders.

The demonstration of extravasation of contrast, either intraparenchymal, perirenal, or pararenal, is one of the most reliable signs of significant injury to the kidney (Tables 4.60–4.62, Figs. 4.40 and 4.41). One infrequently occurring exception is spontaneous urinary extravasation on an excretory urogram. Such extravasation has been demonstrated to occur as a result of fornical microtears. The underlying cause for such tears is acute or chronic ureteric obstruction [152]. However, in the setting of abdominal trauma, extravasation of contrast must be considered diagnostic of renal injury until proved otherwise.

Defects in the renal collecting system or obstruction may be due to preexisting, unrelated renal lesions. However in a setting of abdominal trauma, blood clots, extrarenal hematomas producing strictures, and disruption of the collecting system must be considered.

Ultrasonography of the Kidney. The retroperitoneum is poorly visualized by most radiologic techniques. Ultrasound and computed tomography have increased the ability "to see and diagnose" lesions in the retroperitoneal area. As Pollack and Goldberg [58] indicate, "ultrasound has the unique attribute of being indepen-

TABLE 4.60. Blunt renal injuries

	Minor	Intermediate	Major
Hematuria	Mild, remitting		Severe, unremitting; none
Urography	Normal, delayed/diminished function	?	Nonfunction
Vital signs	Normal, stable		Unstable, unacceptable

Source: Peterson NE (1977) Intermediate-degree blunt renal trauma. J Trauma 17(6): 425–435

TABLE 4.61. Renal trauma series, major blunt injuries

	Pedicle (9)	Shattered (3)
No X-ray	3	1
Nonfunction	6	3
Arteriography	2	1
Severe nonrenal injury	6	3
Extravasation	1	0
Nephrectomy	7	2
Heminephrectomy	1	1

Source: Peterson NE (1977) Intermediate-degree blunt renal trauma. J Trauma 17(6): 425–435

TABLE 4.62. Renal trauma series, intermediate blunt injuries (20)

No IVP	6
Nonfunction	1
Extravasation	8
Parenchymal fracture	19
Arteriogram	8 (7[a])
Serious nonrenal injury	8 (6[b])
Nephrectomy	9
Heminephrectomy	2
Nondefinitive surgery	2[b]

[a] Nonoperative.
[b] No arteriography.
Source: Peterson NE (1977) Intermediate-degree blunt renal trauma. J Trauma 17(6): 425–435

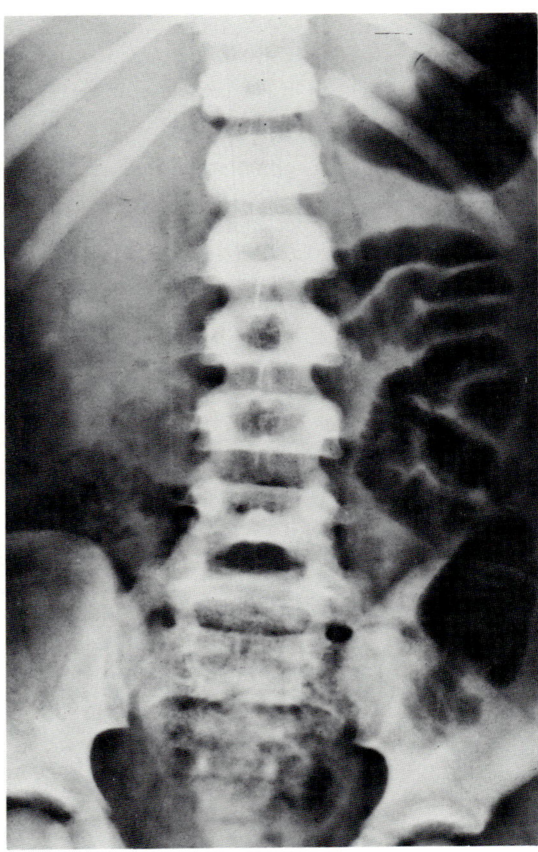

A

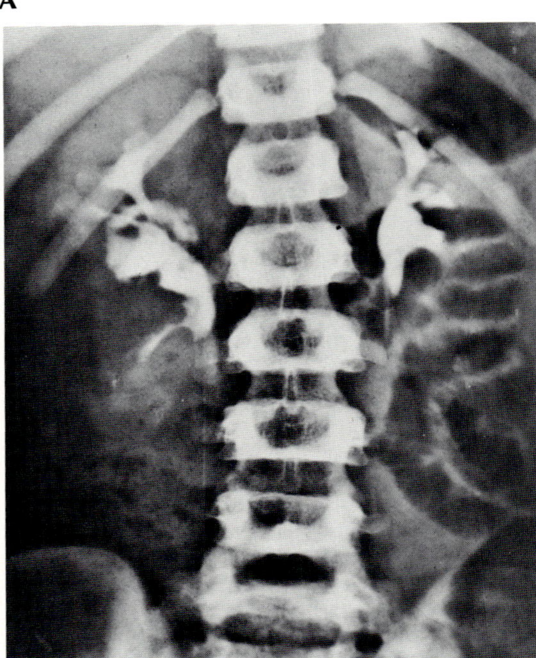

B

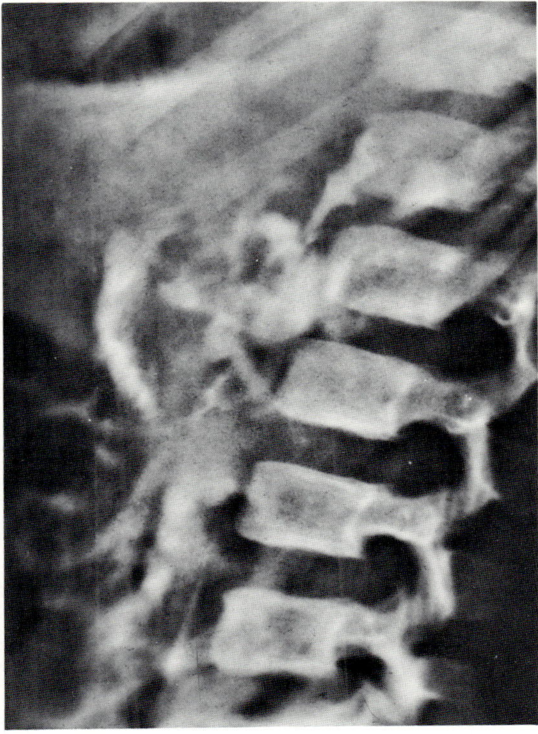

C

FIG. 4.40 A–C. This 6-year-old female was admitted following blunt abdominal trauma. The **(A)** AP supine view of the abdomen reveals a levoscoliosis of the lumbar spine with loss of the right renal and psoas silhouettes. A soft-tissue mass is present in the right flank. There are no fractures. The **(B)** AP and **(C)** lateral views from her excretory urogram reveal contrast extravasation from the right kidney into the perirenal space and lack of visualization of the right lower pole collecting system and ureter. At exploration, a fractured right kidney was found and removed. Courtesy of Dr. Bhatt.

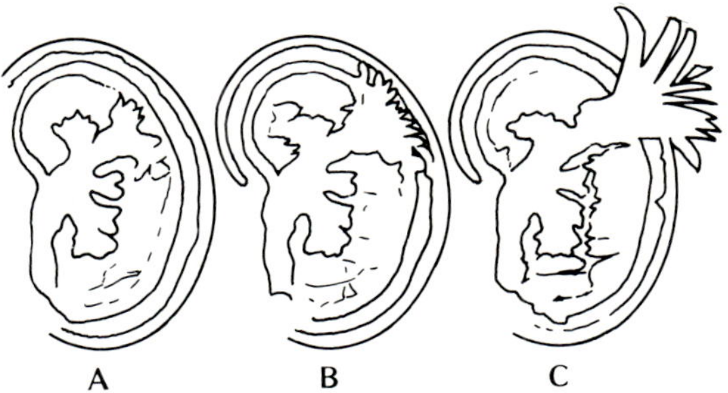

FIG. 4.41. Grading of urinary extravasation. **(A)** Intraparenchymal. **(B)** Extracapsular. **(C)** Retroperitoneal. From Peterson NE (1977) Intermediate degree blunt renal trauma. J Trauma 17(6): 425–435

dent of renal function for its imaging properties. Thus, in the presence of poor renal function, ultrasound appears to be the most satisfactory, non-invasive method of examining the kidneys." As a reasonable routine in evaluating the traumatized patient, ultrasound should be the diagnostic method of choice to follow excretory urography whether the contrast study is positive or negative. While providing additional information about the retroperitoneal areas and the kidneys, ultrasonography can also demonstrate the presence or absence of intraperitoneal fluid and other intraperitoneal abnormalities. Doust et al. [43] state that the advantage of ultrasound studies over conventional radiologic techniques lies in their ability to distinguish fluid-filled structures from solid lesions. Whether due to trauma or some other cause, three major mass-imaging patterns may be demonstrated in the renal area: (a) a cystic mass with a sharply defined, echo-free zone with strong far-wall echoes; (b) a complex mass, similar in its imaging pattern to a cystic mass, except for the presence of echo-generating internal reflecting interfaces; and (c) a solid mass with the capacity to generate internal echoes that increase in number and intensity as the sensitivity of the equipment is increased and that shows much weaker distal-wall echoes due to the greater ultrasound absorption as the beam passes through the mass. Hematomas, which appear as cystic lesions while the blood is fresh, develop the complex pattern when clotting occurs. When hematomas are associated with renal parenchymal injuries such as contusion, the presence of a contused kidney may be determined on ultrasonography by disruption of the renal capsule and the demonstration of extra echoes within the renal parenchyma. Intracapsular hematomas present, on ultrasonography, as cystic lesions that have the tendency to flatten the affected kidney, giving it a characteristic thin, longitudinal configuration. Renal-vein thrombosis often results in enlargement of the kidney and the presence of increased echoes in the area of the renal pelvis associated with hemorrhage into the pelvis. Renal-artery occlusion may be suggested by a combination of nonvisualization of the affected kidney on excretory urography and a slight decrease in size of an otherwise ultrasonically normal kidney. Urinomas may simulate renal or perirenal hemorrhage since these entities are indistinguishable on ultrasound studies. However, the excretory urogram may be helpful by demonstrating extravasation of contrast and/or the classic pattern of a urinoma (mass).

Although ultrasonography may not differentiate the various types of collections of fluid in the retroperitoneum, it is possible to distinguish fluid from a solid mass. In general, collections of fluid tend to enhance the clarity with which the walls of the aorta and the inferior vena cava are detected. Retroperitoneal solid masses, such as lymph nodes, often obscure the walls of the great vessels and usually do not enhance sound-transmission.

Fluid within the peritoneal cavity can be detected by ultrasound. In general, the presence of fluid increases transonicity. Whereas free fluid, such as blood, may show echoes within it due to the presence of clotted material, localized collections of fluid have sharply defined walls and are indented by adjacent organs. Other masses showing a complex cystic pattern, such as inflammatory collections of fluid, have a football-like shape of their own and tend to indent or displace structures around them.

Angiography in Renal Trauma. The first angiographic study of a patient with renal trauma was performed in 1957 [145]. Angiography remains the most accurate diagnostic tool in renal trauma currently available. It can establish the presence, extent, and significance of a traumatic renal lesion. The indications for its use are: nonvisualization of the kidney on excretory urogram; clinical evidence of severe renal trauma with a nondiagnostic excretory urogram or ultrasonogram; the need for evaluation of the vascular supply, extent of injury, and integrity of the opposite kidney prior to surgery for renal trauma; for evaluation of other abdominal viscera; to evaluate penetrating wounds in the area of the kidney; to rule out the presence of a renal tumor; and for evaluation of the late complications of a traumatic renal lesion.

Renal Contusion. The most common renal lesion following trauma is the simple contusion. The diagnosis of renal contusion implies an intact renal parenchyma with some degree of ecchymosis or hematoma contained within an intact renal capsule. Once injury is severe enough to rupture the renal capsule, usually an underlying renal laceration results. However, a renal laceration may occur within an intact renal capsule.

The reported incidence of renal contusion varies with the type and location of the receiving hospital. In a large trauma center such as the Los Angeles General Hospital, the incidence of renal contusion is 5.7% of all cases of renal trauma (10 in 177 cases) whereas at a more specialized center the incidence may be higher. The series reported by Glenn and Howard gives an incidence of 64% [56].

Classically, the angiographic finding in a renal contusion is a swollen kidney with or without slow arterial flow. However, a normal renal angiogram is not uncommon.

Injury to the Renal Pedicle (Fig. 4.42). Injury to the vascular pedicle of the kidney implies severe trauma.

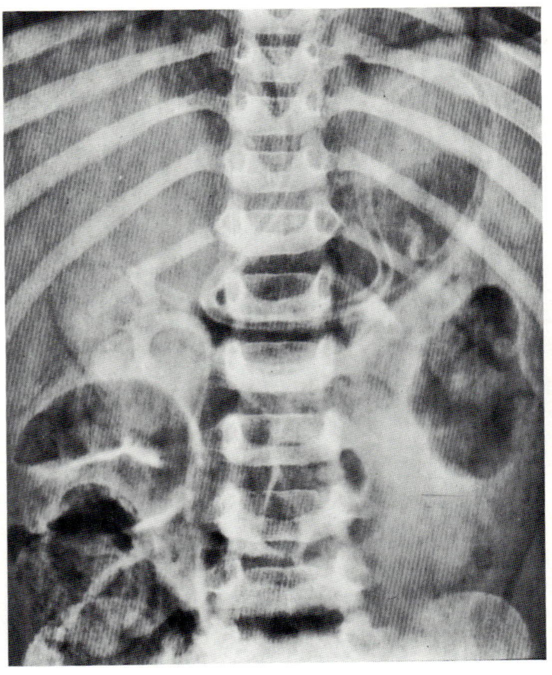

A

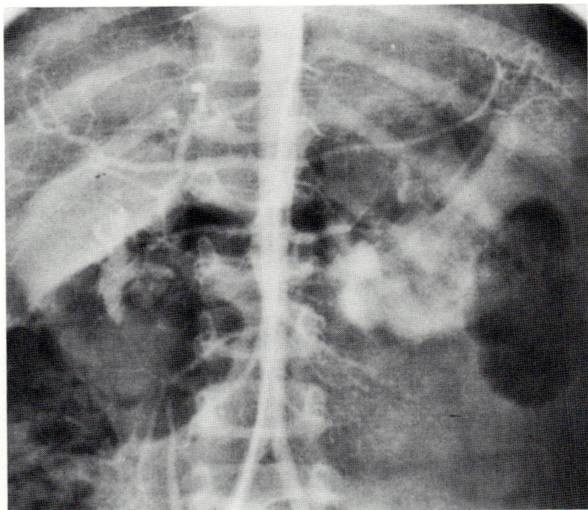

B

FIG. 4.42 A and B. This pediatric patient presented with a history of blunt abdominal trauma. An **(A)** emergency excretory urogram reveals a fracture through the left 9th rib, loss of the left renal and psoas silhouettes, and the suggestion of a left flank mass. There is poor-to-absent visualization of the left kidney. A **(B)** flush aortogram reveals partial transection of the distal left renal artery and poor perfusion of the left kidney. At exploration, a shattered left kidney and partial transection of the left renal artery were found.

Such injury occurs in 6% to 20% of all cases of renal trauma. In most cases, other organs and other segments of the vascular system are traumatized. Anatomically, the renal artery and vein are relatively secure, but if the trauma is severe enough, traction on these vessels can cause partial or complete avulsion. A complete severance of the renal vascular pedicle may lead to shock and, of course, loss of the kidney. Fortunately, partial avulsion or internal trauma of the major vessels is more common.

Partial avulsion of the renal pedicle may result in extravasation of blood or the development of a pseudoaneurysm or arteriovenous fistulization. Trauma to the vessels within the renal parenchyma can lead to extensive cortical necrosis, since the renal vessels are "end arteries" and no effective collateral circulation exists to allow shunting of blood from other sources. In a series of 33 patients with trauma to the renal pedicle reported by Guerriero et al. [61] (Tables 4.63–4.68, Figs. 4.43–4.46), injury to the renal veins required nephrectomy more commonly than did injury to the arteries. The left renal vein was more frequently injured, very likely because of its greater length and its exposed midline position. When this vein was injured, a higher incidence of associated vascular injuries and a much higher overall mortality rate (47%) were noted.

With renal-artery injury, the angiogram may demonstrate evidence of extravasation of contrast. The angiographic findings of thrombosis, however, are more

TABLE 4.63. Type of injury

	No. of patients	Deaths	%
Penetrating	27	10	37
Large caliber or high velocity	12	5	41
Small caliber or low velocity	9	3	33
Stab wound, single	2	0	0
Stab wound, multiple	1	1	100
Shotgun	3	1	33
Blunt	6	2	33
Total	33	12	36

Source: Guerriero WG, Carlton CE Jr, Scott R Jr, Beall ACJ (1971) Renal pedicle injuries. J Trauma 11(1): 53–62

TABLE 4.64. Solitary pedicle injuries

	No. of patients	Nephrectomies	%	Deaths	%
Veins	20	6	30	7	35
Arteries	3	1	33	0	0
Total	23	7	30	7	30

Source: Guerriero WG, Carlton CE Jr, Scott R Jr, Beall ACJ (1971) Renal pedicle injuries. J Trauma 11(1): 53–62

TABLE 4.65. Renal-artery injuries

	Injuries	Deaths	Nephrectomies
Left	7	1	2
Right	7	3	5
Total	14	4	7

Source: Guerriero WG, Carlton CE Jr, Scott R Jr, Beall ACJ (1971) Renal pedicle injuries. J Trauma 11(1): 53–62

TABLE 4.66. Renal-pedicle injuries and associated vascular injuries related to mortality

Injured vessels	No. of patients	Deaths (%)	Deaths from hemorrhage (%)
1	12	17	8
2	11	18	9
3	8	75	50
4	2	100	100

Source: Guerriero WG, Carlton CE Jr, Scott R Jr, Beall ACJ (1971) Renal pedicle injuries. J Trauma 11(1): 53–62

TABLE 4.67. Renal-pedicle and associated visceral injuries

	Injuries	Deaths	%
Liver	18	7	39
Stomach	8	3	38
Colon	7	4	57
Spleen	6	1	17
Small bowel	5	4	80
Common bile duct	3	1	33
Adrenal	2	0	0
Gallbladder	1	0	0

Source: Guerriero WG, Carlton CE Jr, Scott R Jr, Beall ACJ (1971) Renal pedicle injuries. J Trauma 11(1): 53–62

TABLE 4.68. Renal pedicle and injuries to pancreas and duodenum

	No. of patients	Deaths	%
Pancreas	8	2	25
Duodenum	2	0	0
Combined pancreas and duodenum	7	4	57

Source: Guerriero WG, Carlton CE Jr, Scott R Jr, Beall ACJ (1971) Renal pedicle injuries. J Trauma 11(1): 53–62

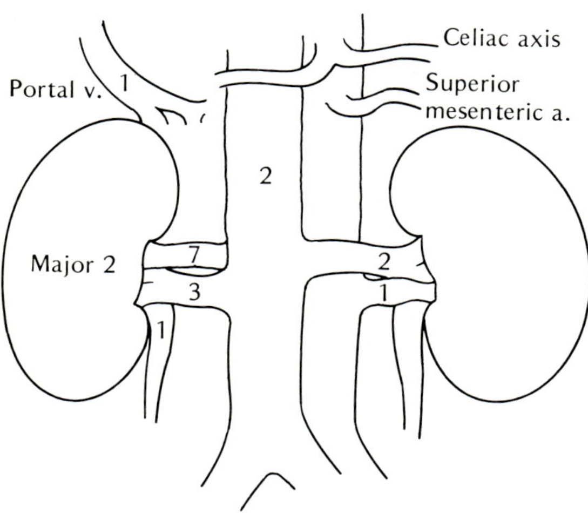

FIG. 4.43. Right renal artery injuries and associated vascular injuries (7 injuries, 3 deaths, and 5 nephrectomies—never injured alone). From Guerriero WG, Carlton CE Jr, Scott R Jr, Beall AC Jr (1971) Renal pedicle injuries. J Trauma 11(1): 53–62

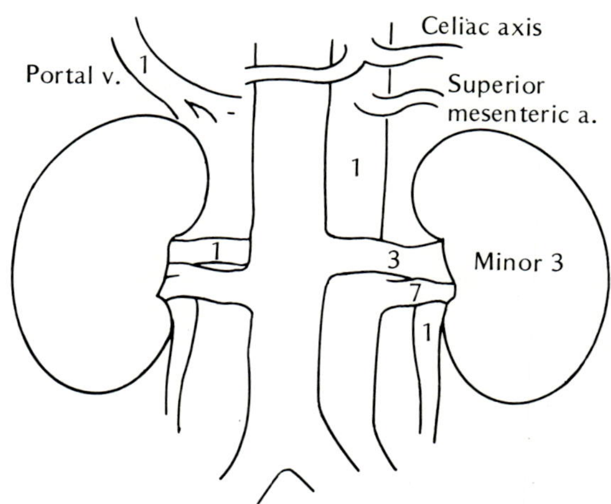

FIG. 4.44. Left renal artery injury and associated vascular injuries (7 injuries, 1 death, 2 nephrectomies, and 3 solitary renal artery injuries). From Guerriero WG, Carlton CE Jr, Scott R Jr, Beall AC Jr (1971) Renal pedicle injuries. J Trauma 11(1): 53–62

commonly observed. Renal-artery thrombosis is demonstrated by abrupt "cut off" of the affected vessel and/or by the demonstration of intraluminal defects. Usually, fusiform dilatation of the renal artery proximal to the thrombosis results.

Angiographic evidence of injury to the renal vein is suggested by the presence of renal enlargement with poor visualization of the parenchyma and of the pelvocalyceal system. Splaying of intrarenal arteries, faint or prolonged nephrographic opacification, and nonvisualization of the renal vein will also occur.

The presence of an intrarenal hematoma is manifested by the demonstration of a poorly marginated defect in the parenchymal phase with stretching and

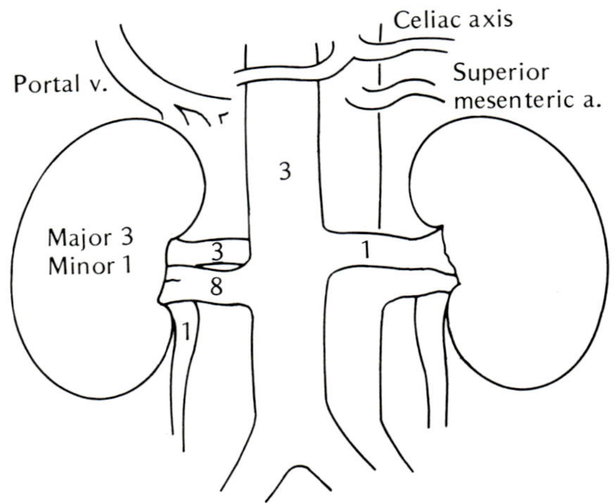

FIG. 4.45. Right renal vein injury and associated vascular injuries (8 injuries, 3 deaths, 6 nephrectomies, and 3 solitary injuries to right renal vein). From Guerriero WG, Carlton CE Jr, Scott R Jr, Beall AC Jr (1971) Renal pedicle injuries. J Trauma 11(1): 53–62

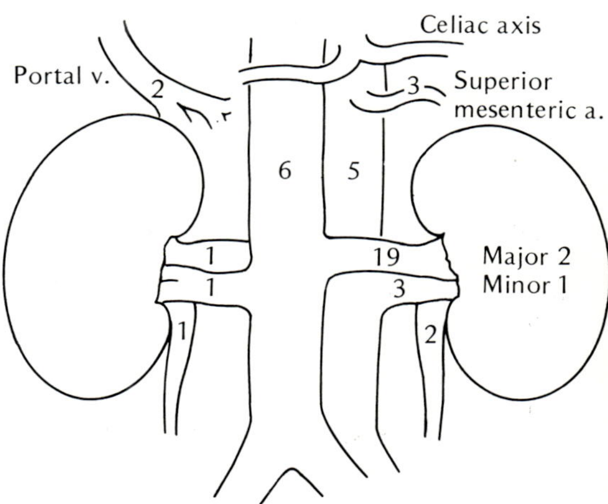

FIG. 4.46. Left renal vein injury and associated vascular injuries (19 injuries, 9 deaths, 5 nephrectomies, and 5 solitary left renal vein injuries). From Guerriero WG, Carlton CE Jr, Scott R Jr, Beall AC Jr (1971) Renal pedicle injuries. J Trauma 11(1): 53–62

displacement of the arteries in this area in the arterial phase.

Fractures and lacerations of the kidney are angiographically demonstrated by separation and stretching of the arterial branches, separation or sequestration of renal fragments, extravasation of contrast material, and, on occasion, the presence of arteriovenous fistulae.

With perirenal hematoma, a parenchymal defect is usually absent. An avascular mass directly adjacent to the renal parenchyma is outlined by displaced and stretched capsular arteries. At the point of contact of the avascular mass with the renal parenchyma, a zone of increased density secondary to compression of the renal parenchyma by the subcapsular hematoma may be observed.

Retroperitoneal Hematoma. The major angiographic findings in retroperitoneal hematoma are stretching and displacement of the lumbar and other retroperitoneal vessels. The hematoma may be suspected on plain films by the presence of a retroperitoneal mass obliterating the psoas density, distortion of the axis of the kidney, and medial displacement of ureters (Fig. 4.47, Tables 4.69–4.71).

Lang [83] has used the angiographic findings to classify the severity of renal injury, thereby determining the management and prognosis. He divides the radiologic features into three separate groups: (a) findings consistent with reversibility, requiring only conservative management; (b) findings which are irreversible but still indicate conservative medical management; and (c) findings suggesting the necessity for surgical intervention (Table 4.72).

TABLE 4.69. Renal trauma and retroperitoneal hematomas: Sex and age of patients

	Sex		Age (years)		
	%	No.		%	No.
Male	78	144	0 to 9	7	13
			10 to 19	22	41
Female	22	41	20 to 29	34	63
	100	185	30 to 39	15	27
			40 to 49	9	17
			50 to 59	8	15
			60 to 69	4	8
			≥70	1	1
				100	185

Source: Holcroft JW, Trunkey DD, Minagi H, Korobkin MT, Lim RC (1975) Renal trauma and retroperitoneal hematomas—Indications for exploration. J Trauma 15(12): 1045–1052

TABLE 4.70. Renal trauma and retroperitoneal hematomas: Mechanism of injury

	%	No.
Blunt trauma	71	131
Motor vehicle accident	35	64
Motor vehicle versus pedestrian	8	14
Assault	14	26
Fall	11	20
Other	4	7
Penetrating trauma	29	54
Gunshot wound	19	35
Stab wound	10	19

Source: Holcroft JW, Trunkey DD, Minagi H, Korobkin MT, Lim RC (1975) Renal trauma and retroperitoneal hematomas—Indications for exploration. J Trauma 15(12): 1045–1052

FIG. 4.47 A and B. This young female was in an automobile accident and received multiple injuries. Her **(A)** admission chest examination shows fractures of the distal left clavicle, the bilateral scapulae, and bilateral ribs. A right pneumothorax is present. A **(B)** retrograde cystogram does not show evidence of contrast extravasation, but there is deformity of the bladder indicative of a perivesical hematoma. In addition, there are multiple, bilateral anterior pelvic fractures, subluxation of the left sacroiliac joint, and dislocation of the right hip. The right psoas and lower right renal silhouettes are absent, suggesting the presence of a retroperitoneal hematoma. A soft-tissue band in the right paracolic gutter *(curved open arrow)* suggests the presence of free intraperitoneal fluid.

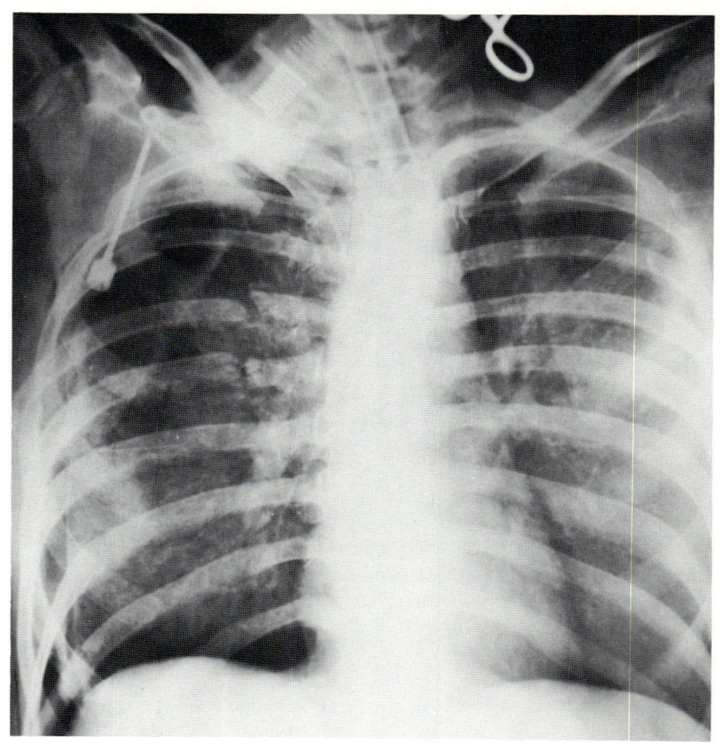

A

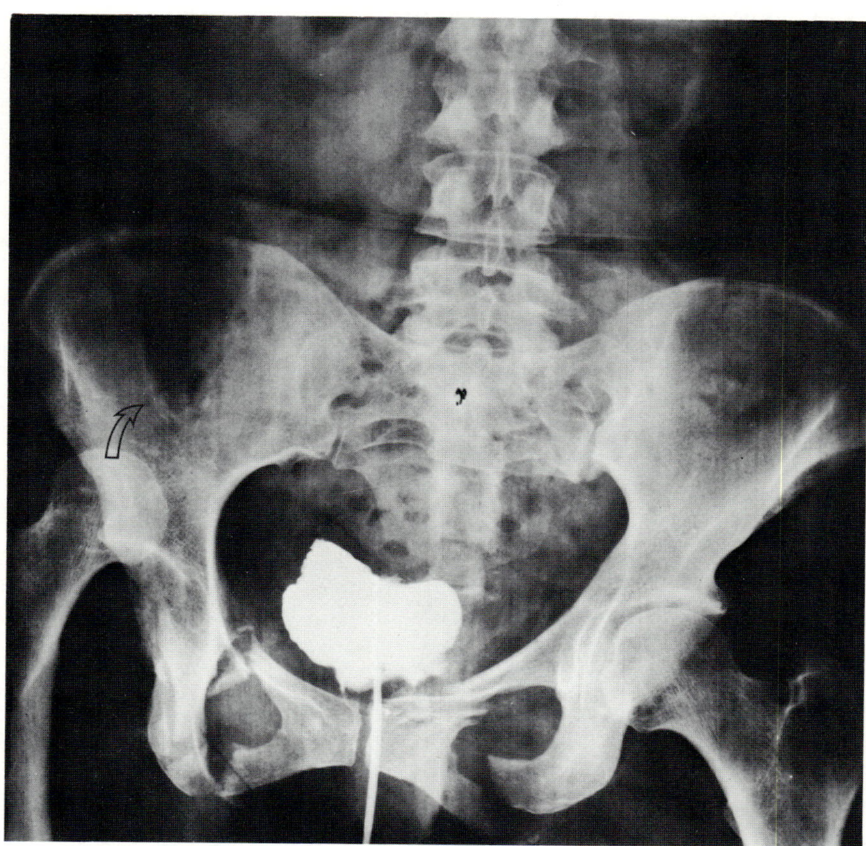

B

The reversible findings consist of slowing of the arterial flow, cortical ischemia, stasis of contrast in small vessels, disassociation of the arterial and venous phases with premature opacification of the medullary veins, and cortical infarcts with prolonged opacification of the dilated arterial segment proximal to the obstruction.

TABLE 4.71. Renal trauma and retroperitoneal hematomas—Roentgen findings in 81 preoperative urograms

	%	No.
Normal urograms	36	29
Abnormal urograms	64	52
Incomplete filling of affected kidney	77	40
Extravasation	23	12
Displaced renal shadow	12	6
Ureteral displacement	10	5
Total nonvisualization of affected kidney	8	4
Obstruction	4	2

Source: Holcroft JW, Trunkey DD, Minagi H, Korobkin MT, Lim RC (1975) Renal trauma and retroperitoneal hematomas—Indications for exploration. J Trauma 15(12): 1045–1052

Findings which usually suggest that the renal lesion can be treated conservatively are the demonstration of unimpaired arterial, parenchymal, and venous circulation in the substance of the kidney adjacent to a fracture (this is usually denoted by a homogeneous staining quality in the parenchymal phase of the arteriogram); minimal separation of the fracture margins (with no evidence of an interposing hematoma); no extravasation of contrast; attenuation and splaying of vessels indicative of intra- and perirenal hematoma without impairment of vascular perfusion of the adjacent parenchyma; and opacification of arteriovenous fistulae without demonstration of significant hemodynamic alteration peripheral to the fistulae.

Features which suggest that surgical management is necessary are marked separation of fracture margins by an interposed hematoma, extravasation of contrast, puddling of contrast in the parenchyma indicating autolysis, hemodynamically significant arteriovenous fistulae (significant siphoning effect resulting in ischemia of the adjacent parenchyma), rupture of the kidney (missing fragments), thrombosis of the main renal artery, severance or avulsion of the main renal arteries, thrombosis of the main renal vein, and severance or avulsion of the main renal vein (Fig. 4.48).

TABLE 4.72. Arteriographic manifestations arranged sequentially to reflect severity of renal injury and its prognostic and management implications

Arteriographic manifestations	Prognosis
1. Slowing of arterial flow	A
2. Cortical ischemia	A
3. Stasis in small veins	A
4. Disassociation of arterial and venous phase	A
5. Premature opacification of medullary veins (shunt mechanism)	A
6. Cortical infarcts; prolonged opacification of the dilated-artery segment proximal to obstruction	A
7. Unimpaired arterial, parenchymal, and venous circulation in parenchyma adjacent to fracture margins (satisfactory and homogeneous staining quality on parenchymal-phase roentgenogram)	B
8. Minimal separation of fracture margins (no interposing hematoma)	B
9. Lack of extravasation of contrast medium (mitigating against active bleeding)	B
10. Attenuation and splaying of vessels indicative of intra- or perirenal hematomas without impairment of vascular perfusion of the adjacent parenchyma	B
11. AV fistulae without hemodynamic significance	B
12. Reduced viability of involved parenchyma (impaired arterial, parenchymal, and venous circulation, mottled staining quality; swiss-cheese appearance)	C (B)
13. Marked separation of fracture margins by interposing hematoma	C
14. Extravasation of contrast medium indicating active bleeding	C (B)
15. Puddling of contrast medium in parenchymal margins indicating autolysis	C
16. Hemodynamically significant AV fistulae (significant siphoning effect and resulting ischemia of adjacent parenchyma)	C
17. Organ rupture (missing fragment of organ)	C
18. Thrombosis of main renal artery	C
19. Severance or avulsion of main renal artery	C
20. Thrombosis of main renal vein	C (B)
21. Severance or avulsion of main renal vein	C

Key: A = Reversible; B = usually managed conservatively (minor permanent deficit or scar); C = necessitating surgical intervention.

Source: Lang EK (1975) Arteriography in the assessment of renal trauma: The impact of arteriographic diagnosis on preservation of renal function and parenchyma. J Trauma 15(7): 553–566

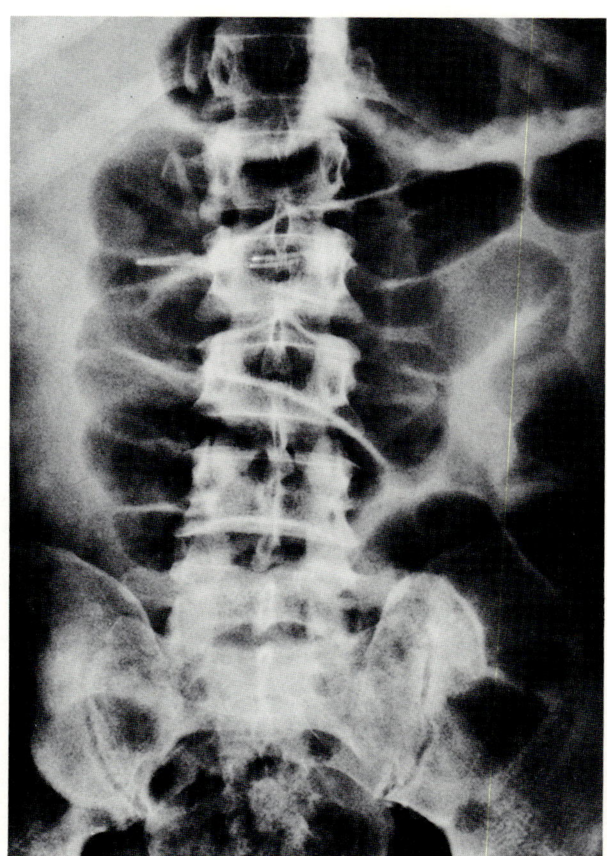

FIG. 4.48 A–C. This 45-year-old male was in an automobile accident and sustained only minimal, obvious trauma to the anterior abdominal wall. However, subsequent to the accident, he noted increasing abdominal girth associated with gross hematuria. His past history was positive for a previous episode of gross hematuria that was said to be due to a ruptured renal cyst. The **(A)** scout film of an excretory urogram shows centralization of bowel loops due to the presence of bilateral flank masses. The **(B)** 15-min film of the excretory urogram shows renal findings consistent with the diagnosis of polycystic disease. Filling defects (blood clots) are present in the right renal collecting system. The **(C)** arterial phase of a selective right renal angiogram reveals a small, nontraumatic aneurysm *(curved open arrow)* arising from the dorsal branch of the renal artery. Distal to this is a site of contrast extravasation *(straight open arrow)* extending from this same dorsal branch to the middle pole collecting system.

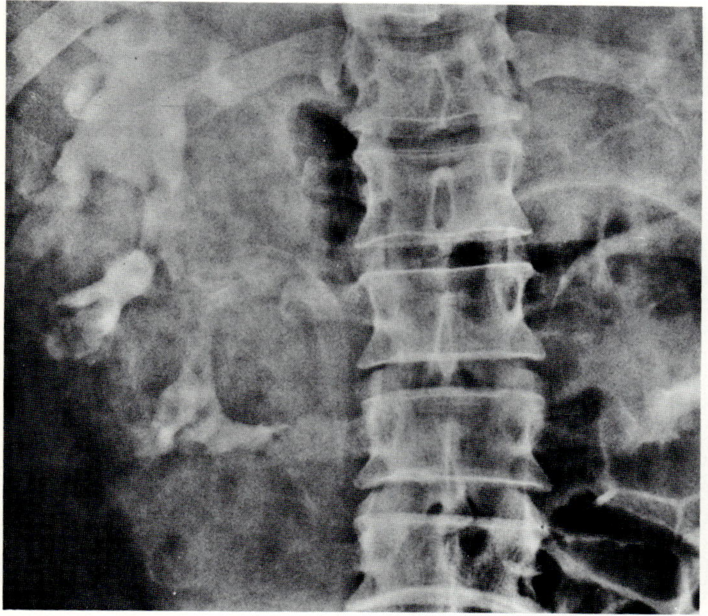

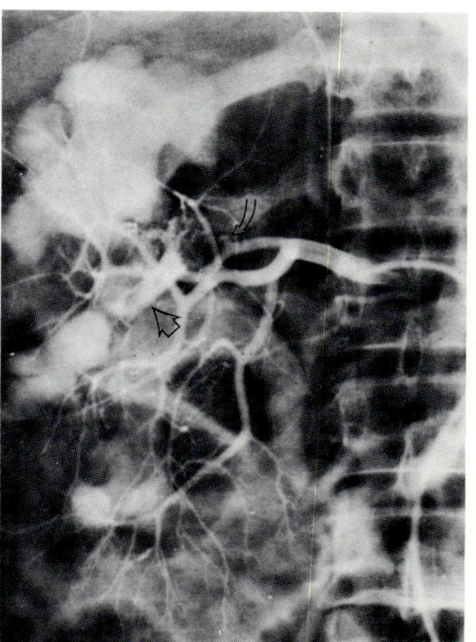

Approximately 5% to 10% of patients who have previously sustained renal trauma will show one of the following late sequelae: calculus formation, persistent urinoma, hydronephrosis, or systemic hypertension. The development of hypertension, representing approximately 4% of the posttraumatic sequelae, is caused by vascular lesions (arterial thrombosis, arteriovenous fistula, segmental infarction, or hematoma) or is the result of renal atrophy and scarring with intrarenal and perirenal calcifications or posttraumatic cyst and aneurysm.

Ureters

The most common cause of ureteral injury is surgical laceration or transection. Penetrating injury is next in frequency, and blunt trauma rarely produces a significant ureteral injury (Table 4.73).

When blunt trauma does occur, it is usually secondary to crush injuries with ureteral lesions produced at the level of L2, L3, and L5 [109]. Tears usually develop at the ureteropelvic junction. If the ureteral injury is isolated and not associated with other genitourinary trauma, hematuria will not occur. A full transection may go undetected until the extravasation of urine produces peritoneal irritation. When unrecognized, the most common presentation of a ureteral injury is a urinary fistula or extravasation of urine into an adjacent area with associated sepsis. If renal function remains intact, these lesions may result in pararenal pseudocysts. Crabtree [116] cites three necessary factors that must be present for the production of a pseudocyst: (a) a transcapsular tear of the renal parenchyma must extend into a calix or the renal pelvis (perforation of the pelvis or ureter alone is often sufficient), (b) the injury must fail to heal or is not sealed by blood clot before any leakage of urine can take place and, (c) ureteral obstruction must be present.

The plain-film radiologic findings suggesting a pararenal pseudocyst include the presence of a soft-tissue mass whose upper border is lateral in the flank as it comes into relationship with the lower pole of the kidney and whose lower border is more medially positioned to overlap the psoas muscle near the level of the iliac crest. The kidney is usually displaced upward, with the lower pole characteristically deviated laterally. The renal outline and upper portion of the psoas muscle remain distinctly outlined by retroperitoneal fat (assuming the absence of significant infiltration of these areas by urine or blood). However, the lower margin of the psoas muscle is obscured by the mass of the pseudocyst. On excretory urography, poor, delayed, or absent function on the side of the lesion is the rule. Hydronephrosis secondary to ureteral compression may also be present. The cystic lesion may

TABLE 4.73. Ureteral injuries, Parkland Memorial Hospital, 1965–1975 (59 cases)

Etiology	
Gunshot wounds	52
Stab wounds	5
Motor vehicle accidents	2
Total	59
Urinalysis of patients with ureteral injury	
Hematuria	32
Gross	(20)
Microscopic	(12)
Normal	19
No urinalysis	8
Infusion pyelographic findings	
Normal	11
Extravasation of contrast material	10
Ureteral dilation	1
Nonvisualizing system	1
Ureteral deviation	1
Bladder displacement	1
Visceral injuries associated with ureteral injury	
Small intestine	41
Large intestine	26
Liver	8
Urinary bladder	6
Duodenum	6
Stomach	4
Gallbladder	2
Pancreas	3
Kidney	2
Spleen	1
Cauda equina	1
Vascular injuries associated with ureteral injury	
Iliac vein	10
Iliac artery	9
Inferior vena cava	9
Hypogastric vein	4
Hypogastric artery	3
Aorta	2
Femoral vein	1
Lumbar vein	1
Mesenteric artery and vein	1
Segmental renal artery	1
Location of ureteral defects	
Upper third	19
Middle third	23
Lower third	17
Total	59

Source: Bright TC, Peters PC (1977) Ureteral injuries due to external violence: Ten years experience with 59 cases. J Trauma 17(8): 616–620

fill with contrast on either excretory urogram or retrograde pyelography. As the ureter courses adjacent to the cyst it is deviated medially, but, on occasion, anterior deviation may occur. The pseudocyst will usually demonstrate the classic pattern on ultrasonography. However, if blood clots are present within the cyst, then a complex cystic pattern will be demonstrated. Angiography will demonstrate changes consistent with a retroperitoneal mass without evidence of either inflammatory or neoplastic hypervascularity. Although angiography is not diagnostic, it may be helpful in evaluating the position and functional state of the kidney on the side of the lesion as well as evaluating the opposite kidney [116].

Urinary Bladder

Before the use of suprapubic diversion, trauma to the bladder resulted in an exceptionally high morbidity and mortality. Infection, peritonitis, and abscess formation were frequent complications and were difficult to treat prior to the use of antibiotics. Chopont in 1792 and Larrey in 1817 advocated tube diversion of the bladder for trauma. It was not until World War I that this technique was widely utilized.

Injury to the urinary bladder is caused by nonpenetrating blunt abdominal trauma in 86% of cases and by penetrating wounds in 14% [22]. Overdistension of the bladder is a predisposing cause to injury from blunt trauma. The most common reasons for distension of the bladder are alcoholism or diseases of the bladder, prostate, or urethra. Four to fifteen percent of patients who have sustained blunt abdominal trauma will develop injuries to the bladder [60]. However, since the bladder is relatively well protected by the bony pelvis, a high association exists between bladder injury and pelvic fractures; 72% of patients with traumatic bladder lesions will have associated pelvic fractures, and 14% of patients with pelvic fractures will demonstrate traumatic lesions of the bladder [22].

Injuries to the bladder are classified as contusions, extraperitoneal ruptures, intraperitoneal ruptures, and combined intra- and extraperitoneal ruptures (Tables 4.74, 4.75) The diagnosis is made by a combination of plain films, cystograms, retrograde cystourethrograms, and excretory urograms. These diagnostic procedures are essential for the complete evaluation of the patient, not only to exclude or to diagnose trauma to the bladder but also to determine the presence (or absence) of associated renal, ureteral, or urethral injuries. In performing retrograde urinary-tract studies, care must be taken that the procedure itself does not worsen the already existing lesion. If evidence of a urethral laceration exists, no attempt should be made to pass a catheter for retrograde studies. However, if the urethra is intact, 150–200 cc of 10% water-soluble contrast should be infused by gravity. Gravity infusion is used to avoid secondary rupture. AP, oblique, and lateral projections of the pelvis are obtained; if no extravasation is demonstrated, additional contrast is injected in order to produce the subjective feelings of distension or until a total of 400 cc has been infused. A repeat radiologic study is performed using AP, lateral, and oblique projections both in the filled and postvoiding states. Cass and Ireland [28] recommend that postvoiding films be obtained after the bladder has been emptied of contrast and washed out with normal saline. Visualization of the bladder in this man-

TABLE 4.74. Cystographic findings in bladder injuries

Contusion	Extraperitoneal rupture	Intraperitoneal rupture
1. Teardrop-shaped bladder 2. Elevation of bladder 3. Obliteration of the soft-tissue planes in the pelvis by hematoma 4. Deviation of the bladder laterally 5. Absence of extravasation of contrast materials	1. Ranges from small lines or streaks to a large stellate or sunburst pattern of extravasated dye 2. Base of the bladder obscured by dye	1. Hourglass pattern when the extravasated contrast medium layer is in the dependent portion of the peritoneal cavity 2. Gas-containing small-bowel loops are surrounded by opaque contrast material 3. Colon is outlined by the contrast medium in an irregular fashion, resulting in a scalloped appearance 4. Opaque linear bands along the peritoneal reflections of the paracolic recesses 5. Contrast medium may outline portions of the diaphragm, liver, and spleen

Source: Brosman SA, Fay R (1973) Diagnosis and management of bladder trauma. J Trauma 13(8): 687–694

TABLE 4.75. Patients with bladder injuries

	Blunt	Penetrating
Contusion	35	
Extraperitoneal	22	2
Intraperitoneal	10	4
Combined	11	6
Total	78	12

Source: Brosman SA, Fay R (1973) Diagnosis and management of bladder trauma. J Trauma 13(8): 687–694

ner is essential since 11% to 15% of bladder ruptures cannot be demonstrated on excretory urograms [22]. Cass and Ireland [28] also note that normal cystograms with bladder rupture have been reported especially with penetrating wounds and with extraperitoneal rupture.

Plain-film examination of the patient with bladder injury may reveal fractures of the bony pelvis, displacement or obliteration of the normal pelvic fat lines (particularly the obturator line), or a soft-tissue haze over the pelvis secondary to the accumulation of blood and other fluids. Other signs of fluid accumulation may also be present.

CONTUSION OF THE URINARY BLADDER

Contusion, with or without a mucosal tear, is the most common type of injury to the bladder and is usually caused by blunt trauma. The presence of a perivesical hematoma should be included as one of the manifestations of contusion. It is important to remember that a perivesical hematoma may "leak" blood into the peritoneal cavity and produce a positive paracentesis without frank laceration of the peritoneum. The radiologic manifestations of perivesical hematoma are a teardrop shape to the bladder, elevation of the bladder secondary to the perivesical hemorrhage, obliteration of the soft-tissue planes in the pelvis by the hematoma, lateral deviation of the bladder, and absence of extravasation of contrast [22].

EXTRAPERITONEAL RUPTURE OF THE BLADDER

This form of rupture (Fig. 4.49) is four times more common than intraperitoneal rupture [22], 80% of these tears occurring in the presence of pelvic fractures. The most common mechanism for the development of this injury is a direct puncture by the bony edges of the associated pelvic fractures with avulsion of the ligamentous moorings of the bladder. The most common site for this laceration is on the anterolateral surface of the bladder near its neck [28,150,183].

The plain-film findings are similar to those described with contusions of the bladder. Retrograde studies define the presence of this lesion by demonstrating extravasation of contrast. The nature and extent of this extravasation will depend on the size and location of the tear of the bladder, the amount of paravesical hemorrhage, and the time-lapse between injection and exposure of the roentgenogram. The extravasation may present as a small, feathery streak or have the appearance of a more characteristic large stellate or sunburst pattern. Since the base of the bladder is usually torn, extravasation results in obscuration of the base of the bladder. The contrast may extend between lacerated muscle bundles or into the paravesical or pararectal spaces. The bladder usually assumes a teardrop appearance. In some instances, where the laceration is not in its usual location, the filled contrast films may appear to be normal. Postevacuation films are needed before a definite statement concerning absence of extravasation can be made. Extravasation on the postvoiding film will appear as an amorphous mass of contrast outside of the normal confines of the bladder.

INTRAPERITONEAL RUPTURE OF THE BLADDER

This form of rupture is one-fourth as frequent as extraperitoneal rupture and is usually due to a direct blow on the dome of the distended bladder (Fig. 4.50) [22,23,150]. As with extraperitoneal rupture, the diagnostic examination of choice is the retrograde cystogram. When positive, this examination will reveal extravasation of contrast into the most dependent portion of the pelvic peritoneal cavity, producing an hourglass configuration of the visualized contrast. The superior portion of the hourglass represents the extravasated contrast, and the inferior portion represents the intact bladder. The superior aspect of the bladder is usually obscured by the contrast, since it is at this site that rupture most frequently occurs. Coating of large and small bowels by contrast; the demonstration of opaque bands of contrast along the peritoneal reflections and into the paracolic gutters; and the outlining of the liver, spleen, or diaphragm by the intraperitoneal accumulation of contrast may be observed.

COMBINED INTRA- AND EXTRAPERITONEAL RUPTURE

Such rupture (Fig. 4.51) is usually produced by a penetrating missile (e.g., knife, bullet, bone spicule). A definite correlation exists between the severity of pelvic injury and the frequency of combined rupture of the bladder. The radiologic findings represent a composite of those described for both intra- and extraperitoneal rupture.

Urethra

Urethral injuries are observed primarily in the male. The location and short length of the female urethra

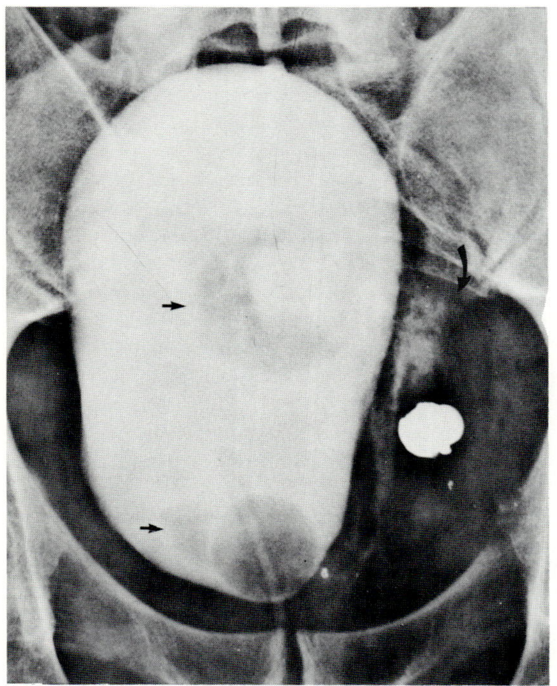

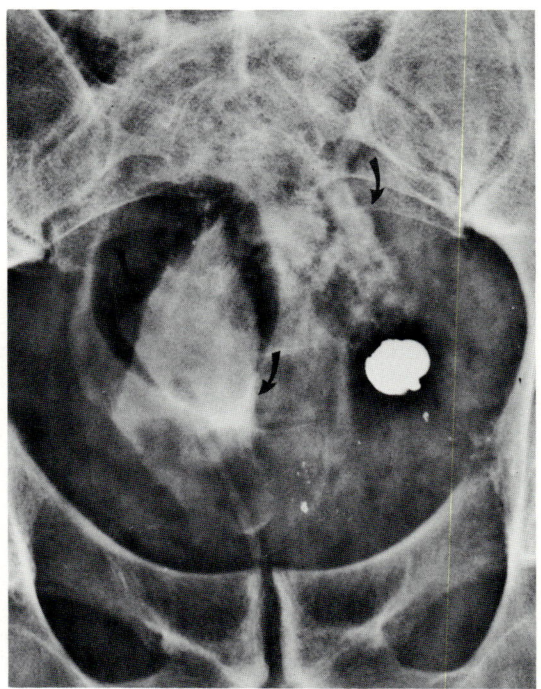

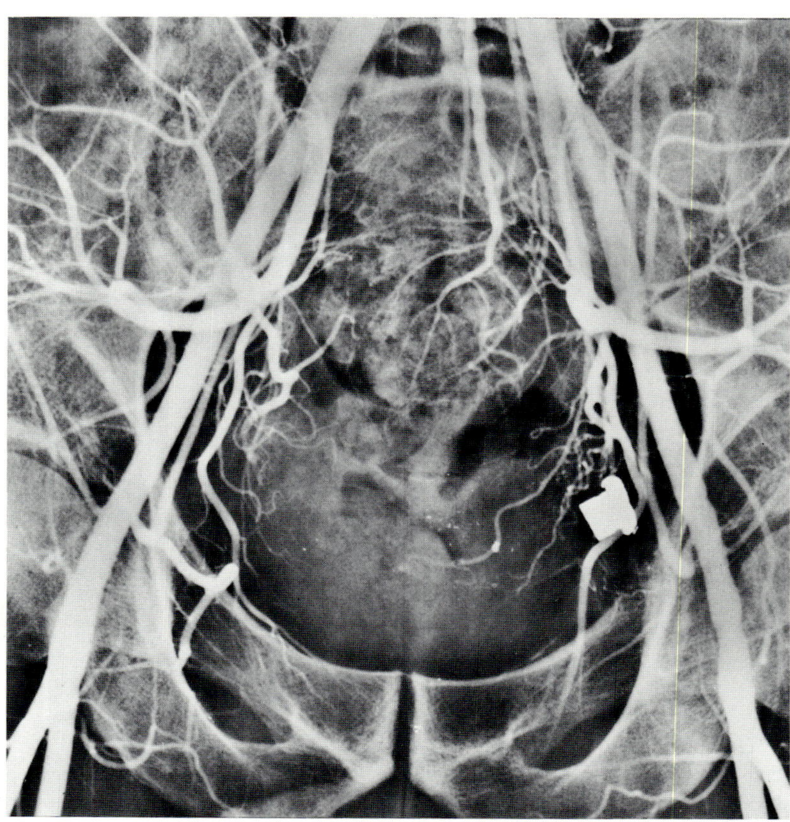

FIG. 4.49 A–C. This 41-year-old male received a gunshot wound to the right buttock. Intravenous pyelography revealed that the bilateral upper collecting systems were normal. The **(A)** bladder is displaced to the right and contains filling defects *(solid arrows)*. There is faint, retroperitoneal contrast extravasation *(curved arrows)* that is better seen on the **(B)** postvoiding film. **(C)** Pelvic angiography did not reveal any evidence of significant vascular injury.

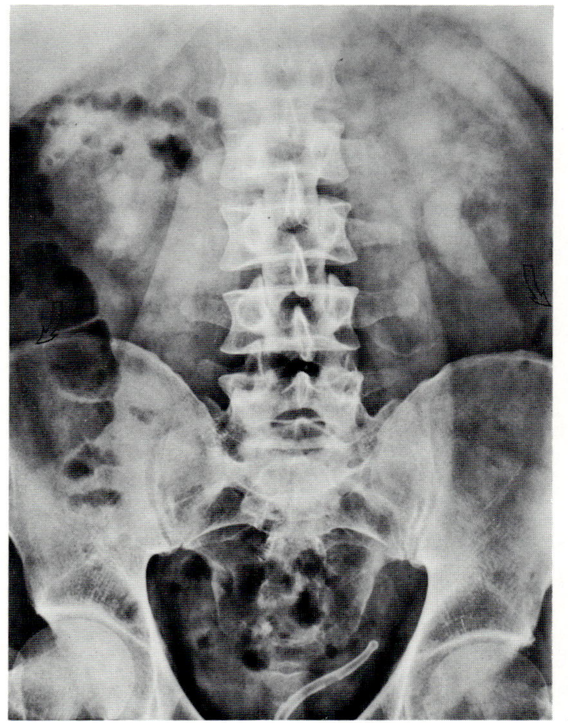

A

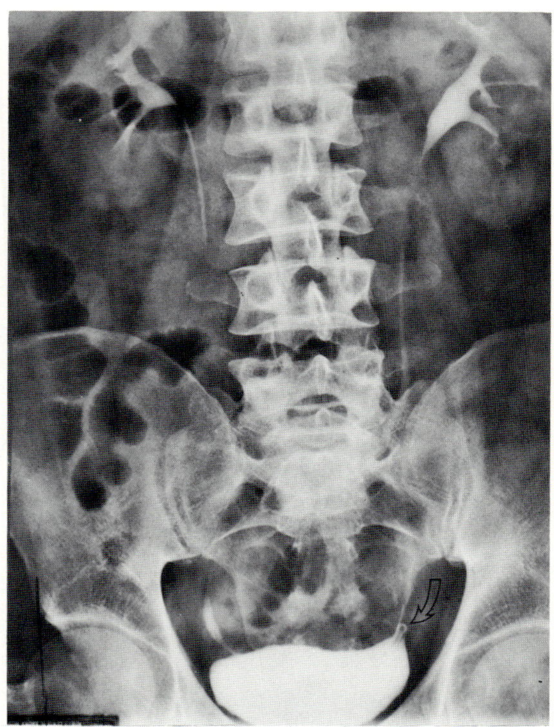

B

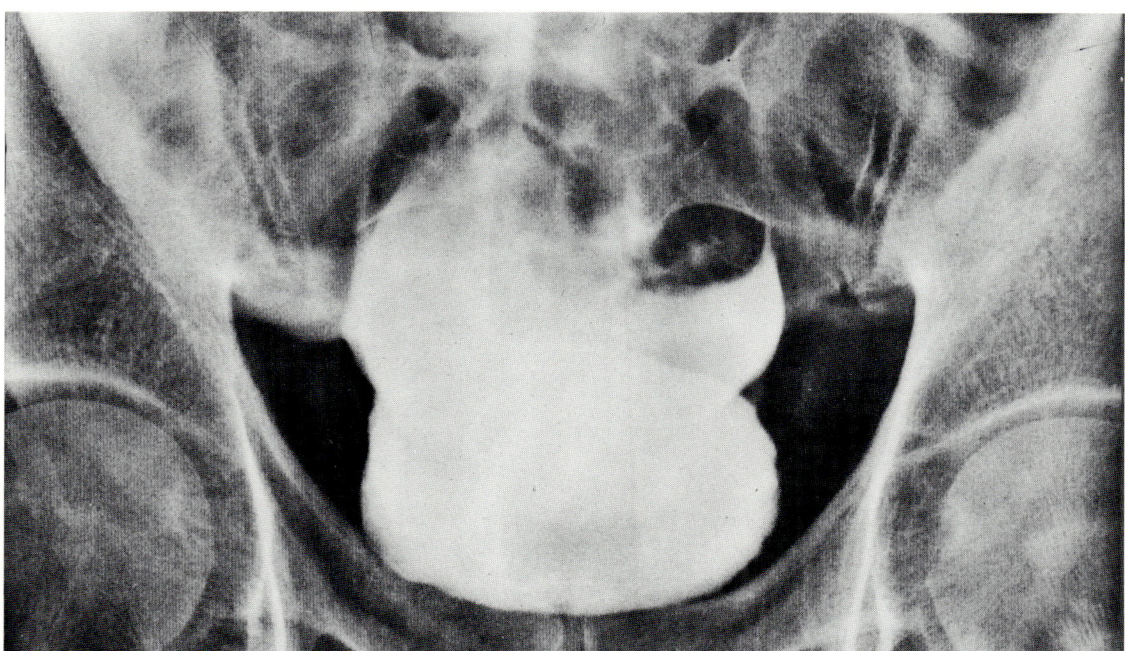

C

FIG. 4.50 A–C. This 40-year-old male was assaulted on the street and sustained blunt trauma to the head and body. The **(A)** scout film of his excretory urogram reveals an indwelling bladder catheter whose position appears abnormal. There is bulging of the flanks with soft-tissue densities *(open arrows)* in the bilateral paracolic gutters consistent with the presence of intraperitoneal fluid. The **(B)** 15-min film of the excretory urogram suggests perforation of the catheter tip through the left bladder wall *(open arrow)*, but there is no contrast extravasation. A **(C)** retrograde cystogram reveals intraperitoneal contrast extravasation. *(Continued)*

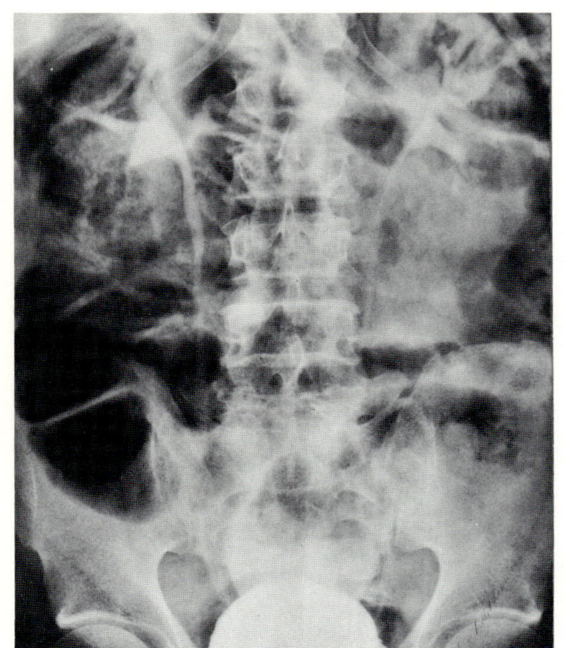

D

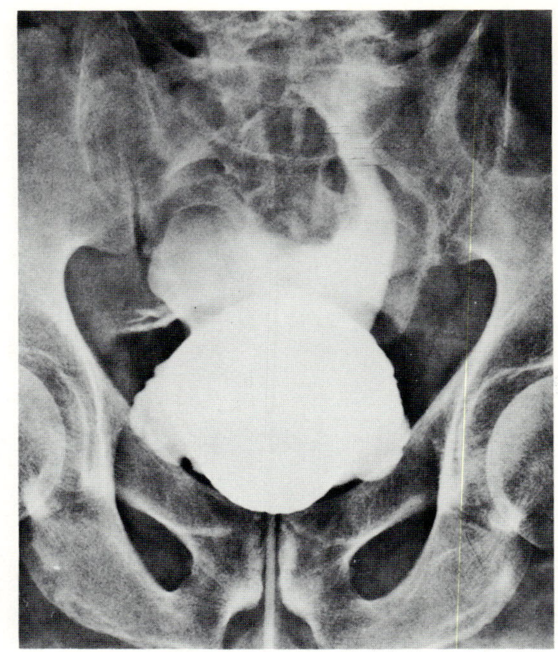

E

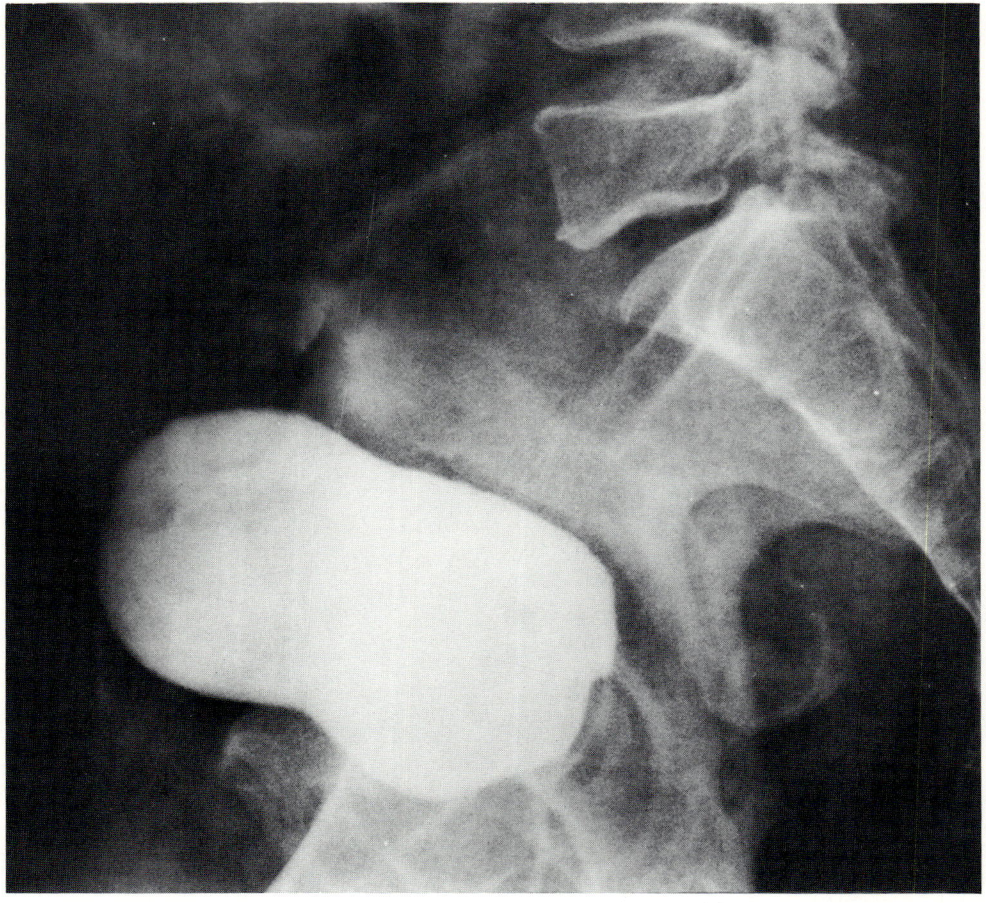

F

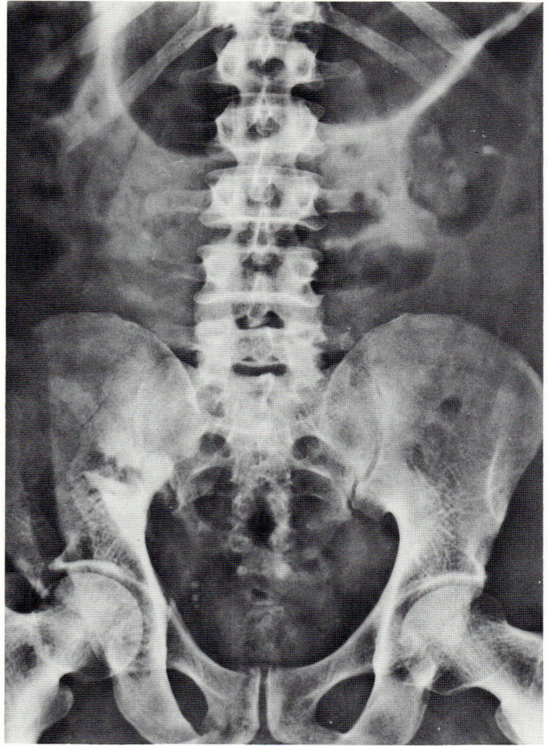

G

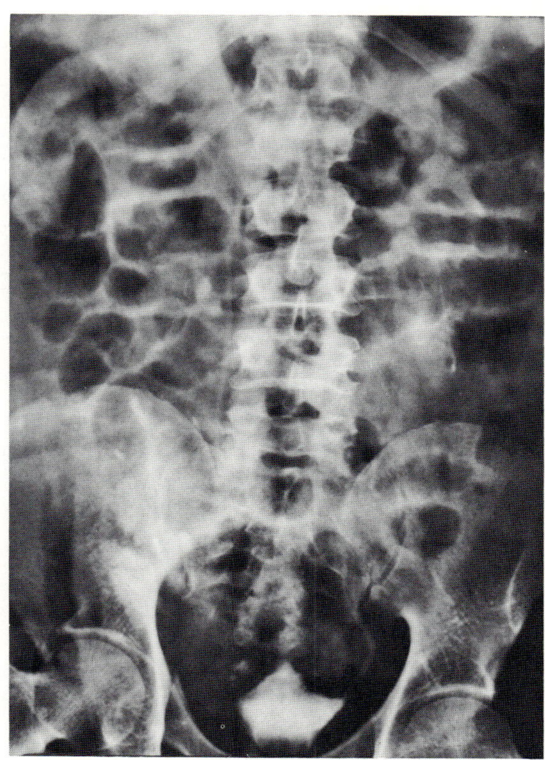

H

FIG. 4.50 D–F. This 49-year-old male was admitted with the history of having fallen on the abdomen and being unable to void since the fall. At the time of his admission, blood was expressed from the urethra. The **(D)** 10-min film of the excretory urogram reveals normal kidneys and upper ureters, but there is a faint suggestion of intraperitoneal contrast extravasation in the pelvis. The **(E)** AP and **(F)** lateral films from the retrograde cystogram show intraperitoneal contrast extravasation from the bladder.

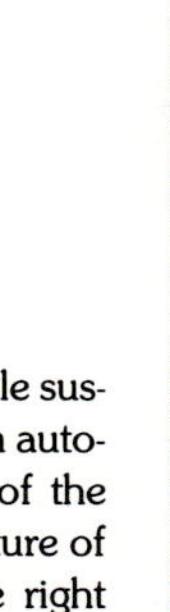

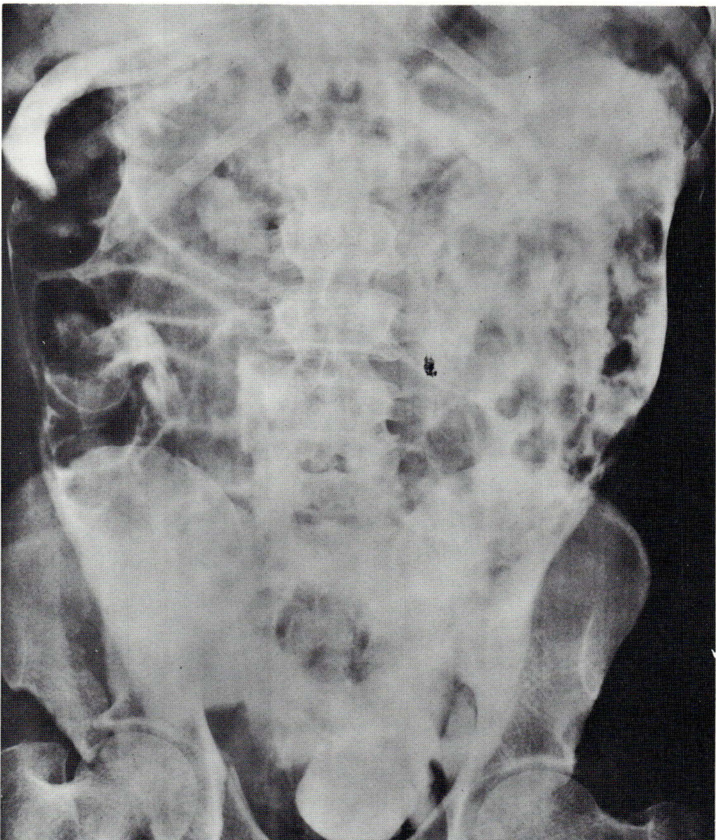

I

FIG. 4.50 G–I. This 40-year-old male sustained blunt trauma as the result of an automobile accident. The **(G)** AP view of the abdomen reveals a comminuted fracture of the right ileum and fractures of the right superior and inferior pubic rami. The **(H)** 20-min film from his excretory urogram shows normal appearing kidneys and ureters. There is poor filling of a deformed bladder and the suggestion of intraperitoneal spread of contrast material. The **(I)** retrograde cystogram reveals extensive intraperitoneal contrast extravasation.

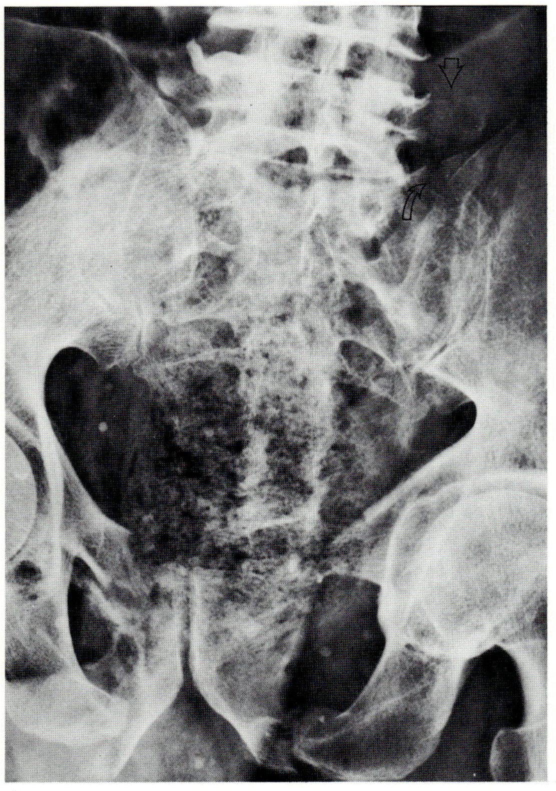

A

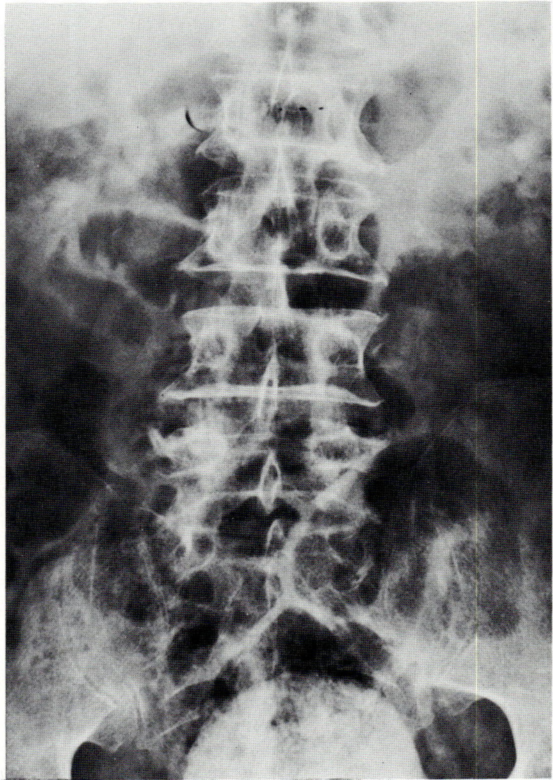

B

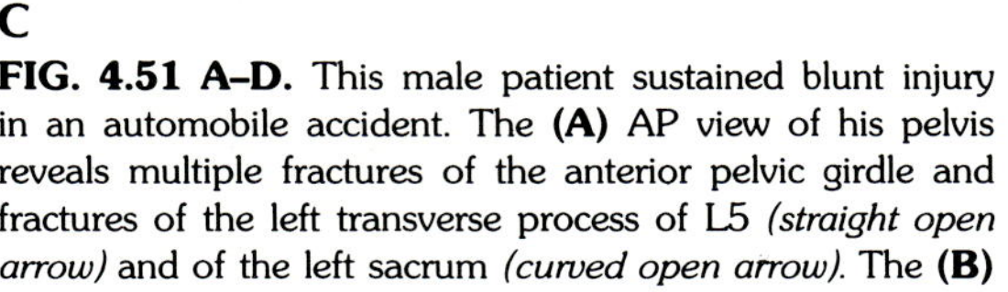

C

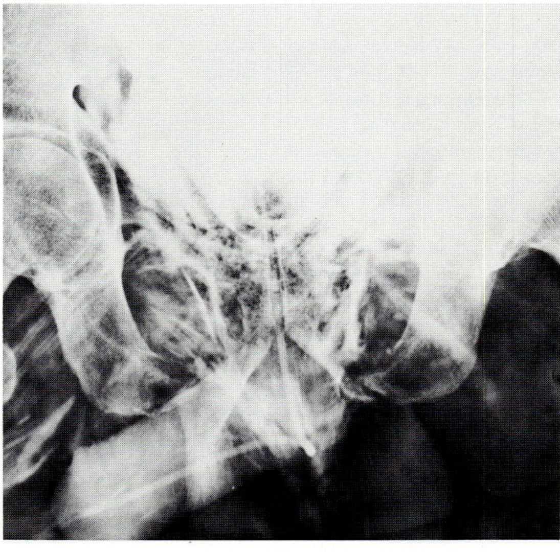

D

FIG. 4.51 A–D. This male patient sustained blunt injury in an automobile accident. The **(A)** AP view of his pelvis reveals multiple fractures of the anterior pelvic girdle and fractures of the left transverse process of L5 *(straight open arrow)* and of the left sacrum *(curved open arrow).* The **(B)** excretory urogram fails to reveal any evidence of injury to the kidneys, ureters, or bladder. The **(C)** and **(D)** retrograde cystogram shows perivesical, retroperitoneal, and intraperitoneal *(straight solid arrow)* contrast extravasation. Courtesy of Dr. Bhatt.

account for its low incidence of injury. If the urethral injury is above the urogenital diaphragm, fracture of the pelvis is usually present, particularly of the pubic and ischial bones; injuries to the urethra below the urogenital diaphragm usually occur without associated skeletal lesions. In addition, the urogenital diaphragm tends to act as a barrier which limits and defines the extravasation of contrast in urethral injuries. Rupture above the diaphragm usually results in extravasation into the perivesical and retroperitoneal soft tissues, whereas rupture below this diaphragm results in extravasation into the perineum and scrotum [108] (Fig. 4.52).

Urethral injury is defined either by the demonstration of extravasation of contrast on excretory urogram or extravasation demonstrated during retrograde studies. Plain-film examination demonstrates pelvic fractures and distortion and/or obliteration of the normal extraperitoneal fat lines, including those around the bladder.

Posterior urethral injuries occur in approximately 15% of patients with pelvic fractures. These injuries should be diagnosed by the demonstration of extravasation either on excretory urogram or retrograde studies. The lesions are significant because of the high frequency of late sequelae which include urethral stricture, impotence (noted in 20% to 30% of patients), and impairment of urinary control.

Injuries to the bulbous portion of the urethra are usually not associated with pelvic fractures. These lesions most frequently occur as a result of a straddle injury (Fig. 4.53).

The penile urethra is the portion of the urethra most infrequently injured, since its mobile nature allows it to withstand traumatic forces more easily. Mild contusion is the most frequent injury sustained. However, in penile erection, penile urethral lacerations may occur. As with other urethral injuries, the diagnosis is made either by excretory urogram with postvoiding films or on retrograde studies.

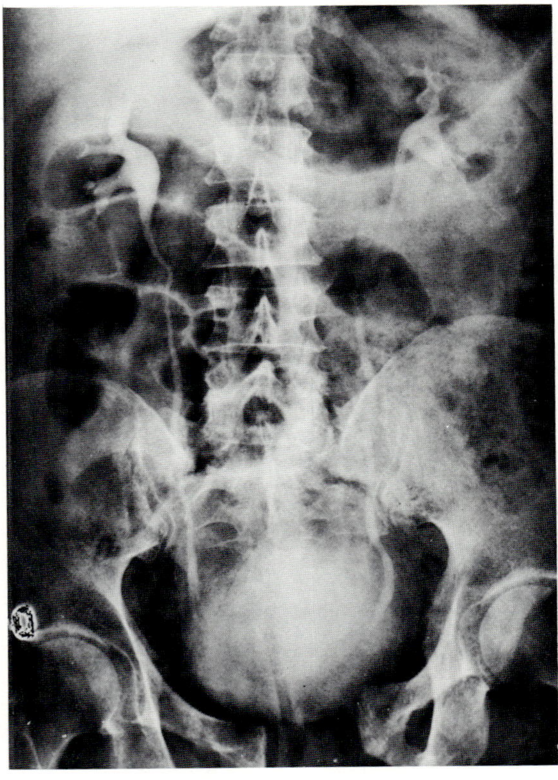

A

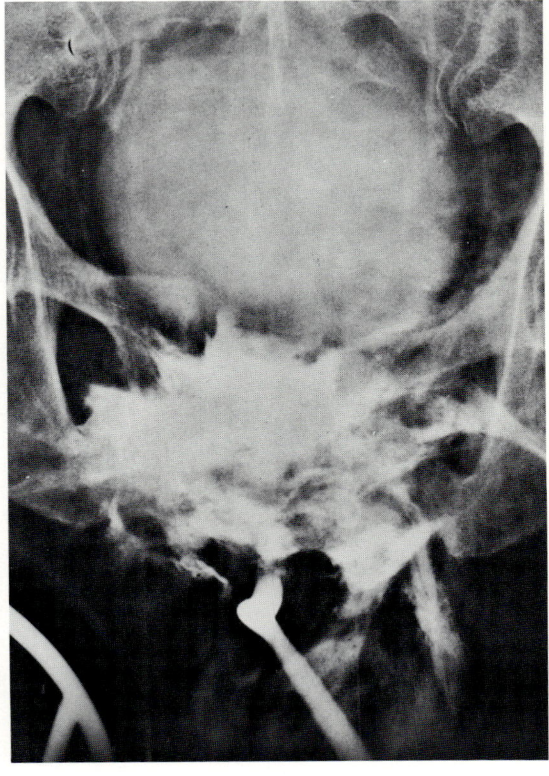

B

FIG. 4.52 A and B. This blunt trauma patient was found to have separation of the symphysis pubis and a left femoral shaft fracture. The **(A)** excretory urogram revealed apparently normal kidneys, ureters, and bladder. A **(B)** retrograde urethrogram demonstrated contrast extravasation from the posterior urethra. The accumulation of contrast in the scrotum suggests urethral injury below the urogenital diaphragm, injury of the urogenital diaphragm, or both.

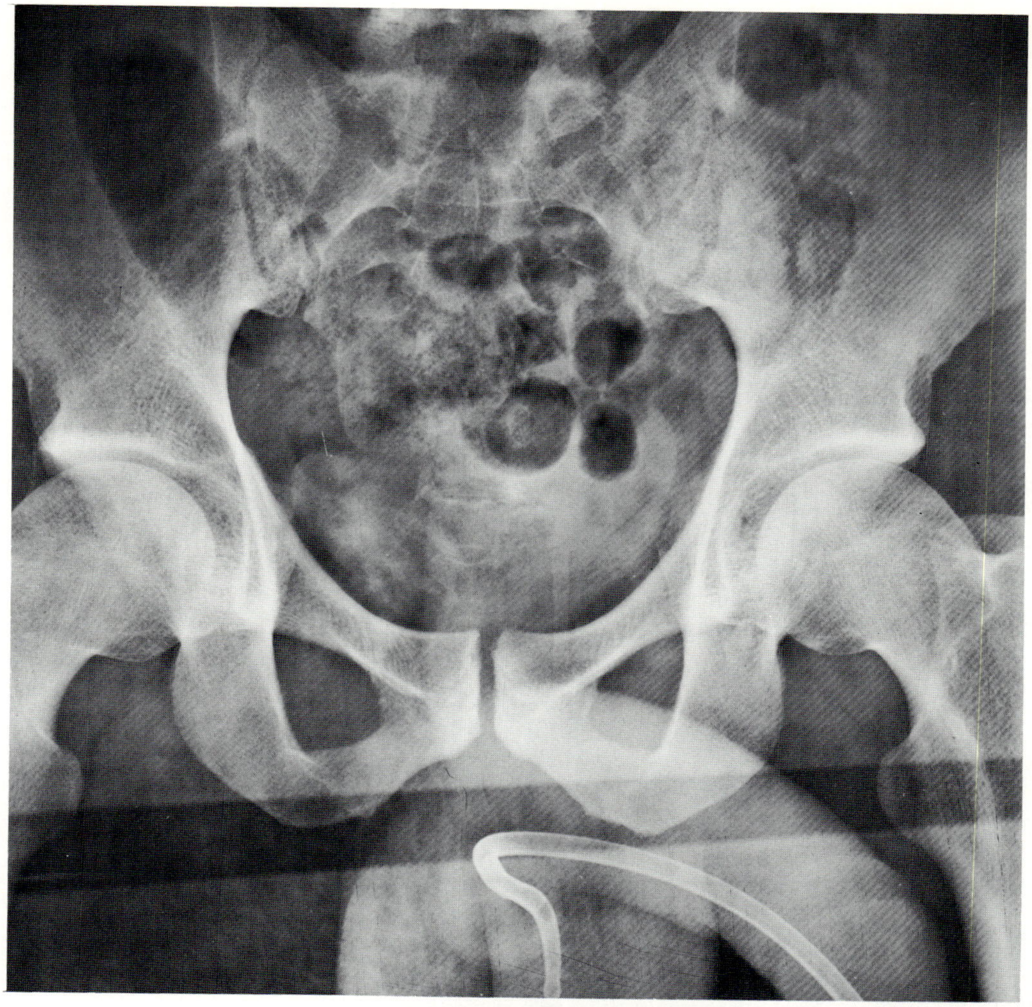

A

FIG. 4.53 A and B. This young male fell in a straddle fashion on a tennis-net post while trying to return a difficult shot. The **(A)** AP view of the pelvis fails to reveal any evidence of fracture, but there is soft-tissue swelling of the scrotum and penis. Attempts to pass a urethral catheter resulted in positioning of its tip in the scrotum. Following catheter removal, a **(B)** retrograde urethrogram defines a laceration of the bulbous urethra with contrast extravasation into the scrotum. Courtesy of Dr. Bhatt.

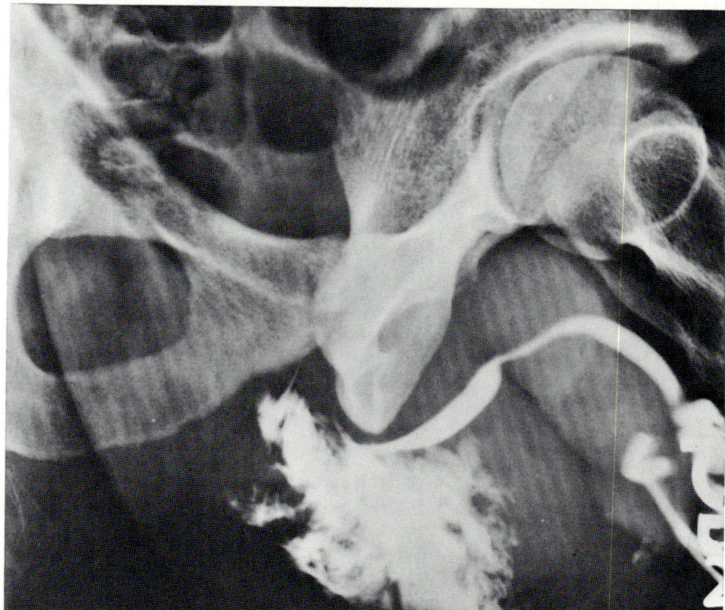

B

PELVIC FRACTURES

The bony pelvis in a semirigid, skeletal ring with points of relative elasticity at the symphysis pubis and at the two sacroiliac joints. The pelvis acts as a protective envelope for such soft-tissue structures as the rectosigmoid, the reproductive organs, the lower urinary tract, and a complex of large and small vascular structures. A force sufficient to disrupt this bony envelope can produce significant soft-tissue injury by the direct impact of the force itself or by the secondary lacerating effect of the fracture fragments. Although fractures of the pelvis do not have a high incidence relative to other skeletal fractures, they are important in terms of interest, complications, and possible mortality. The chief factors affecting morbidity and mortality are hemorrhage, rupture of the bladder or urethra, and associated injuries.

Classification and Mortality

Conolly and Hedberg have divided pelvic fractures into major and minor groups. A major fracture is defined as one that involves the line of transmission of weight from the spine to the acetabulum or one that involves the rami on both sides of the symphysis pubis (Fig. 4.54). The remaining fractures are classified as minor [33]. Bleeding results not only from disruption of the arterial and venous plexus within the pelvis but also from the fractured bones themselves. The degree of blood loss usually is proportional to the number of fractures of the pelvis. Of 200 evaluated by Conolly and Hedberg, 109 had major fractures, with 28 deaths. Minor fractures occurred in 91 patients with 2 deaths. Of the 30 patients who succumbed, 3 died from massive intrapelvic hemorrhage and 11 from renal failure secondary to shock (Table 4.76). Braunstein et al. have estimated that 60% of deaths following pelvic trauma result from complications of blood loss alone [20]. Margolies et al. also report that massive extraperitoneal hemorrhage is the leading cause of death after pelvic fracture [100]. Rothenberger et al. have listed etiology of pelvic fracture, mortality statistics, and causes of death, either directly or indirectly, as a result of pelvic fracture [155] (Tables 4.77, 4.78).

Associated Injuries and Mortality

Lang [83] notes that in the past, massive extraperitoneal hemorrhage was attributed to bleeding from lacerated iliac veins; it is only recently that arterial hemorrhage has been identified as the most common cause for this complication. A significant correlation exists between certain types of pelvic fracture and arterial injury: Fractures adjacent to the sacroiliac joint frequently result in tears of the iliolumbar artery; disruption of the ilium or separation of a sacroiliac joint can result in injury of the common or external iliac vessels; fractures of the pubic rami may affect the obturator and internal pudendal arteries; disruption of the posterior segment of the pelvis in children and adults can result in avulsion of the superior gluteal artery; and Malgaigne fractures (fracture of the hemipelvis with separation of the symphysis pubis or fractures of the pubic rami with fractures through the ilium or sacrum or dislocation of the sacroiliac joint) are associated with the highest rate of fatal hemorrhage.

Thaggard et al. believe that injury to the lower urinary tract is so frequent with fractures of the pelvis that such injury should be considered to be present until proved otherwise. They report injury to the urinary bladder in 6% and urethral injury in nearly 10% of cases. The urethral injuries were found to occur almost exclusively in males and were observed with

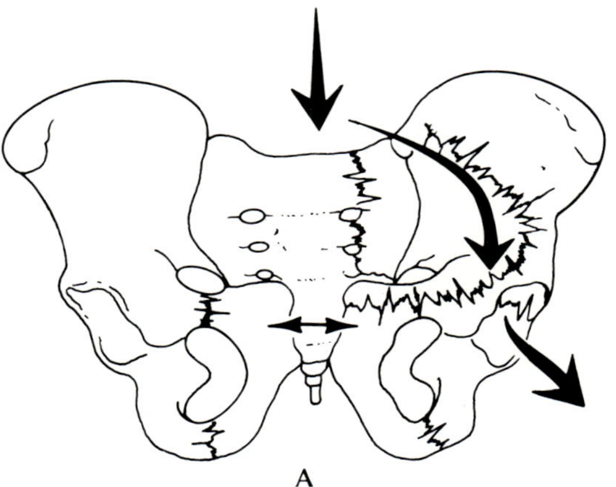

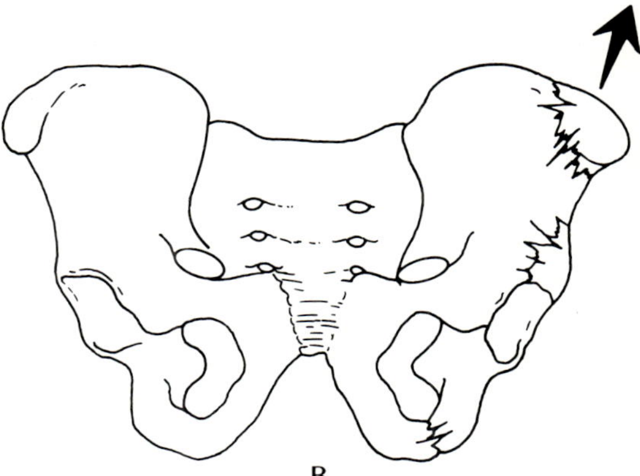

FIG. 4.54 A and B. (A) Major fracture (weight-bearing); **(B)** minor fracture (non-weight-bearing). From Conolly WB, Hedberg CA (1969) Observations on fractures of the pelvis. J Trauma 9(2): 104–111

TABLE 4.76. Associated injuries in 200 cases of fracture of the pelvis

		Associated injuries							
Type of fracture	Total no. of patients	No. of patients	Urinary	Retro-perito-neal hemor-rhage	Fracture	Abdom-inal	Intra-thoracic	Central nervous system	Mor-tality (num-ber)
Sacrum	0	0	0	0	0	0	0	0	0
Hemipelvis	21	21	7	16	18	7	5	11	17
Acetabulum	49	37	7	7	26	4	2	1	8
Bilateral pubic rami	34	29	14	5	15	2	2	7	3
Symphysis pubis separation	5	4	2	0	1	0	0	0	0
Subtotal	109	91	30	28	60	13	9	19	28
Avulsion	1	0	0	0	0	0	0	0	0
Ilium	8	5	1	1	3	2	0	0	0
Unilateral pubic rami	82	52	1	0	38	2	6	7	2
Subtotal	91	57	2	1	41	4	6	7	2
Total	200	148	32	29	101	17	15	26	30

Source: Conolly WB, Hedberg CA (1969) Observations on fractures of the pelvis. J Trauma 9(2): 104–111

TABLE 4.77. Pelvic fracture: Etiology

Etiology	No. of patients	No. of deaths	Mortality (%)
Vehicular	233	23	10
Pedestrian	162	35	22
Motorcycle	48	7	15
Minor fall	82	2	2
Major fall	32	4	13
Other blunt	44	1	2
Penetrating	3	0	0
Total	604	72	12

Source: Rothenberger DA, Fischer RP, Strate RG, Velasco R, Perry JJ (1978) The mortality associated with pelvic fractures. Surgery 84: 356–361

TABLE 4.78. Cause of death in 72 patients with pelvic fracture

Cause of death (No. of patients)	Pelvic fracture primary cause of death	Pelvic fracture significant secondary cause of death	Pelvic fracture not related to death
Shock/coagulopathy (30)	18	10	2
Head/spinal cord injury (15)	0	4	11
Sepsis (9)	4	0	5
Cardiorespiratory failure/ pulmonary emboli (7)	0	2	5
Renal failure (6)	4	0	2
Miscellaneous (5)	0	1	4
Total	26 (36%)	17 (24%)	29 (40%)

Source: Rothenberger DA, Fischer RP, Strate RG, Velasco R, Perry JJ (1978) The mortality associated with pelvic fractures. Surgery 84: 356–361

TABLE 4.79. Relationship of type of pelvic fracture and bladder injury

Pelvic ring fracture	Contusion	Intraperitoneal rupture	Extraperitoneal rupture
	(24)	(16)	(16)
Anterior			
Unilateral	7 }54%	5 }38%	4 }38%
Bilateral	6 }	1 }	2 }
Anterior and posterior			
Unilateral	5 }25%	4 }25%	2 }19%
Bilateral	1 }	— }	1 }
Protrusio acetabulum	—	—	1 }12%
Symphyseal separation	—	—	1 }
Combined, prot. acetab/sym. sep. ± ant./post.	4 (17%)	5 (31%)	3 (19%)
Others, not known	1 (4%)	1 (6%)	2 (12%)

Source: Cass AS, Ireland GW (1973) Bladder trauma associated with pelvic fractures in severely injured patients. J Trauma 13(3): 205–212

TABLE 4.80. Associated injuries with bladder trauma

Associated injury	Fractured pelvis present			No fractured pelvis		
	Contusion	Intraperitoneal rupture	Extraperitoneal rupture	Contusion	Intraperitoneal rupture	Extraperitoneal rupture
	(24)	(16)	(16)	(7)	(7)	(3)
Number of patients with associated injuries	18	10	14	3	4	2
Fractured ribs	2	3	6	1	2	0
Ruptured diaphragm	1	1	2	—	—	—
Lacerated spleen	3	2	4	—	1	—
Lacerated liver	1	1	2	1	1	—
Bowel perforation	1	1	1	1	—	1
Fractured skull	6	1	1	—	—	—
Fractured spine	—	1	4	1	—	—
Fractured extremities	14	8	10	2	1	1
Other (vascular, head)	3	3	5	1	—	1
Deaths	4	4	9	1	1	1
Mortality rate %	22	40	64	33	25	50

Source: Cass AS, Ireland GW (1973) Bladder trauma associated with pelvic fractures in severely injured patients. J Trauma 13(3): 25–212

major diastasis of the symphysis pubis or fractures in the area of the pubic rami [180]. Brosman and Paul [23] report that 72% of patients with trauma to the bladder had associated pelvic fracture. However, only 15% of patients with pelvic fractures also had significant injury of the bladder. Cass and Ireland report an overall mortality rate ranging from 29.8% to 44.2%, with multiple severe injuries including a fractured pelvis and trauma to the lower urinary tract [28] (Tables 4.79, 4.80). However, the bladder injuries themselves are rarely lethal. It is the combination of bladder, pelvic, and associated injuries that lead to the high mortality rate in these cases. Conolly and Hedberg [33] found rupture of the bladder or urethra in 27% of their group of major pelvic fractures and in 50% of those patients sustaining fractures involving both pubic rami (Table 4.76). They state that early diagnosis and prompt treatment of urologic injuries not only are life-saving but also reduce the frequency of late complications.

Conolly and Hedberg [33] found that associated injuries complicated the course of treatment in 90% of major and 60% of minor fractures (Tables 4.81, 4.82). Trunkey and Blaisdall [185] correlated mortality with the severity of fracture. Mortality was 21.7% for comminuted or crush injury to the pelvis, 11.4% for unstable fractures, and 4.5% for stable fractures. Rothenberger et al. [155] who reported a mortality for pelvic fractures of 12%, made the observation that major abdominal injuries were four times more frequent in patients who died than in the survivors (Tables 4.77, 4.78). Pelvic fracture was the sole major injury in only one patient who expired.

The experience at Morrisania City Hospital over a 4-year period was reviewed by the authors, and the mortality, incidence of multisystem injuries, and the frequency of exploratory laparotomy were considerably below the figures in reports from other institu-

TABLE 4.81. Soft-tissue injuries associated with fractures of the pelvis in 200 patients

Type of injury	No. of patients
Brain injury	18
Thorax	
Pneumothorax	4
Hemothorax	5
Flail chest	4
"Wet lung"	2
Abdomen	
Ruptured liver	7
Ruptured spleen	8
Ruptured small bowel	2
Ruptured large bowel	2
Lacerated rectum	1
Urinary	
Lacerated kidney	2
Ruptured bladder	10
Urethral injury	18
Genital	
Lacerated vagina	1
Avulsed testis	2
Lumbosacral nerve plexus injury	2
Retroperitoneal hematoma	29
Injury to iliac vessels	4

Source: Conolly WB, Hedberg CA (1969) Observations on fractures of the pelvis. J Trauma 9(2): 104–111

TABLE 4.82. Causes of death in 200 patients with fractures of the pelvis

	No. of patients
Renal failure secondary to shock	11
Massive intrapelvic hemorrhage	5
Multiple injuries and shock	5
Cerebral laceration	3
Bronchopneumonia	3
Died during anesthesia	1
Fat embolism	1
Coronary occlusion	1
Total	30

Source: Conolly WB, Hedberg CA (1969) Observations on fractures of the pelvis. J Trauma 9(2): 104–111

TABLE 4.83. Pelvic fractures, Morrisania City Hospital, 1967–1971

	No.	%
Causative agent for injury		
Struck by vehicle	71	57.2
Passenger in auto accident	5	4.0
Fall from height (major)	13	10.4
Fall from height (minor)	29	23.3
Miscellaneous penetrating injury	4	3.2
No obtainable history	2	1.6
Total	124	
Patients admitted in shock BP<100, systolic	12	9.6
Mortality	9	7.2
Patients explored	6	4.8
Patients having tap/lavage	8	6.4
Patients with hematuria	47	37.9
Patients with bladder displacement by hematoma	9	7.2
No. of patients with major GU injury	3	2.4

tions. The relatively low mortality and morbidity in the authors' experience are probably related to the inner-city location of Morrisania Hospital and, subsequently, a lower incidence of high-speed automobile trauma. The relevant factors for this experience are listed in Table 4.83. Of the 124 patients, 47 had either microscopic or gross hematuria. Only 12 patients had genitourinary-tract injuries of sufficient severity to produce abnormalities on radiologic evaluation with contrast.

Exploratory Laparotomy

Several important questions are involved in the assessment of patients suffering pelvic fractures and suspected injury to intraabdominal organs. The abdominal physical findings may be obscured by the symptoms produced by the pelvic, retroperitoneal, and perivesical hematomas; and it may be difficult to determine when exploratory laparotomy is necessary (Fig. 4.55). Only 5 patients in the authors' series of 124 had significant visceral injury associated with the pelvic fracture; 17 patients had associated abdominal injuries in the Conolly and Hedberg series [33] and of the 35 patients explored by Hawkins et al. [65] in a series of 192 patients, 30 patients had significant injuries requiring repair (Table 4.84).

Exploratory laparotomy for pelvic fractures must be approached cautiously. Smith et al. [168] note that early surgical exploration of the blood-filled extraperitoneal pelvic space is complicated by the difficulty in localizing and controlling a specific bleeding site. Furthermore, opening the pelvic peritoneum destroys the most important mechanism for tamponade. In addition, Margulies and Stoane [101] state that aside from destroying the tamponade effect, exploration of the pelvic retroperitoneal area increases the risk of later sepsis. An idea of the degree of difficulty associated

TABLE 4.84. Abdominal-organ injuries associated with 35 patients with pelvic fractures who underwent laparotomy

No associated injury found	5
Ruptured bladder	13
Ruptured urethra	6
Vascular injury	5
Liver laceration	4
Ruptured spleen	4
Bowel laceration	3
Ruptured gallbladder	1
Pancreatic laceration	1

Source: Hawkins L, Pomerantz M, Eiseman B (1970) Laparotomy at the time of pelvic fracture. J Trauma 10: 619–623

with exploration of such an injury is suggested by the view of Ravitch, who said that no surgical exploration should be performed for direct control of bleeding until 20 units of blood have been administered. The problem with this approach, as Trunkey and Blaisdall and others have noted, is that the combination of shock, massive soft-tissue injury, extensive fractures, and multiple transfusions set the stage for intravascular coagulation, acute thromboembolic complications, possible pulmonary damage, and acute renal failure. The mortality from these complications is extremely high. Thus it would seem that a less conservative approach than that of Ravitch must be followed. The indications for laparotomy outlined by Hawkins [65] are applicable in most instances. They include:

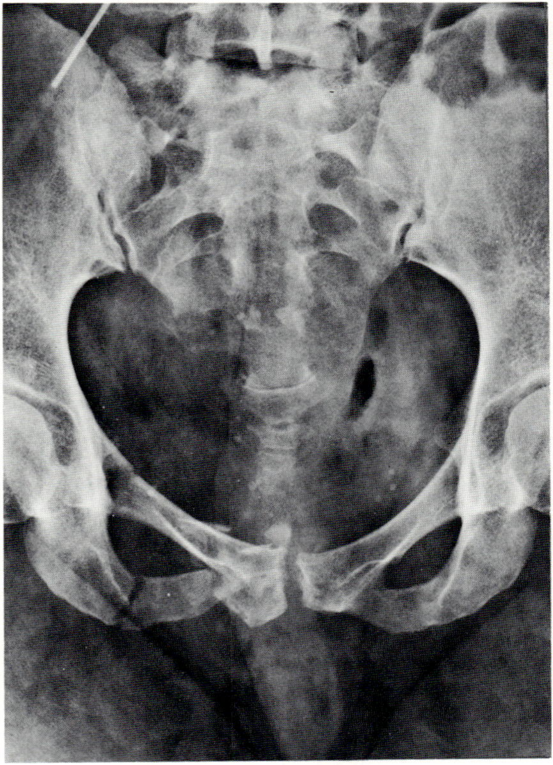

A

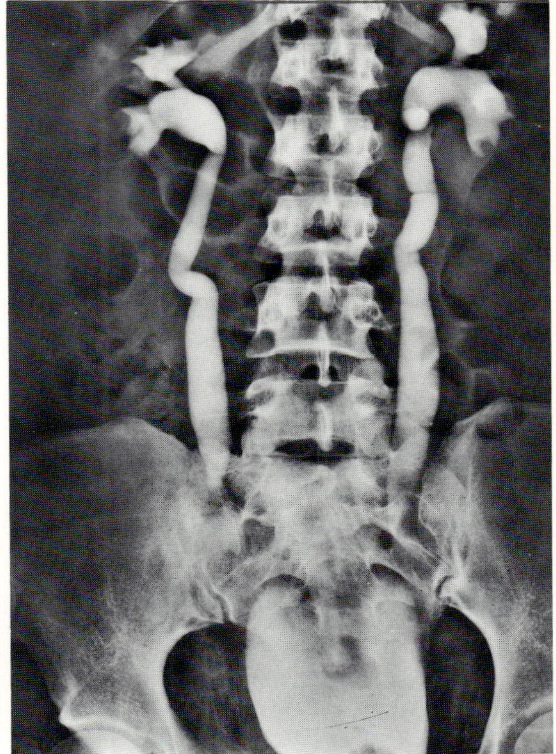

B

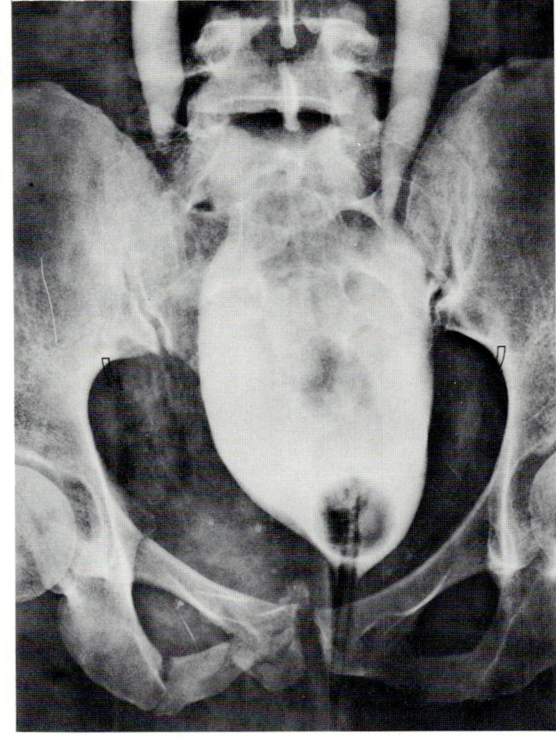

C

FIG. 4.55 A–C. The **(A)** AP view of the pelvis of this victim of blunt trauma reveals multiple fractures of the anterior pelvis with loss of normal soft-tissue planes. A **(B)** 20-min film of the excretory urogram shows compression of the bladder and distal ureters resulting in mild obstructive changes of the kidneys and proximal ureters. The **(C)** filled bladder film confirms the previous findings and suggests minimal contrast extravasation *(curved open arrows)*. At exploration, there was no evidence of viscus perforation. Courtesy of Dr. Bhatt.

1. Classic evidence of free intraperitoneal bleeding or visceral perforation.
2. Bladder perforation into the peritoneal cavity as demonstrated by cystography. Such perforation is uncommon, since most series suggest that extraperitoneal perforation is more common with pelvic fractures. Laparotomy adds little to the extraperitoneal cystomy that is usually required in patients with this type of bladder rupture.
3. Evidence of expanding, pulsatile, suprapubic hematoma.
4. Severity in location of the trauma.
5. Radiologic demonstration of bony fragments driven into the pelvic cavity or evidence of major pelvic fracture.
6. Blood loss exceeding 2500 cc that cannot be ascribed to associated injuries.

The abdominal organs injured in 35 patients who had abdominal exploration for pelvic fractures reported by Hawkins et al. are listed in Table 4.84.

Paracentesis and lavage can be of aid in determining whether or not laparotomy should be performed. Tap/lavage was used in eight patients in our experience and was positive in only one. In most of the patients explored in the authors' series, the indications were clear and not related to the tap/lavage procedure. Laparotomy was avoided, based on the tap/lavage, in seven cases. In 20 of the 35 patients explored by Hawkins et al. [65], the paracentesis and lavage supported their decision for surgery. Rothenberger et al. [155] reviewed 604 patients with pelvic fractures and found that only 3 had false-positive lavages in the series.

Radiographic Diagnosis

GENERAL EVALUATION

The initial diagnosis and categorization of the severity of fractures after a pelvic injury can be established radiologically. However, it should be clear that the complexity of this type of injury may require various diagnostic procedures to establish the extent of associated injuries (and the course of treatment). Subsequent standard radiologic studies, physical examination, urinalysis, examination of the stool for blood, sigmoidoscopy, and paracentesis with lavage may individually or in combination permit a full picture of the injury to be obtained.

Diagnostic radiology is an important modality in the management of such patients. By a careful review of the pelvic films, the radiologist may not only define the sites of fracture and suggest the possibility of associated soft-tissue injury, but he may also be able to determine the extent of retroperitoneal hemorrhage. Harris et al. have given excellent description of the soft-tissue anatomy of the normal, nontraumatized patient. They note that the extraperitoneal, perivesical space is bounded above by the pelvic peritoneal reflection, laterally by the obturator internus and levator ani muscles, anteriorly by the anterior pubic arch, posteriorly by the sacrum, and inferiorly by the urogenital diaphragm. The urogenital diaphragm is a dense, tough, fibromuscular, triangularly shaped structure extending from the pubic symphysis to the level of the ischial tuberosities posteriorly. Laterally, it is firmly attached to the ischial pubic rami. The urethral traverses the urogenital diaphragm [62].

The perivesical space is filled with loose areolar or adipose tissue which also extends in a thin layer over the dome of the urinary bladder separating the bladder from the pelvic peritoneum. Posteriorly, this areolar tissue is continuous with the posterior pararenal fat and, laterally, with the properitoneal fat that constitutes the flank stripe. Because of the contrast afforded by the perivesical fat and its reflections over regional muscle masses, it is possible to define even a minimal amount of extraperitoneal fluid (blood or urine). The radiologic signs of pelvic extraperitoneal effusion include:

1. Displacement of the urinary bladder
2. Loss of definition or obliteration of the normal soft-tissue shadows within the pelvis
3. Elevation of the pelvic peritoneum as indicated by cephalad displacement of small-bowel loops out of the pelvis

As fluid continues to accumulate in the extraperitoneal space, it will extend laterally and superiorly into the properitoneal fat of the flank (the flank stripe), causing obliteration of this stripe and medial displacement of its medial wall, i.e., parietal peritoneum. It is important to distinguish retroperitoneal pelvic accumulation of fluid from intraperitoneal accumulations. This is done by noting the persistence of the curvilinear lucent stripe representing the areolar tissue between the dome of the bladder and the pelvic peritoneum and/or noting the persistence, on the frontal projection of the soft-tissue shadow cast by the obturator internus muscle and its aponeurosis (Fig. 4.56). Clear definition of these structures exclude extraperitoneal-fluid accumulation.

In addition, Peltier and others have noted the usefulness of the infusion pyelogram coupled with cystoscopy in determining not only injury to the urinary system but also the presence and amount of retroperitoneal hemorrhage. The degree of ureteral or bladder displacement or deformity has been found to correlate reasonably well with the amount of blood accumulated in the retroperitoneum [137].

Angiographic Evaluation

In view of the admitted difficulty encountered when attempting surgical exploration in patients with pelvic hematomas, Margolies et al. and Ring et al. have advocated the use of abdominal and pelvic angiography in the early management and treatment of patients with severe pelvic fractures [100,151]. It has been demonstrated that significant diagnostic information in those patients who are stable enough to undergo angiography can be obtained (Fig. 4.57). In addition, because of the difficulty associated with the surgical management of bleeding vessels in the pelvis, angiography can be used to diagnose the site and to provide control of the hemorrhage. Occlusion of one or both hypogastric arteries by balloon catheter tamponade, autologous clot or muscle embolization, gelfoam embolization, or angiographic adhesive material have all been found to be beneficial in controlling bleeding in

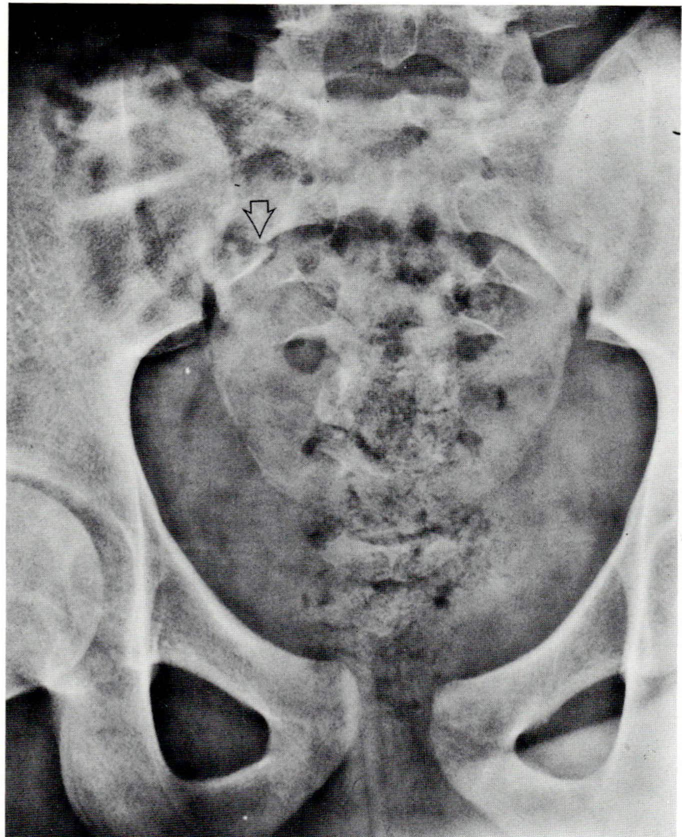

A

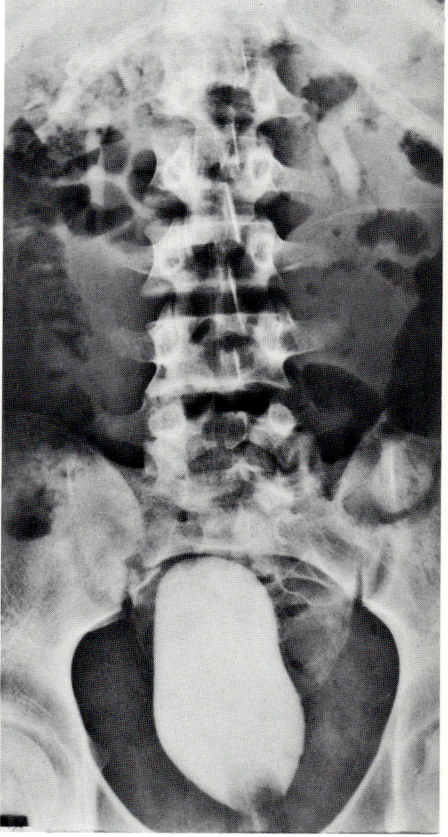

B

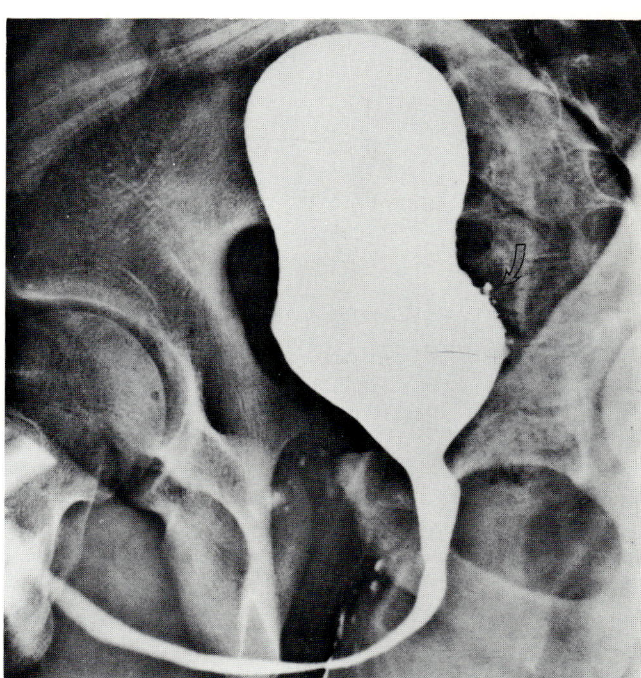

C

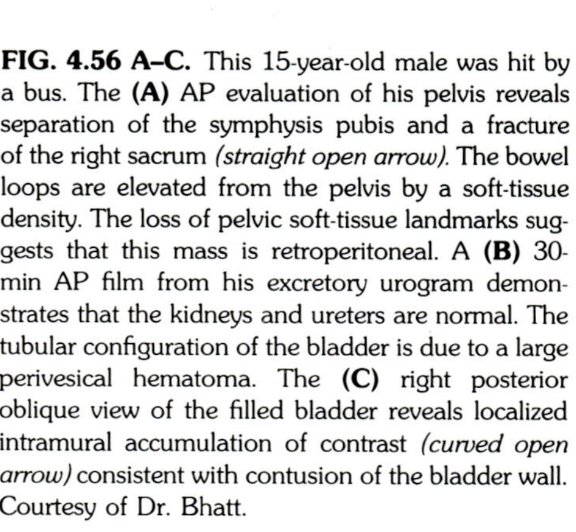

FIG. 4.56 A–C. This 15-year-old male was hit by a bus. The **(A)** AP evaluation of his pelvis reveals separation of the symphysis pubis and a fracture of the right sacrum *(straight open arrow)*. The bowel loops are elevated from the pelvis by a soft-tissue density. The loss of pelvic soft-tissue landmarks suggests that this mass is retroperitoneal. A **(B)** 30-min AP film from his excretory urogram demonstrates that the kidneys and ureters are normal. The tubular configuration of the bladder is due to a large perivesical hematoma. The **(C)** right posterior oblique view of the filled bladder reveals localized intramural accumulation of contrast *(curved open arrow)* consistent with contusion of the bladder wall. Courtesy of Dr. Bhatt.

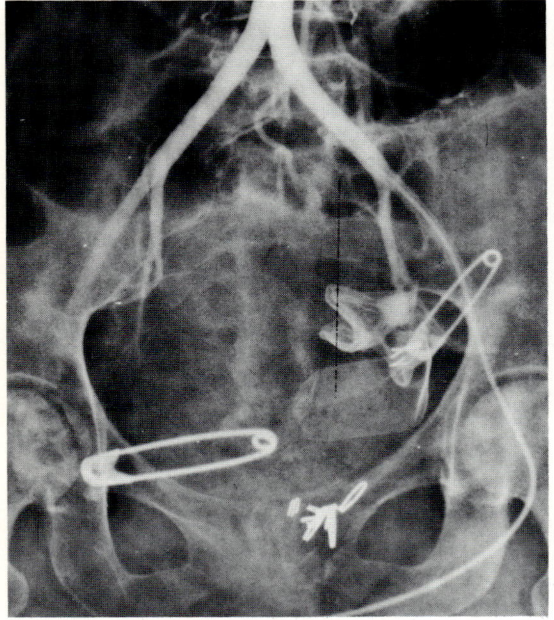

A

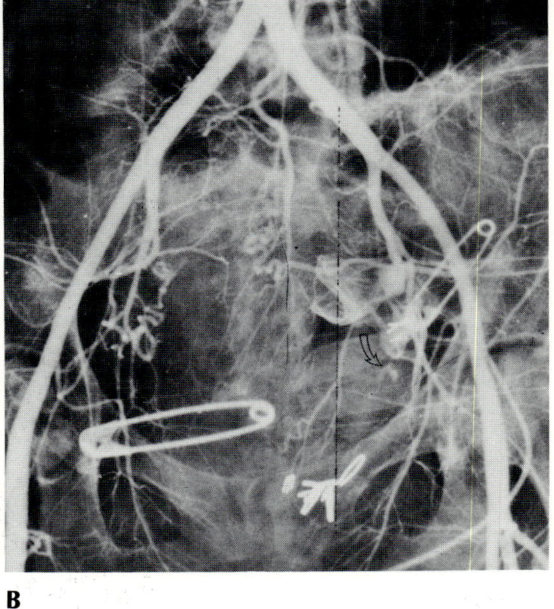

B

C

FIG. 4.57 A–C. This 36-year-old female, with a history of lupus erythematosus, was admitted after she jumped from her second-story apartment window. Pelvic fractures were stabilized, and a pelvic hematoma was drained through a suprapubic tube. However, the patient's hematocrit continued to fall, and pelvic angiography was performed to localize the bleeding site. The **(A)** early arterial phase reveals drainage tubes in situ, metallic staples at the site of symphysis pubis injury, pelvic soft-tissue densities consistent with intra- and retroperitoneal-fluid accumulation, and aseptic necrosis of the bilateral femoral heads but no evidence of a bleeding site. The **(B)** intermediate and **(C)** late arterial phases reveal a site of bleeding *(curved open arrow)* from one of the branches of the left internal iliac artery.

pelvic fractures [100]. In performing such endovascular therapeutic procedures, it is imperative that angiography of the opposite hypogastric artery is carried out to exclude continued bleeding from collateral vessels. Superselective catheterization of bleeding vessels is not necessary to obtain such control. Occlusion of the hypogastric artery itself is all that is needed and is associated with a very low morbidity. Unlike gastrointestinal bleeding, vasopressin has not proved effective in controlling posttraumatic hemorrhage in the pelvis. The reason for this probably rests on the large size of the vessels involved in bleeding with pelvic fractures as contrasted with the relatively small vessels involved in gastrointestinal bleeding. An appropriate plan for rapid assessment of patients with pelvic fracture is described by McAvoy and Cook (Fig. 4.58).

Pelvic fractures represent a traumatic entity that requires the best efforts of the radiologist, the orthopedic surgeon, the general surgeon, and frequently the internist. The presence of pelvic fractures demands a multidisciplinary approach to the traumatized patient. Whether endovascular catheter vessel occlusion, exploratory laparotomy, or pulmonary and renal support are required, all of the modern techniques of diagnosis and therapy related to trauma may be needed for these patients.

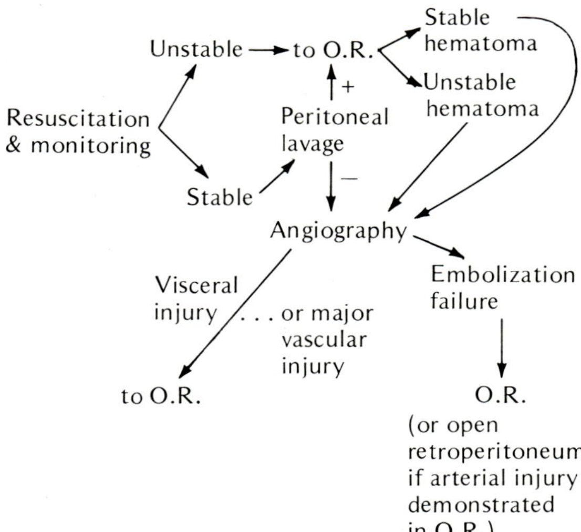

FIG. 4.58. Proposed triage plan for patients with pelvic fractures and massive bleeding. From McAvoy J, Cook JH (1978) A treatment plan for rapid assessment of the patient with massive blood loss and pelvic fractures. Arch Surg 113: 986–990

REFERENCES

1. Aakhus T, Enge I (1971) Angiography in rupture of the liver. Acta Radiol (Stockh) 2: 535–362
2. Abeshouse BS (1935) Rupture of the kidney, pelvis. Surg Gynecol Obstet 60: 710
3. Abrams HL (ed) (1971) Angiography, Vols. I and II. Little, Brown and Company, Boston
4. Adams JT, Elebute EA, Schwartz SI (1966) Isolated injury to the pancreas from penetrating trauma in children. J Trauma 6: 86–98
5. Allen RB, Curry CJ (1957) Abdominal trauma, a study of 297 consecutive cases. Am J Surg 93: 398
6. Allen RE Jr, Blaisdell FW (1972) Injuries to the inferior vena cava. Surg Clin North Am 52: 699–710
7. Altner PC (1964) Constrictive lesions of the colon due to blunt trauma to the abdomen. Surg Gynecol Obstet 118: 1257–1262
8. Bach RD, Frey CF (1971) Diagnosis and treatment of pancreatic trauma. Am J Surg 121: 20–29
9. Balasegaram M (1976) The surgical management of hepatic trauma. J Trauma 16(2): 141–148
10. Bartrum RJ Jr, Crow HC (1977) Gray-Scale Ultrasound: A Manual for Physicians and Technical Personnel. W. B. Saunders Company, Philadelphia
11. Bassett FA III, Silver D (1966) Arterial injury associated with fractures. Arch Surg 92: 13–19
12. Baudet R (1907) Ruptures de la Rate. Med Pract 3: 565–581
13. BeKassy SM, Dave KS, Wooler GH, Ionescu MI (1972) "Spontaneous" and traumatic rupture of the diaphragm. Ann Surg 177: 32–324
14. Bell D, Cockshott WP (1965) Angiography of traumatic arterio-venous fistulae. Clin Radiol 16: 241–247
15. Benjamin CI, Engrav LH, Perry JF Jr (1976) Delayed rupture or delayed diagnosis of rupture of the spleen. Surg Gynecol Obstet 142: 171
16. Bergquist D, Dahlgren S, Hedelin H (1978) Rupture of the diaphragm in patients wearing seat belts. J Trauma 18: 781
17. Bernatz PE, Burnside AF Jr, Clagett OJ (1958) Problems of the ruptured diaphragm. JAMA 168: 877
18. Boijsen E, Judkins MP, Simay A (1966) Angiographic diagnosis of hepatic rupture. Radiology 88: 66–81
19. Bollinger JA, Fowler EF (1956) Traumatic rupture of spleen with special reference to delayed splenic rupture. Am J Surg 91: 561–570
20. Braunstein PW, Skudder PA, McCarroll JR (1964) Concealed hemorrhage due to pelvic fracture. J Trauma 4: 832–838
21. Bright TC, Peters PC (1977) Ureteral injuries due to external violence: 10 years experience with 59 cases. J Trauma 17(8): 616–620
22. Brosman SA, Fay R (1973) Diagnosis and management of bladder trauma. J Trauma 13: 687–694
23. Brosman SA, Paul JG (1976) Trauma of the bladder. Surg Gynecol Obstet 143: 605–608
24. Campbell MF (1970) Injuries of the Urogenital Tract, 3rd ed. W. B. Saunders Company, Philadelphia
25. Cantor MO (1970) Abdominal Trauma. Charles C Thomas, Springfield, Ill.
26. Carlson RI, Dickey WL, Gobbel WG, Daniel RA (1958) Dehiscence of the diaphragm associated with fractures of the pelvis or lumbar spine due to non-penetrating wounds of the chest and abdomen. J Thorac Surg 36: 254–261
27. Carter R, Brewer LA III (1971) Strangulating diaphragmatic hernia. Ann Thorac Surg 12: 281
28. Cass AS, Ireland GW (1973) Bladder trauma associated with pelvic fractures in severely injured patients. J Trauma 13(3): 205–212
29. Cass AS, Ireland GW (1974) Renal injuries in children. J Trauma 14(8): 719–722
30. Cerise EJ, Scully JH (1970) Blunt trauma to the small intestine. J Trauma 10(1): 46–50
31. Clark OH, Lim RC, Margarettey W (1975) Spontaneous delayed splenic rupture—Case report of a five year interval between trauma and diagnosis. J Trauma 15: 245
32. Cleveland HC, Reinschmidt JD, Waddell WR (1963) Traumatic pancreatitis: An increasing problem. Surg Clin North Am 43(2): 401
33. Conolly WB, Hedberg EA (1969) Observations on fractures of the pelvis. J Trauma 9(2): 104–111
34. Corica A, Powers SR Jr (1975) Blunt liver trauma: An analysis of 75 treated patients. J Trauma 15: 751–756
35. Cosgrove MD, Mendez R, Morrow JW (1973) Traumatic renal arterio-venous fistula. Report of 12 cases. J Urol 101: 627–631
36. Culotta RJ, Howard JM, Jordan JL (1965) Traumatic injuries of the pancreas. Surgery 40: 320
37. DeBakey ME, Simeone FA (1946) Battle injuries of the arteries in World War II: An analysis of 2,471 cases. Ann Surg 123: 534–579
38. DeFore WW Jr, Mattox KL, Jordan Gl, Beall AC Jr (1976) Management of 1,590 consecutive cases of liver trauma. Arch Surg 111: 493–497

39. DeWeerd JH (1959) Management of injuries to the bladder, urethra and genitalia. Surg Clin North Am 39: 973
40. DiVincenti FC, Rives JD, LaBorde EJ, Fleming ID, Cohn I (1968) Blunt abdominal trauma. J Trauma 8: 1004–1013
41. Domrich H (1938) Versuche Über die Funktion Verletzker Nieren. Ztschr f Urol 32: 78
42. Donovan AJ, Turrell F, Berne CJ (1972) Injuries of the pancreas from blunt trauma. Surg Clin North Am 52(3): 649–665
43. Doust BD, Quiroz F, Stewart JJ (1977) Ultrasonic distinction of abscesses from other intraabdominal fluid collections. Radiology 125: 213–218
44. Drezner AD (1975) Decreasing morbidity after liver trauma. Am J Surg 129(4): 483–489
45. Drowse JL, Kihn RB (1963) Renal injuries. Diagnosis, management and sequelae in 67 cases. Br J Surg 50: 353–361
46. Emanuel B, Weiss H, Gollin P (1977) Renal trauma in children. J Trauma 17(4): 275–278
47. Epstein LJ, Lempke RE (1968) Rupture of the right hemidiaphragm due to blunt trauma. J Trauma 8: 19–28
48. Esho JO, Ireland GW, Cass AS (1973) Renal trauma and pre-existing lesions of the kidney. Urology 1: 134–135
49. Evans JP (1973) Traumatic rupture of the ileum. Br J Surg 60(2): 119
50. Felson B, Levin EJ (1954) Intramural hematoma of duodenum: Diagnostic roentgen sign. Radiology 63: 823–831
51. Fiss TW, Cigtay OS, Miele AJ, Twigg HL (1975) Perforated viscus presenting with gas in the soft tissues. (Subcutaneous emphysema.) Am J Roentgenol 125(1): 226–233
52. Fitzgerald JB, Crawford E, DeBakey ME (1960) Surgical considerations of abdominal injuries, analysis of 200 cases. Am J Surg 20: 100
53. Freeman T, Fischer RP (1976) The inadequacy of peritoneal lavage in diagnosing acute diaphragmatic rupture. J Trauma 16(7): 538–542
54. Frey CF, Trollope M, Harpster W, Snyder R (1973) A fifteen year experience with automotive hepatic trauma. J Trauma 13: 1039–1049
55. Garvey JW, Delany HM (1974) Giant cyst of the spleen. J Trauma 14: 974
56. Glenn JF, Howard BM (1966) The injured kidney. JAMA 173: 1189–1195
57. Gold RE, Redman HC (1972) Splenic trauma: Assessment of problems in diagnosis. Am J Roentgenol 116: 413–418
58. Goldberg BB (ed) (1977) Abdominal Gray Scale Ultrasonography. John Wiley & Sons, New York
59. Gould RJ, Thorwarth WT (1963) Retroperitoneal rupture of duodenum due to blunt, non-penetrating abdominal trauma. Radiology 80: 743–747
60. Griswold RA, Collier HS (1961) Collective review: Blunt abdominal trauma. Surg Gynecol Obstet 112: 309–329
61. Guerriero WG, Carlton CE Jr, Scott R Jr, Beall A Jr (1971) Renal pedicle injuries. J Trauma 11: 53–62
62. Harris JH Jr, Loh CK, Perlman HC, Rotz CT Jr (1977) The roentgen diagnosis of pelvic extraperitoneal effusion. Radiology 125: 343–350
63. Harrison RC, Debas HT (1972) Injuries of stomach and duodenum. Surg Clin North Am 52(3): 635–648
64. Hassani N (1976) Ultrasonography of the Abdomen. Springer-Verlag, New York
65. Hawkins L, Pomerantz M, Eiseman B (1970) Laparotomy at the time of pelvic fracture. J Trauma 10: 619–623
66. Hegarty MM, Bryer JV, Angorn IB, Baker LW (1978) Delayed presentation of traumatic diaphragmatic hernia. Ann Surg 188(2): 229–233
67. Hill LD (1972) Injuries of the diaphragm following blunt trauma. Surg Clin North Am 52(3): 611–624
68. Holland ME, Hurwitz LM, Charles MM (1966) Traumatic lesions of the urinary tract. Radiol Clin North Am 4(2): 433–450
69. Howell HW, Bartizal JF, Freeark RJ (1976) Blunt trauma involving the colon and rectum. J Trauma 16: 624
70. Howell JF, Burrus GR, Jordan GL Jr (1968) Surgical management of pancreatic injuries. J Trauma 1: 32–40
71. Jacobson G, Carter R (1951) Small intestinal rupture due to non-penetrating abdominal injury: Roentgenological study. Am J Roentgenol 66: 52–64
72. Jacobson SJ, DeNardo G (1971) Splenosis demonstrated by splenic scan. J Nucl Med 12: 570–572
73. Jarrett F, Bernhardt LC (1978) Right sided diaphragmatic injury: Rarity or overlooked diagnosis. Arch Surg 113(6): 737–739
74. Joseph TP, Wyllie GG, Savage JP (1977) The non-operative management of splenic trauma. Aust NZ J Surg 47: 180
75. Kakos GS, Grosfeld JL, Morse TS (1971) Small bowel injuries in children after blunt abdominal trauma. Ann Surg 174(2): 238–241
76. Kaufman JJ, Brosman SA (1972) Blunt injuries of the genitourinary tract. Surg Clin North Am 52(3): 747–760
77. Kazmin MH, Brosman SA, Cockett AJK (1969) Diagnosis and early management of renal trauma: A study of 120 patients. J Urol 101: 783
78. Kerry RL, Glas WW (1962) Traumatic injury of the pancreas and duodenum: A clinical and experimental study. Arch Surg 85: 813–816
79. Kessler E, Stein A (1976) Diaphragmatic hernia as a long term complication of stab wounds of the chest. Am J Surg 132: 34–39
80. Kindling PH, Wilson RF, Watt AJ (1969) Hepatic trauma with particular reference to blunt injury. J Trauma 9(1): 17–26
81. Katzen BM, Levy N (1978) Splenosis simulating an intramural gastric mass. Radiology 126: 45–46
82. LaMura J, Pin Chung-Fat S, San Filippo AJ (1977) Splenorrhaphy for the treatment of splenic rupture in infants and children. Surgery 81: 487–501

83. Lang EK (1975) Arteriography in the assessment of renal trauma. J Trauma 15: 553–566
84. Lang EK (1976) The role of arteriography in trauma. Radiol Clin North Am 14(2): 353–370
85. Larenson SG Jr, Cohen A (1971) Management of rectal injury. Am J Surg 122: 226–230
86. Leandoer JL, Tremann JA, Oishi RH, Manchioro TL (1972) Bilateral renal artery thrombosis following blunt trauma. Report of two cases. J Trauma 12: 166–169
87. Levin DC, Watson RC, Sos TA, Baltaxe HA (1973) Angiography in blunt hepatic trauma. Am J Roentgenol 119(1): 95–101
88. Lim RC Jr, Glickman MG, Hunt TK (1972) Angiography in patients with blunt trauma to the chest and abdomen. Surg Clin North Am 52(3): 551–565
89. Linke CA, Cockett ATK, Frank IN, Davis RS (1975) Recent advances in the diagnosis and management of blunt renal trauma. J Urol 113: 750–754
90. LoCicero J, Tajima T, Drapanas T (1975) A half century of experience in the management of colon injuries: Changing concepts. J Trauma 15(7): 575–579
91. Love L (1970) Arterial trauma. Semin Roentgenol 5: 267–284
92. Love L (1975) Radiology of abdominal trauma. JAMA 231(13): 1377–1380
93. Love L, Greenfield GB, Braun TW, Moncado R, Freeark RJ, Baker RJ (1968) Angiography of splenic trauma. Radiology 91: 96–102
94. Lowe RJ, Boyd DR, Folk FA, Baker RJ (1972) The negative laparotomy for abdominal trauma. J Trauma 12: 853–860
95. Lowe RJ, Saletta JD, Read DR, Radhakrishnan J, Moss GS (1977) Should laparotomy be mandatory or selective in gun shot wounds of the abdomen? J Trauma 17: 903–907
96. Lowsley OS, Kerwin TJ (1956) Clinical Urology. Williams & Wilkins, Baltimore
97. Lubbers EJ (1977) Injury of the duodenum caused by a fixed three-point seatbelt. J Trauma 17(12): 960–963
98. Lucas CE, Ledgerwood AM (1975) Factors influencing outcome after blunt duodenal injury. J Trauma 15: 839–846
99. Mandal AK, Boitano MA (1978) Reappraisal of low velocity gun shot wounds of the aorta and inferior vena cava in civilian practice. J Trauma 18(8): 580–585
100. Margolies MN, Ring EJ, Waltman AC, Kerr WS, Baum S (1972) Arteriography in the management of hemorrhage from pelvic fractures. N Engl J Med 287(7): 317–321
101. Margulies M, Stoane L (1967) Hepatic angle in roentgen evaluation of peritoneal fluid. Radiology 88: 51–57
102. Martin JD (1969) Trauma to the Thorax and Abdomen. Charles C Thomas, Springfield, Ill.
103. Mattixm KD, Whisennand HH, Espada R, Beall CA Jr (1975) Management of acute combined injuries to the aorta and inferior vena cava. Am J Surg 130: 720–724
104. Maul KI, Fallahzadeh H, Mays ET (1978) Selective management of post-traumatic obstructing intramural hematoma of the duodenum. Surg Gynecol Obstet 146: 221–224
105. McAlhany JC Jr, Black HC Jr, Hanback LD Jr, Yarbrough DR III (1971) Renal arteriovenous fistula as a cause of hypertension. Am J Surg 122: 117
106. McAvoy JM, Cook JH (1978) A treatment plan for rapid assessment of the patient with massive blood loss and pelvic fractures. Arch Surg 113: 986–990
107. McCort JJ (1973) Abdominal trauma. In: Margulis AR, Burhenne HJ (eds) Alimentary Tract Roentgenology, Vol. I. C. V. Mosby Company, St. Louis, pp. 228–270
108. McCort JJ (1964) Radiographic examination in blunt abdominal trauma. Radiol Clin North Am 2: 121–143
109. McCort JJ 91966) Radiographic Examination in Blunt Abdominal Trauma. W. B. Saunders Company, Philadelphia
110. McCort JJ (1962) Rupture or laceration of the liver by non-penetrating trauma. Radiology 78: 49–57
111. McCune RP, Roda CP, Eckert C (1976) Rupture of the diaphragm caused by blunt trauma. J Trauma 16(7): 531–537
112. McKenzie AD, Bell GA (1972) Non-penetrating injuries of the colon and rectum. Surg Clin North Am 52: 735–740
113. Meyers HI (1968) The radiologic evaluation of patients with non-penetrating abdominal trauma. Surg Clin North Am 48: 1205
114. Meyers MA (1976) Dynamic Radiology of the Abdomen. Normal and Pathologic Anatomy. Springer-Verlag, New York
115. Meyers MA (1974) Radiographic features of spread and localization of extraperitoneal gas and their relationship to its sources: An anatomical approach. Radiology 111: 17–27
116. Meyers MA (1975) Uriniferous perirenal pseudocyst. New observations. Radiology 117: 539–545
117. Miller DW Jr, Kelly DL (1972) Splenic trauma. Arch Surg 105: 561–563
118. Mitchell JP (1963) Injuries to the urinary tract. Proc R Soc Med 56: 1046–1050
119. Moore JB, Moore EE (1977) Lower gastrointestinal bleeding. An unusual presentation for blunt abdominal trauma. J Trauma 17: 961–963
120. Morrow JW, Mendez R (1970) Renal trauma. J Urol 104: 649
121. Morse TS (1975) Renal injuries. Pediatr Clin North Am 22(2): 379
122. Morton JR, Jordan GL (1968) Traumatic duodenal injuries: Review of 131 cases. J Trauma 8(2): 127–137
123. Mullen JT (1974) Editorial. The magnitude of the problem of trauma. J Trauma 14(12): 1070–1072
124. Nahum H, Levesque M (1973) Angiography in hepatic trauma. Radiology 109: 557–563
125. Naylor R, Coln D, Shires GT (1974) Morbidity and mortality from injuries to the spleen. J Trauma 14(9): 773–778
126. Neely WA, Hardy JD, Arts CP (1961) Arterial injuries in civilian practice. A current reappraisal with analysis of forty-three cases. J Trauma 1: 424–439
127. Nelson JF (1966) The roentgenologic evaluation of abdominal trauma. Radiol Clin North Am 4(2): 415–431

128. Nick WV, Zollinger RW, Pace WG (1967) Retroperitoneal hemorrhage after blunt abdominal trauma. J Trauma 7: 652–658
129. Nick WV, Zollinger RW, Williams RD (1965) The diagnoses of traumatic pancreatitis with blunt abdominal injuries. J Trauma 5: 495–502
130. Northrup WF, Simmons RL (1972) Pancreatic trauma: A review. Surgery 71(1): 27–43
131. O'Donnell VA Jr, Lou MA, Maxwell TM (1975) Penetrating wounds of the abdomen. J Natl Med Assoc 67(2): 155–157
132. Olsen WR (1974) Delayed rupture of the spleen as an index of diagnostic accuracy. Surg Gynecol Obstet 138: 82
133. Olsen WR, Folley TZ (1977) A second look at delayed splenic rupture. Arch Surg 112: 422–425
134. Orkin LA (1953) The diagnoses of urological trauma in the presence of other injuries. Surg Clin North Am 33: 1473–1495
135. Osborn DJ, Glickman MG, Graja V, Ramsby G (1973) The role of angiography in abdominal nonrenal trauma. Radiol Clin North Am 11: 579–592
136. Paster SB, VanHouten FX, Adams DF (1974) Percutaneous balloon catheterization: A technique for control of arterial hemorrhage caused by pelvic trauma. JAMA 230: 573–575
137. Peltier LF (1965) Complications associated with fractures of the pelvis. J Bone & Joint Dis 47: 1060–1069
138. Penberthy GC (1952) Acute abdominal injuries. Surg Gynecol Obstet 94: 626
139. Perry JF (1965) A five year survey of 152 acute abdominal injuries. J Trauma 5: 53–61
140. Peterson NE (1977) Intermediate degree blunt renal trauma. J Trauma 17(6): 425–435
141. Petty AH (1973) Abdominal injuries. Ann R Coll Surg Engl 53: 167–177
142. Pontius GV, Kilbourne BC, Paul EG (1956) Nonpenetrating abdominal trauma. Arch Surg 72: 800–811
143. Prince JC, Pearlman CK (1969) Thrombosis of the renal artery secondary to trauma. J Urol 102: 670–674
144. Rasaretnam R, Thavendran A (1974) Rupture of the retroperitoneal duodenum after blunt abdominal trauma. Br J Surg 61: 893–895
145. Redman HC, Reuter SR, Bookstein JJ (1969) Angiography in abdominal trauma. Ann Surg 169: 57–66
146. Reuter SR, Redman HC (1972) Gastrointestinal Angiography. W. B. Saunders Company, Philadelphia
147. Reynolds BM, Balsano NA (1971) Venography in pelvic fractures. A clinical evaluation. Ann Surg 173: 104–106
148. Rich NN, Spencer FC (1978) Vascular Trauma. W. B. Saunders Company, Philadelphia
149. Richardson JD, Belin RP, Griffen WO Jr (1972) Blunt abdominal trauma in children. Ann Surg 176: 213–216
150. Richter MW, Lytton B, Myerson D, Gruja V (1973) Radiology of genitourinary trauma. Radiol Clin North Am 11: 593–631
151. Ring EJ, Athanasoulis C, Waltman AC, Margolis MN, Baum S (1973) Arteriographic management of hemorrhage following pelvic fracture. Radiology 109: 65–70
152. Rittenberg GM, Schabel SI, Nelson RP (1978) Bilateral spontaneous urinary extravasation in ureteral obstruction. Radiology 172: 648
153. Rohner TJ Jr (1971) Experience with renal injuries from penetrating trauma in Viet Nam. J Trauma 11: 118
154. Rosoff L, Cohen JL, Telfer N, Halpern M (1972) Injuries of the spleen. Surg Clin North Am 52(3): 667–685
155. Rothenberger DA, Fischer RP, Strate RG, Velasco R, Perry JJ (1978) The mortality associated with pelvic fractures. Surgery 84: 356–361
156. Roy AD (1974) Abdominal injuries. Br Med J 4:335–336
157. Rusche CF (1948) Injury of the ureter due to gun shot wounds. J Urol 60: 63–72
158. Rushe CF, Morrow JW (1970) Injury to the ureter. In: Campbell MF (ed) Urology, Vol. I. W. B. Saunders Company, Philadelphia, pp. 834–850
159. Rutlow IM (1978) Rupture of the spleen in infectious mononucleosis. Arch Surg 113: 718–720
160. Sandblom P (1948) Hemorrhage into the biliary tract following trauma. Traumatic Hemobilia Surg 24: 571–586
161. Sanders RC (ed) (1975) Symposium on B-scan ultrasound. Radiol Clin North Am 13(3): 417–434
162. Schaner EG, Balow JE, Doppman JL (1977) Computed tomography in the diagnoses of subcapsular and perirenal hematoma. Am J Roentgenol 124: 83–88
163. Schrock TR, Christiansen N (1972) Management of perforating injuries of the colon. Surg Gynecol Obstet 135: 65
164. Schwartz SS, Boley SJ, McKinnon WM (1959) The roentgen findings in traumatic rupture of the spleen in children. Am J Roentgenol 82: 505–509
165. Scott R, Carlton CE Jr, Goldman M (1969) Penetrating injuries of the kidney. An analysis of 181 patients. J Urol 101: 247–253
166. Scott R Jr, Gordon HL, Carlton CE Jr, Scott BF, Beach PD (1972) Current Controversies in Urologic Management. W. B. Saunders Company, Philadelphia
167. Sinclair MC, et al. (1974) Injury to hollow abdominal viscera from blunt trauma in children and adolescents. Am J Surg 128(5): 693–698
168. Smith K, Ben-Menachem Y, Duke JH, Hill GL (1976) The superior gluteal: An artery at risk in blunt pelvic trauma. J Trauma 16(4): 273–279
169. Snyder CJ (1972) Bowel injuries from automobile seat belts. Am J Surg 123: 312–316
170. Sperling L, Rigler LG (1937) Traumatic retroperitoneal rupture of duodenum. Radiology 29: 521–524
171. Steele M, Lim RC (1975) Advances in management of splenic injuries. Am J Surg 130: 159–169
172. Steichen FM (1975) Hepatic trauma in adults. Surg Clin North Am 55(2): 387–407
173. Stivelman RL, Glanbitz JP, Crampton RS (1963) Laceration of the spleen due to nonpenetrating trauma. One hundred cases. Am J Surg 106: 888–891
174. Strauch GO (1973) Major abdominal trauma in 1971. Am J Surg 125: 413–418
175. Sturm TJ, Perry FJ Jr, Cass A (1975) Renal artery

and vein injury following blunt trauma. Ann Surg 182(6): 696–698
176. Tadavarthy SM, Knight L, Ovitt TW, Snyder C, Amplatz K (1974) Therapeutic transcatheter arterial embolization. Radiology 112: 13–16
177. Talbot WA, Shuck JM (1975) Retroperitoneal duodenal injury due to blunt abdominal trauma. Am J Surg 130: 654–666
178. Tan DT, Kim HS, Richmond D (1975) Gastric mucosal lacerations from blunt trauma to the abdomen. Am J Gastroenterol 63(3): 226–228
179. Terry JH, Self MM, Howard JM (1956) Injuries of the spleen. Report of 102 patients. Surgery 40: 615–619
180. Thaggard A, Harle TS, Carlson V (1978) Fractures and dislocations of bony pelvis and hip. Semin Roentgenol 13(2): 117–133
181. Thal AP, Wilson RF (1964) A pattern of severe blunt trauma to the region of the pancreas. Surg Gynecol Obstet 119: 733
182. Ting YM, Reuter SR (1973) Hollow viscus injury in blunt abdominal trauma. Am J Roentgenol 119: 408–413
183. Toxopeus MD, Lucas CE, Krabbenhoft KL (1972) Roentgenographic diagnoses in blunt retroperitoneal duodenal rupture. Am J Roentgenol 115(2): 281–288
184. Trimble C, Eason FJ (1972) A complication of splenosis. J Trauma 12(4): 358–361
185. Trunkey DD, Blaisdall FW (1975) Abdominal vascular injuries. West J Med 123(4): 321–324
186. Tunell WP, Knost J, Nance FC (1975) Penetrating abdominal injuries in children and adolescents. J Trauma 15(8): 720–725
187. Tynberg PLH, Hoch WH, Persky L, Zollinger RM (1973) The management of renal injuries coincident with penetrating wounds of the abdomen. J Trauma 13(6): 502–508
188. Van Wagoner FA (1961) Died in hospital. A three year study of deaths following trauma. J Trauma 1: 401–408
189. Wanebo HJ, Hunt TK, Mathewson C (1969) Rectal injuries. J Trauma 9(8): 712–722
190. Wang CC, Robbins LL (1956) Roentgenologic diagnoses of ruptured spleen. N Engl J Med 254: 445–449
191. Waterhouse K, Gross M (1969) Trauma to the genitourinary tract. A 5 year experience with 251 cases. J Urol 101: 241–253
192. Watkins GI (1960) Blunt trauma to abdomen. Arch Surg 80: 187–191
193. Watnick M, Spindola-Franco H (1973) Traumatic visceral pseudoaneurysms. J Can Assoc Radiol 24: 62–64
194. Weens HS, Newman JH, Florence TJ (1946) Trauma of the lower urinary tract. A roentgenologic study. N Engl J Med 234: 357–364
195. Westcott JL, Smith JR (1975) Mesenteric and colon. Injuries secondary to blunt trauma. Radiology 114(3): 597–600
196. White PH, Benfield JR (1972) Amylase in the management of pancreatic trauma. Arch Surg 105: 158–163
197. Wilkinson AE (1973) Abdominal injuries. S Afr J Surg 11: 217–223
198. Williams RD, Sargeant FT (1963) The mechanism of intestinal injury in trauma. J Trauma 3: 288–296
199. Williams RD, Zollinger RM (1959) Diagnostic and prognostic factors in abdominal trauma. Am J Surg 97: 575–581
200. Wilson DH (1962–63) Incidence, etiology, diagnosis and prognosis of closed abdominal injuries. A study of 265 cases. Br J Surg 50: 381–389
201. Wilson H, Sherman R (1961) Civilian penetrating wounds of the abdomen. I. Factors in mortality and differences from military wounds in 494 cases. Ann Surg 53: 639–649
202. Wilson RF, Tagett JP, Pucelik JP, Walt AJ (1971) Pancreatic trauma. J Trauma 7(5): 643–651
203. Wiot JF (1966) Intramural small intestinal hemorrhage—A differential diagnosis. Semin Roentgenol 1: 219–233
204. Woodruff JH Jr, Cockett ATK, Cannon R, Swanson LE (1967) Radiologic aspects of renal trauma with emphases on arteriography and renal isotope scanning. J Urol 97: 184
205. Woolley MM, Mahour GH, Sloan T (1978) Duodenal hematoma in infancy and childhood. Changing etiology and changing treatment. Am J Surg 136: 8–14
206. Worth MH Jr (1976) Abdominal trauma. JAMA 235(8): 853–854
207. Wyman AC (1954) Traumatic rupture of the spleen. Am J Roentgenol 72: 51–63
208. Yajko RD, Seydel F, Trimble C (1975) Rupture of the stomach from blunt abdominal trauma. J Trauma 15(3): 177–183
209. Yeh HC, Wolf BS (1977) Ultrasonography in ascites. Radiology 124: 783–790
210. Zabrinski EJ, Harkins HN (1943) Delayed splenic rupture: A clinical syndrome following trauma. Report of 4 cases with an analysis of 177 cases collected from literature. Arch Surg 46: 186–213

Index